PRAISE FOR
THE ALZHEIMER'S ANTIDOTE

"Magnificent. . . . *The Alzheimer's Antidote* harvests our most highly regarded scientific research to create an empowering, user-friendly game plan that rewrites our health destiny as it relates to the brain. And this is a program for everyone, whether already diagnosed, at high risk, or even if there is no family history of this disease. . . . In these pages are your highly empowering tools that will allow *you* to gain control over your genetic and cognitive destiny."

—**David Perlmutter**, MD, author of *Grain Brain*,
#1 *New York Times* bestseller (from the Foreword)

"There are few things people fear more than cancer, with the possible exception of neurodegenerative diseases such as Alzheimer's disease (AD). Not only does AD ultimately cut lives short, it effectively steals who the person 'is' long before they die. Traditional treatment methods have been lackluster at best, but there is hope. *The Alzheimer's Antidote* is a scientifically sound method of nutrition and lifestyle that combats AD at a molecular level. If you or someone you know suffers from AD, I highly recommend this book."

—**Rob Wolf**, *New York Times* bestselling author of
The Paleo Solution and *Wired to Eat*

"Amy Berger elegantly explains how Alzheimer's, a devastating disease that has touched virtually every American family (or soon will), is much more than just a normal manifestation of growing old, and its management must include much more than just cholinesterase-inhibiting drugs. She delves deep into Alzheimer's as a complex metabolic disease, one that can be greatly reduced, and likely avoided completely, with the right combination of lifestyle modifications within our control. Berger offers comprehensive treatment approaches that go way beyond what most patients are told by their physicians. This book is long overdue and a must-read for health care providers and laypeople alike."

—**David M. Brady**, ND, CCN, DACBN, author of Amazon bestseller
The Fibro Fix; vice president for health sciences and director of
the Nutrition Institute, University of Bridgeport

"Amy Berger brings a fresh, new perspective to the rising problem of Alzheimer's disease. She proposes a natural treatment that has, in my opinion, a far greater chance of clinical success than standard medications. *The Alzheimer's Antidote* is a terrific book."

—**Jason Fung**, MD, author of *The Obesity Code*

"A growing body of research suggests brain insulin resistance is strongly linked to Alzheimer's disease (AD). In *The Alzheimer's Antidote*, Amy Berger provides a clear understanding of the pathology of AD and explains how a low-carb, high-fat lifestyle can improve cognitive function and increase quality of life by providing an alternate fuel source for the Alzheimer's brain to use: ketone bodies. This exceptionally well-written, well-researched book is a must-read for family members and caregivers of people with AD."

—**Franziska Spritzler**, RD, CDE

"Real hope and real help are finally here. Amy Berger expertly explains the fascinating connection between diet and dementia, in plain English and from every conceivable angle, arming you with the scientific understanding and practical strategies you need to change the course of your future. *The Alzheimer's Antidote* will completely change the way you think and feel about Alzheimer's disease."

—**Georgia Ede**, MD, psychiatrist and nutrition specialist

THE
Alzheimer's
ANTIDOTE

Using a Low-Carb, High-Fat Diet to

Fight Alzheimer's Disease, Memory Loss,

and Cognitive Decline

AMY BERGER, MS, CNS, NTP

Chelsea Green Publishing
White River Junction, Vermont

Disclaimer
This book is intended as information, not medical advice. You must not rely on the information in this book as an alternative to medical advice from your doctor or other professional health care provider. If you have any specific questions about any medical matter, you should consult your doctor or other professional health care provider. If you think you may be suffering from any medical condition, you should seek immediate medical attention. You should never delay seeking medical advice, disregard medical advice, or discontinue medical treatment because of information in this book.

Project Manager: Angela Boyle
Developmental Editor: Makenna Goodman
Copy Editor: Deborah Heimann
Proofreader: Eileen M. Clawson
Indexer: Shana Milkie
Designer: Melissa Jacobson

Printed in the United States of America.
First printing February, 2017.
10 9 8 7 6 5 4 3 2 1   17 18 19 20 21

Our Commitment to Green Publishing
Chelsea Green sees publishing as a tool for cultural change and ecological stewardship. We strive to align our book manufacturing practices with our editorial mission and to reduce the impact of our business enterprise in the environment. We print our books and catalogs on chlorine-free recycled paper, using vegetable-based inks whenever possible. This book may cost slightly more because it was printed on paper that contains recycled fiber, and we hope you'll agree that it's worth it. Chelsea Green is a member of the Green Press Initiative (www.greenpressinitiative.org), a nonprofit coalition of publishers, manufacturers, and authors working to protect the world's endangered forests and conserve natural resources. *The Alzheimer's Antidote* was printed on paper supplied by Thomson-Shore that contains 100% postconsumer recycled fiber.

Library of Congress Cataloging-in-Publication Data
Names: Berger, Amy.
Title: The Alzheimer's antidote : using a low-carb, high-fat diet to fight Alzheimer's disease,
    memory loss, and cognitive decline / Amy Berger, MS, CNS, NTP.
Description: White River Junction, VT : Chelsea Green Publishing, [2017]
    | Includes bibliographical references.
Identifiers: LCCN 2016050356| ISBN 9781603587099 (paperback) | ISBN 9781603587105 (ebook)
Subjects: LCSH: Alzheimer's disease—Prevention—Popular works. | Alzheimer's disease—Diet
    therapy—Popular works. | Self-care, Health—Popular works. | BISAC: HEALTH & FITNESS /
    Diseases / Alzheimer's & Dementia. | MEDICAL / Nutrition. | COOKING / Health & Healing / Low
    Carbohydrate. | COOKING / Health & Healing / General.
Classification: LCC RC523.2 .B48 2017 | DDC 616.8/310654—dc23
LC record available at https://lccn.loc.gov/2016050356

Chelsea Green Publishing
85 North Main Street, Suite 120
White River Junction, VT 05001
(802) 295-6300
www.chelseagreen.com

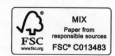
MIX
Paper from
responsible sources
FSC® C013483

To individuals with Alzheimer's disease,
mild cognitive impairment, and other forms
of dementia and cognitive decline, I present this
information to you, your loved ones, and your caregivers
with my sincerest wishes that it helps you reclaim
what has been so devastatingly taken from you.

CONTENTS

PART THREE

Lifestyle Factors to Support
Healthy Neurological Function

PART FOUR

Setting Yourself Up for Success:
Beyond Diet and Lifestyle

FOREWORD

Alzheimer's disease, like so many other degenerative conditions, is highly influenced by factors over which each of us has control. Unfortunately, however, we have been coerced to shift the responsibility for our health and wellness to professionals and, as such, upon the coin of medical commerce—the prescription. The pervasive mentality is one that portrays a paradigm in which our lifestyle choices produce no consequence in terms of our health destiny. And should we happen upon a disease of any sort, our misguided belief holds that highly successful medical developments will certainly get us back on our feet.

But this misplaced reliance has failed us miserably across a wide panorama of diseases, most notably Alzheimer's. For there exists no pharmaceutical, magic-bullet cure for this pernicious process. Moreover, despite what advertisers may portray on the evening news, there is no pharmaceutical intervention that has any meaningful effect even in terms of reducing the progression of this disease.

And yet, prescriptions for "Alzheimer's medications" are written for millions of Americans by physicians who are quite probably aware of their lack of efficacy, likely only as an attempt to placate patients' distraught family members who feel compelled to "do something."

The absence of any medical treatment for Alzheimer's disease may well explain the lack of attention this devastating condition receives. Our awareness of breast cancer, for example, is raised by pervasive pink ribbons, walkathons, and other events ostensibly organized to "find a cure." Ironically, this campaign is, in large part, funded by companies that develop and sell highly profitable proprietary treatments for this disease. Absent meaningful treatment, efforts to raise awareness of a disease that, like breast cancer, primarily targets women, but may be associated with a death rate ninefold higher, are subdued.

What follows in the pages you are about to read is a different story. Amy
Berger has done a magnificent job summarizing our most leading edge
research that demonstrates the game changing role that lifestyle factors play
in not only determining Alzheimer's risk but also in paving the way for
actual clinical improvement in individuals already manifesting the disease.

As such, *The Alzheimer's Antidote* stands in contrast to the pessimistic
outlook generally delivered to patients and their loved ones when the diagnosis is made. It challenges us to relinquish tightly held beliefs and embrace
the notion that dietary fat, for example, is not the villain that it has been
portrayed to be. And that by welcoming healthful fats back to the table, we
are enhancing the way brain cells power themselves—a fundamental flaw
in Alzheimer's disease.

Cholesterol, long demonized as a cause of so many health issues, is
finally and rightfully celebrated as being an important player in building,
maintaining, and repairing delicate brain cells.

Sugar and carbohydrates, which continue to represent the foundation
of the American diet, are finally called out for their devastating effects on
the health of the brain, with a clear explanation as to their association with
Alzheimer's disease.

The amyloid hypothesis—which holds that the accumulation of a specific
protein, *beta-amyloid*, plays an important causative role in Alzheimer's
disease—is rightfully and factually challenged as well. Indeed, research
efforts to develop a blockbuster drug focused on ridding the brain of
beta-amyloid in hopes of curing Alzheimer's disease have almost uniformly
intensified the rate of cognitive decline in human subjects.

Most importantly, *The Alzheimer's Antidote* harvests our most highly
regarded scientific research to create an empowering, user-friendly game
plan that rewrites our health destiny as it relates to the brain. And this is
a program for everyone, whether already diagnosed, at high risk, or even
if there is no family history of this disease. Alzheimer's risk is certainly
increased for those with a diagnosed family member, the 28 million
Americans with diabetes, and people whose diets favor carbohydrates in
comparison to fat, but Alzheimer's risk approaches an astounding 50% for
all of us if we reach 85 years of age.

Reductionism, as applied to nutritional science, focuses on the roles of
macronutrients, including fat, carbohydrate, and protein, as well as micronutrients, such as vitamins and minerals, in terms of cellular metabolism.

But we now know that our food choices have a much more profound role that highly influences brain health.

The foods we consume actually interact with our DNA, changing the expression of our genes moment to moment, for better or worse. In this sense, food is information, and the instructions our food choices provide to our DNA regulate processes like inflammation, detoxification, and the production of antioxidants, all of which are pivotal for the health or decay of the brain.

And it is from this perspective that the dietary recommendations in this book become most valuable. For the dietary plan that Amy Berger so eloquently delivers, a diet that welcomes healthful fat back to the table while virtually eliminating sugar and refined carbohydrates, is one that specifically targets gene expression to calm inflammation, help the body rid itself of potentially brain-damaging toxins, and amplify the production of brain protective antioxidants.

These gene pathways exist in all of us, ready to participate in protecting, enhancing, and even restoring brain functionality. And in these pages are your highly empowering tools that will allow *you* to gain control over your genetic and cognitive destiny.

David Perlmutter, MD
Board-certified neurologist and
fellow, American College of Nutrition

ACKNOWLEDGMENTS

The act of writing is, at least for me, one that must be conducted in silence and solitude. My ability to access, understand, and interpret the body of research that underpins this book, however, was most definitely a team effort. I would like to acknowledge the many researchers, clinicians, academics, and extraordinarily scientifically literate laypeople who have contributed to my ever-deepening understanding of the biochemical and physiological principles and mechanisms discussed herein and their implications for guiding us toward nutrition and lifestyle strategies to combat some of our most challenging states of compromised health. I will inevitably and inadvertently forget key individuals who belong in these categories, so to anyone who knows they've made meaningful contributions to my ongoing education and professional development, please know that I value your guidance and support, and if your name does not appear below, it is unintentional.

For their prolific research in the fields of Alzheimer's disease, brain fuel metabolism, ketones, and low-carbohydrate and ketogenic diets as metabolic therapy across a wide range of health conditions, I am indebted to the following individuals, as well as their colleagues, collaborators, and graduate students: Stephen Cunnane, PhD; Dominic D'Agostino, PhD; Thomas Seyfried, PhD; Richard Veech, PhD; Yoshihiro Kashiwaya, PhD; Mary Newport, MD; Theodore VanItallie, PhD; Samuel Henderson, PhD; Stephanie Seneff, PhD; Jeff Volek, PhD, RD; Stephen Phinney, MD, PhD; Eric Westman, MD; Richard Feinman, PhD; Eugene Fine, MD; Colin Champ, MD; and Dale Bredesen, MD.

I would like to recognize the following physicians for supporting and encouraging my work, as well as for employing low-carbohydrate or ketogenic diets in their practices, along with the other lifestyle strategies I suggest herein. These doctors regularly *remove* pharmaceutical medications from patients' regimens rather than add them, and on a daily basis they improve the lives of those with type 2 diabetes, heart disease, obesity, and more, largely by recommending the *opposite* of what the public has been led to believe constitutes a healthy diet: Jason Fung, MD; Theodore Naiman, MD; Jeffry Gerber, MD; Mark Cucuzzella, MD; and Eric Thorn, MD. I feel an additional kinship with nutritionists and dietitians doing similar work using low-carbohydrate and ketogenic diets to help those who are debilitated and demoralized by chronic modern illnesses reclaim the health and vitality that are their birthright: Franziska Spritzler, RD; Miriam Kalamian, CNS; Kelley Pounds, RN; Beth Zupec-Kania, RD; and Patricia Daly.

For sharing my work on their blogs, websites, podcasts, and in their print publications, thereby allowing me to bring this potentially life-changing information to a much larger audience than I would have reached on my own, my thanks to Robb Wolf, Jimmy Moore, Sally Fallon Morell, Christine Lehmann, Paul Burgess, Mackay Rippey, and Scott Miners.

For their work in helping medical and nutrition professionals and the public alike question our most deeply held beliefs regarding dietary cholesterol, saturated fat, vegetable oils, cereal grains, and more, I would like to acknowledge Gary Taubes; Nina Teicholz; Adele Hite; Loren Cordain, PhD; Mark Sisson; and the late Mary Enig, PhD.

As is so often the case in research pursuits—be they in nutrition or other fields—outsiders provide a fresh perspective to those who have been eyeball-deep in matters for years and who, albeit unintentionally, might have developed tunnel vision, myopia, and unhealthy attachments to particular points of view. It is these outsiders who sometimes put the final nails in the coffins of incorrect dogma, as their livelihoods don't depend on defending a failing status quo, and their professional reputations are not intertwined with an established viewpoint that is crumbling. As a nutrition professional, I am routinely impressed by and indebted to laypeople who, purely for the pursuit of knowledge and following personal passions—or, more often, with the goal of improving their own health or that of loved ones when conventional medical care has failed them—share their findings with the rest of us. They are proof that credentials aren't always what they're made out to be, and sometimes, the best, most logical, and most *helpful* ideas come from unlikely places. My thanks to the following individuals for contributing to my understanding of human physiology, metabolism, blood glucose regulation, and ketone dynamics, and for sharing their low-carb successes with the public: Marty Kendall, L. Amber O'Hearn, R.D. Dikeman, Jeff Cyr, Raymund Edwards, Mike Julian, Luis Villaseñor,

Tyler Cartwright, and Bob Briggs. Special thanks to Ivor Cummins, who deserves the spotlight for resurrecting the pioneering work of Joseph Kraft, MD, and Kenneth Brookler, MD, and for bringing to light the primacy of chronically elevated insulin, rather than solely blood glucose, in driving the vast majority of illnesses that rob people of quantity and quality of life in the modern age.

I am grateful to my colleagues at Designs for Health, Inc., for their patience and flexibility with my schedule to allow me time to complete this manuscript. My knowledge of micronutrients, botanicals, pharmaco-dynamics, and the human factors that complicate any dietary and lifestyle therapy grows deeper with every day that I research and write. I am proud to be associated with DFH, which stays faithful to its motto of *science first*. Special thanks to Suzanne Copp and David Brady, ND, for their support and encouragement.

During my initial nutrition education, I was fortunate to have been seated in the classrooms of several dedicated and talented professors. The biochemistry courses of two of these educators, in particular—Charles Saladino, PhD, and Margaret Carroll, PhD—instilled in me a fascination for the fundamental ways in which the human body works, and a desire to share that fascination with others. It is thanks to them that yours truly—whose brain is naturally inclined toward the humanities, literature, and languages—is able to make sense of the scientific literature.

I am indebted to Mike Sheridan for helping to make an early electronic version of this book available on Amazon, which allowed me to bring this important information to a wider audience. We worked well together, and I'm happy to confirm this for other authors who are not tech-savvy and need assistance in bringing their work into the twenty-first century.

My deepest gratitude to Ellen Davis, MS, a colleague and dear friend, whose support and encouragement always come at just the right time—which is always! It is because of Ellen's website—www.ketogenic-diet-resource.com—the single most comprehensive clearinghouse I'm aware of for information regarding ketogenic diets—that you are holding this book in your hands or reading it on a screen right now. This book originated in ebook format, which Ellen designed. I am a writer; words are my craft. Regarding layout and design, I am as unskilled as anyone can be. Without Ellen's assistance and tireless dedication to spreading the word about the life-changing effects of reduced carbohydrate diets, the initial iteration of this book would have never made it beyond a Microsoft Word file languishing on my home computer. Knowing how critical it was for this little-known perspective on cognitive decline and dementia to be available to the public, Ellen was kind enough to host it on her site, which is where the current publisher encountered it.

When I was conducting the initial research into Alzheimer's disease as a metabolic condition—one with a metabolic solution—I never could have predicted the direction things would go. Thanks to Margo Baldwin and Makenna Goodman at Chelsea Green Publishing, for recognizing the urgency of getting this information to the people who need it most, and for trusting me to deliver it.

And finally, my heartfelt gratitude to my family and friends, who have always believed in me far more than I've believed in myself. I was unable to help my own mother with her health struggles, but it is my sincere hope that, through this book, I will help someone else's.

INTRODUCTION

In the current landscape of conventional medicine and pharmaceutical drugs, a diagnosis of Alzheimer's disease is essentially a death sentence. Pharmaceutical treatments developed to date have been woefully ineffective, and modern medicine has little else to offer in the fight against this debilitating condition. The best advice doctors and therapists have to offer is to keep the mind active, such as by taking up new hobbies or learning foreign languages. To imply that something as devastating as Alzheimer's disease can be prevented by crosswords and Sudoku puzzles is irresponsible and downright insulting. The lack of progress regarding Alzheimer's treatment is discouraging and disheartening, given the emotional, psychological, and financial tolls this disease exacts from its victims and their caregivers.

Cognitive decline is not inevitable as we age, and if it does occur, we do not have to sit idly by and wait helplessly while it progresses. Based on the theory of the etiology of Alzheimer's as outlined in this book, there might be ways to prevent, delay, and possibly even reverse the course of this devastating degenerative disease.

The reason the strategies you will read about herein aren't more widely discussed is that they aren't well known beyond small groups of researchers and medical practitioners who study them in laboratories and implement them for their patients. Even many physicians—including neurologists and geriatric specialists, the experts whom we rely on to be the most knowledgeable on these issues—are generally unfamiliar with this extremely promising therapeutic avenue. We cannot blame them for this lapse in knowledge, however. The research I have done and the strategies discussed in this book are unconventional, and in some ways, they're relatively new. They don't have decades of "gold standard" randomized, double-blind, placebo-controlled studies backing them up. But as they say in scientific circles, "Absence of evidence does not imply evidence of absence." The reason we don't have piles upon piles of scientific evidence proving the efficacy of the methods discussed here is not because they're ineffective, but because they're unconventional. Few doctors have the courage to step outside the normal standards of care and accepted courses of action to try something different, even though the same-old conventional courses of action continue to yield the same-old results: namely, *no* results. No improvement for the Alzheimer's sufferers, and no relief for their loved ones and caregivers.

This is heartbreaking—and absolutely unnecessary. A review of the medical literature to date makes a strong case that Alzheimer's disease is largely a problem of brain fuel metabolism—meaning, it results from a disturbance in the brain's capacity to generate energy. And if Alzheimer's disease is a metabolic problem, then the most promising avenue for address-ing the root cause of the condition—and therefore potentially slowing and reversing it—is a metabolic strategy that restores energy utilization in the brain. Specifically, this relates to a dietary overhaul and lifestyle modifica-tions to alter fuel metabolism throughout the body but, in particular, in the brain. Seems pretty straightforward, right? Then why hasn't conventional medicine adopted this belief?

Alzheimer's disease was first classified as a unique medical entity over a century ago by Dr. Alois Alzheimer. In the hundred-plus years that have passed since then, a staggering body of knowledge has accumulated regard-ing the metabolic aberrations that underlie the condition. Despite what you might read in mass-market health publications or hear on the TV news, we do, in fact, know a great deal about what is causing this frightening form of cognitive decline. Unfortunately, the fascinating research being conducted in laboratories and universities around the world takes years—decades, sometimes—to trickle down to the medical community as a whole, where neurologists and geriatricians would be made aware of it. And it takes even longer before such findings are incorporated into standards of care. (Moreover, it's not in the interests of pharmaceutical companies to devote research efforts to proving the efficacy of dietary changes and lifestyle inter-ventions that don't require multimillion-dollar laboratories and that cannot be patented and sold for a king's ransom.)

Fortunately, we need not wait decades for the slow-moving behemoth that is the conventional medical community to catch up. We can take action right now to reclaim our own health or help our loved ones do the same. The weight of the scientific evidence strongly indicates there are steps we can take to slow, prevent, and potentially reverse cognitive impairment and decline resulting from metabolic derangement impacting the brain.

Alzheimer's disease and its precursor, called mild cognitive impairment (MCI), are multifactorial conditions that require multifactorial solutions. The disease process is complex, but that doesn't mean potential solutions must be equally complex. In fact, with an understanding of the biochemical and physiological aberrations underlying the neurodegenerative changes that result in Alzheimer's and MCI, the solutions are self-evident and quite elegant.

If you have been fighting the ravages of this disease yourself, or if you are a caregiver watching a loved one's painful transformation into someone unrecognizable, I present this information to you so that you'll see there is hope. There is a way out of the fog. Continue reading, come to understand the science and the logic behind the recommendations in this book, have the courage to implement them, and start making your way out, now.

To medical professionals, researchers, and academics who might be reading this, please note that, by necessity and out of consideration for my intended audience—individuals with cognitive impairment or Alzheimer's disease, and their loved ones and caregivers—I have simplified my explanations of some of the relevant biochemical and physiological mechanisms. It is my sincere hope, though, that I have not oversimplified anything to the point of inaccuracy. I have tried to respect the cautionary principle that is frequently, though perhaps erroneously, attributed to Albert Einstein: "Everything should be made as simple as possible, but not simpler."

A Note to Caregivers

As you will soon see, the dietary and lifestyle interventions I recommend require close monitoring, and they also require near-complete control over the affected individual's food supply and daily routine. Most of their meals will need to be prepared from whole, unprocessed foods, so that you can control the ingredients and your efforts to help your loved one will not be stymied by the hidden sugars and starches in packaged foods. Therefore, the nutritional plan outlined in this book will be easiest to implement if your loved one lives with you, or if they have a live-in aide whom you can educate regarding the requirements of this approach and who can monitor food intake and daily actions to make sure there is no trickling in of prohibited foods or engaging in behaviors that will hinder progress.

This strategy will be difficult—if not impossible—to implement if your loved one lives in a managed care facility or other assisted living situation where food is provided for them.

Unfortunately, in these situations, the food is typically of poor quality, and it is also usually high in carbohydrates, relatively low in good quality protein, and devoid of natural, health-promoting fats. This is especially true in conventional care facilities that receive federal or state funds. The dietitians who design the meal plans for these facilities—well-intentioned though they surely are—are beholden to government guidelines regarding what constitutes a "healthy diet." This means they must limit the amount of cholesterol and fat the meals provide. As you will learn in this book, however, these are precisely two of the nutrients a struggling, damaged brain needs most desperately.

Due to budget reasons, the foods in these facilities are typically low-cost packaged foods full of sugars and starches: white bread, jams and jellies, fruit cups, fruit juices, pastries, breaded chicken patties, and so on. The vegetables provided are often starchy; again, due to cost. (Starchy vegetables [corn, potatoes, peas] are more cost-effective and less perishable than nutrient-rich greens and other vibrantly colored fresh produce that spoils more readily.) To make matters worse, due to over sixty years of misguided attacks on saturated fat and cholesterol, the animal foods that are provided in these facilities will lack the critical vitamins and minerals the body needs for repair and regeneration, because they will typically be low- or no-fat; for example, skim milk, margarine instead of butter, skinless chicken, reduced-fat cheeses, nonfat yogurt, and imitation meat products made from soybeans, corn, and wheat protein.

But don't lose heart! If your loved one lives in a special care facility, don't be discouraged. Perhaps you can approach the management—including and especially the staff dietitians—and broach the subject of this nutritional intervention with them. In fact, I encourage you to do so. We must open this dialogue, and the sooner, the better. These professionals are in the unique position of being able to affect many (sometimes hundreds of) residents. By encouraging them to start thinking differently about their approach to Alzheimer's and other forms of neurological degeneration, perhaps we can begin to turn the tide on these horrible illnesses, for which the conventional care model has proven to be a failure.

Even for those of you who provide care in your own home for a loved one affected by dementia, implementing this strategy will be a challenge. Although I believe it can be effective, it is certainly not easy. Alzheimer's disease is a complex, multifactorial condition, and it therefore necessitates a multifactorial approach to address it. If your loved one is relatively young, has very mild cognitive impairment, and is still able to take care of themselves to a large extent, that will take much of the burden off you. For the very elderly or those with advanced, severe, and longstanding illness, you might find it all but impossible to make an impact. The confusion, belligerence, and other behavioral disturbances that often accompany advanced dementia can make dietary changes a virtual impossibility. If this is the case with your loved one, I still encourage you to read on and gain a deeper understanding of how and why this illness might have developed, not only in order to implement potential prevention and mitigation strategies in your own life, but also because you might find pearls of information here and there that you *can* implement to help your loved one. You have felt powerless in this fight for too long. Now is the time to take hold of the tools that are available to you and use them. You might not be able to do *everything*, but don't let that stop you from doing *something*.

If your loved one lives with you (or another relative or friend who is willing to take on the responsibility of food preparation), it will be easier for them to stick to the diet if someone else in the household (or more than one other person) adopts the diet along with them. This nutritional approach is effective for myriad diverse health conditions, so even those who are not struggling with Alzheimer's but who might be living with heart disease, type 1 or type 2 diabetes, metabolic syndrome, obesity, chronic fatigue, gastroesophageal reflux disease (GERD), polycystic ovarian syndrome (PCOS), mood disturbances, and more might benefit greatly by being a "diet buddy" to the Alzheimer's sufferer. (See chapter 23 for other conditions for which low-carbohydrate or ketogenic diets have proven effective.)

Your loved one might have compromised digestive function or changes in their sense of taste and smell that will interfere with their getting the best impact from the dietary recommendations provided herein. Workarounds for some of these issues are provided in chapter 21.

Again, I have no illusions as to the difficulty of implementing this strategy for individuals of advanced illness and severe cognitive impairment. It will not be an easy row to hoe. But I encourage you to implement as many of the recommendations as you are able to. I believe they hold incredible potential to improve your loved one's quality of life, as well as your own.

PART ONE

The Metabolic Origins of Alzheimer's Disease

In part one, we will explore the metabolic origins of Alzheimer's disease and make connections between our modern diet and lifestyle and the development of this condition. We'll address key factors related to Alzheimer's, including brain fuel metabolism, chronically elevated insulin, neuron structure, beta-amyloid plaques, and the ApoE4 genotype. We'll also explore the logic behind why a low-carbohydrate nutritional plan might be effective for stemming the tide of memory loss and cognitive decline.

CHAPTER 1

The Origins of Alzheimer's and a Strategy to Fight It

From aluminum to pesticides, environmental toxins, and genetically modified foods, several possible causes of Alzheimer's disease (AD) have been put forward, many of which involve potentially harmful substances entering the body from the outside and negatively affecting cognitive function. And many different strategies have been recommended to keep the mind active and healthy, such as crossword puzzles, learning a musical instrument or a new language, or taking up hobbies that encourage the formation of new neural pathways. But what if the true underlying cause of AD is a systemic metabolic problem coming from the inside? If that were the case, then the solution would be a metabolic one—a multifaceted strategy that alters several biochemical pathways in the body and, in particular, restores proper fuel metabolism in the brain—and no amount of word games or memorizing foreign idioms would be likely to have a significant impact. It is important, of course, to keep cognitive function robust and active as we age and to challenge ourselves to keep learning, but to imply that Alzheimer's is mostly a result of letting one's mind get "lazy" is scientifically irresponsible and, frankly, a cop-out. Something else is at work—something that affects cognitive function and neuronal impulse transmission in the brain at the most basic level.

Identifying the fundamental causes of AD is imperative and grows more critical every day. Financial costs for health care related to AD are expected to reach into the trillions of dollars by mid-century, and this economic shock pales in comparison to the emotional toll this debilitating disease exacts from its victims and their loved ones and caregivers.[1] It is also of paramount importance that we uncover the causes of AD because addressing the problem at its source is the only hope we have of preventing, slowing the progression of, and possibly even reversing this frightening form of neurodegeneration. And because we have not yet been able to address the root cause, the vast majority of pharmaceutical drugs targeting individual symptoms of the condition piecemeal have failed to demonstrate beneficial effects. In fact, some initially promising drugs have actually made the signs and symptoms of AD *worse*.[2]

A dive into the scientific literature regarding the causes of AD reveals a wealth of information indicating that the condition results from metabolic abnormalities that start outside the brain. These abnormalities affect the entire body, but the signs are often missed—or worse, ignored—until damage to the brain is so deep and widespread that it begins to cause cognitive decline that interferes with everyday living and renders formerly strong, independent, capable people unable to care for themselves.

The research is unambiguous: AD results primarily from a failure of parts of the brain to harness sufficient energy from glucose. As a consequence of this insufficient fueling, neurons in the affected brain regions degrade and degenerate, leading to a loss of communication among them. This breakdown in neuronal communication results in the confusion, memory loss, and behavioral changes characteristic of Alzheimer's disease. The connection between glucose handling, insulin signaling, and AD is so strong that many researchers now refer to AD as "diabetes of the brain," or "type 3 diabetes."[3] Although type 2 diabetes and AD are closely associated, we must not be fooled into believing that type 2 diabetes causes AD. Many people with type 2 diabetes will never go on to develop AD, and many Alzheimer's patients are not diagnosed diabetics. The relationship between the two is more like that of physiological cousins; that is, they result from the same underlying metabolic disturbances, but they manifest differently depending on which parts of the body are affected. In type 2 diabetes, for example, insulin resistance and disturbed carbohydrate metabolism affect the muscles, organs, and periphery (the rest of the body aside from the brain and central nervous system); in Alzheimer's disease, damage is mostly localized to the brain.

The Role of the Modern Diet

If Alzheimer's is ultimately the result of metabolic disturbances similar to those seen in type 2 diabetes—namely, insulin resistance and hyperinsulinemia (elevated levels of insulin in the bloodstream for extended periods of time)—then the same causes as are seen in type 2 diabetes are likely to be behind AD. While there are many factors that contribute to dysregulated insulin signaling, one of the most powerful is a diet that is mismatched to basic human physiology.

The pattern of eating that has become the "standard American diet" and that has morphed and spread into the "modern Western diet" in many other parts of the world, is very different from the one on which our human ancestors are theorized to have evolved.[4] Although the current commonly accepted dietary recommendations from government health agencies and medical organizations are slowly shifting, over a half-century of fear-mongering regarding saturated fats and dietary cholesterol in the modern industrialized world has led to recommendations to consume a diet low in total fat and cholesterol, with an emphasis on carbohydrates—specifically, grains, such as wheat, corn, and rice—as the primary source of calories. The few fats that are recommended are vegetable oils (such as soybean and corn oil), which are high in fragile, easily oxidized polyunsaturated fatty acids; we have been cautioned away from the saturated fats found predominantly in animal foods and tropical plants (such as butter, coconut, and palm oils), which are more chemically stable and better suited for cooking.[5]

The modern industrial diet is also generally lower in phytonutrients and antioxidant-rich dark green and brightly colored vegetables and fruits than the diet our robust, healthy ancestors likely consumed. The majority of the plant foods we now consume are starchy carbohydrate sources, such as wheat, potatoes, and corn. This evolutionarily discordant diet has been linked to conditions as diverse as heart disease, acne, obesity, poor eyesight, polycystic ovarian syndrome (PCOS), and cancer.[6] When the physiological and biochemical effects of these foods, coupled with a lack of micronutrient-rich vegetables and whole, unprocessed, naturally occurring fats start affecting cognitive function later in life, we can add Alzheimer's disease to the list of conditions likely caused by this dietary derailment.

With epidemics of hypertension, diabetes, heart disease, and metabolic syndrome threatening human health on a global scale, the effects of this highly refined diet so poor in vitamins, minerals, and naturally occurring fats upon the physical body are undeniable. But the physiological insults of this diet don't stop at the boundary that separates the brain from the rest of the body (called the "blood-brain barrier"). The brain is an extremely energy-hungry organ: Although it typically accounts for just 2 percent of total body weight, the brain uses around 20 percent of the body's glucose and oxygen.[7] Considering the brain's disproportionate consumption of fuel, anything that interferes with fuel delivery or processing in the brain will have dramatic effects on memory, emotions, behavior, and cognition.

Metabolic syndrome (MetSy) is an especially important piece of this puzzle. MetSy is a conglomeration of markers that indicate the body is improperly handling carbohydrates.[8] (A person's body responds with abnormally high levels of insulin or blood glucose for a prolonged period upon consumption of starchy and sugary foods.) These markers include abdominal obesity (the apple shape of an enlarged midsection with relatively thinner arms and legs); elevated triglycerides (fats in the blood); elevated numbers of small, dense low-density lipoprotein (LDL) particles; reduced high-density lipoproteins (HDLs); elevated fasting blood glucose and insulin levels; hypertension (high blood pressure); and elevated hemoglobin A1c (a long-term measurement of blood glucose levels).[9] Many of these conditions go hand in hand with type 2 diabetes, and there is reason to suspect that mild cognitive impairment—the precursor to AD—could well be added to the diseases they lead to.

Most, if not all, of the features of MetSy can be ameliorated by reducing the amount of carbohydrate in the diet.[10] This is because MetSy is the result of long-term insulin resistance secondary to overconsumption of total food—refined carbohydrates, in particular—compounded by the relentless stress of modern life, poor quality and quantity of sleep, and insufficient physical activity, all of which contribute to a breakdown in the body's ability to properly process carbohydrates and other fuels. Other lifestyle and dietary factors beyond carbohydrate intake contribute to insulin resistance and MetSy, but excessive carbohydrate consumption is one of the most powerful drivers.

It is important to note here that being diagnosed with MetSy or type 2 diabetes is not required for a subsequent diagnosis of Alzheimer's disease. (We will explore this in more detail in chapter 2.) Due to genetics, environmental factors, or just the way things play out in the body, cognitive impairment or Alzheimer's disease might be the only observable manifestation of insulin resistance and carbohydrate intolerance. Therefore, even if all the numbers on one's bloodwork are in the "normal" ranges, the possibility of problems with carbohydrate handling and elevated insulin should not be dismissed outright. And it is much more likely that at least some of the features of MetSy *will* be present when the labwork is evaluated more closely. They might have been present for years, in fact, but the signs were missed because clinicians were looking for them mainly from the perspective of weight loss, heart disease, or diabetes, and not from the perspective of a connection to brain health and cognitive function.

The scientific literature shows that the brain is no more protected from metabolic and environmental assaults than the rest of the body. In fact, there is reason to believe that, due to its high energy demands, accelerated oxygen consumption, high concentration of long-chain polyunsaturated fatty acids (which are susceptible to damage by oxidation), and decreased capacity for regeneration (ability to create new cells), the brain is especially vulnerable to the detrimental effects of the modern diet and lifestyle.

If we look to type 2 diabetes as a model for energy usage in a body that has lost the ability to handle carbohydrates properly, we see that not only can the body no longer be fueled effectively by carbohydrates but also chronically elevated insulin levels prevent the body's other premier fuel sources—fats and ketones—from reaching high enough levels in the bloodstream to sustain the body. People with type 2 diabetes often experience problems with fatigue, chronic pain, and poor energy levels. This is because, despite often (but not always) being overweight, at a cellular level, they're actually starving. The same idea is at work in the Alzheimer's brain: At its heart, AD is a fuel shortage in the brain. It is the result of the widespread starvation and death of neurons secondary to hyperinsulinemia (excessive amounts of insulin in the blood), insulin resistance, and a reduced capacity to metabolize glucose.

What Is the Evidence?

Like any other modern chronic illness, Alzheimer's disease doesn't develop overnight. Measurable and subjective signs and symptoms appear years before a diagnosis is made. Cognitive function declines by degrees. (In fact, as I've said, "mild cognitive impairment" often precedes full-blown Alzheimer's.) What we consider the normal foibles and forgetfulness of older age might well be the earliest signs that the brain is struggling to fuel itself.

One of the primary hallmarks of AD is a reduction in the rate at which the brain uses glucose (called the cerebral metabolic rate of glucose, or CMRglu). Compared to healthy people, AD patients have shown up to 45 percent reductions in CMRglu, with some researchers claiming that this is the *predominant abnormality* in AD.[11] Notably, this reduced fuel usage is localized to regions of the brain involved in memory processing and learning, while areas dedicated to visual and sensorimotor processing are unaffected—meaning that cognitive function is affected, but not a person's ability to walk, see, pick things up, or otherwise move around. Positron emitting tomography (PET) scans of people at risk for developing AD show that this decline begins in younger years, long before symptoms of AD are present, and it seems to be the very first step in a long chain of events whose eventual end is AD. This drop in glucose usage as a triggering factor is particularly insidious because there are no overt signs that the change is occurring. The brain might spend decades compensating for and overcoming this fuel shortage before it has progressed to the point where signs and symptoms become evident. It is noteworthy that subjects tested in younger years are cognitively normal; they show no signs of Alzheimer's disease. Therefore, this slow decline in CMRglu can be seen as a kind of canary in the coal mine—preclinical evidence that something has gone awry long before damage has progressed to the point of overt signs and symptoms.

The decline in brain glucose metabolism can be detected in those at risk (based on genetic type or family history) as young as in their twenties and thirties, decades before noticeable manifestation of AD. This makes dietary and lifestyle interventions a lifelong concern, and not just something to tack onto an Alzheimer's diagnosis at age eighty, in desperation. The brain might be able to compensate for and overcome this suboptimal fuel delivery for years, which allows cognitive function to remain normal. And when cognitive function is normal in individuals in their forties or fifties, there's no reason to seek a PET scan to measure the brain's glucose usage. However, the occasional fuzzy-headedness and "brain fog" we tend to associate with normal aging—*Where did I leave my keys? Don't I have an appointment somewhere on Thursday?*—might be the brain's way of letting us know it is beginning to lose the ability to harness energy from glucose effectively. We can joke about having "senior moments," and we all have times when we walk into a room and forget why we went there, but as these things happen more frequently and in more disturbing ways as we age, they are no laughing matter.

At one time, Alzheimer's disease was flippantly referred to as "old timer's disease," because it typically struck the elderly. Now, however, individuals ever younger are being diagnosed with MCI and AD. No longer is cognitive impairment limited to those in their twilight years. Moreover, we might expect that a certain degree of memory loss and confusion is normal in people of very advanced age. But what are we to make of things when people in their fifties and sixties—or younger—begin to show the signs and symptoms of cognitive decline?

A decline in cerebral glucose metabolism has obvious ramifications. In the context of a standard diet containing the three main types of fuel sources (called *macronutrients*—proteins, fats, and carbohydrates), glucose (which derives predominantly from carbohydrates) serves as the brain's primary fuel. Therefore, if the brain's ability to use this fuel is compromised, neuronal cells will struggle to perform their functions and might eventually starve. To emphasize again: At its core, AD is the deterioration and death of brain cells via starvation.

Another piece of the puzzle linking AD to chronically elevated insulin levels is what is known as beta-amyloid (Aβ) plaques in the brain. (We'll cover Aβ in more detail in chapter 6.) Aβ plaques are protein fragments that accumulate in the brain, solidify, and interfere with cells' ability to communicate with each other. Aside from the reduced utilization of glucose, these plaques are one of the defining signatures of AD. The appearance of Aβ protein fragments is a normal process that occurs even in healthy people, but their formation into larger, insoluble masses represents a quintessential feature of AD.[12]

Aβ is found in healthy human brains, but in AD patients it accumulates far beyond the levels seen in healthy people.[13] This is noteworthy because, at low levels, the body can easily clear away Aβ proteins. But at higher levels they coalesce into plaques. Think of it this way: Everyday household trash isn't a problem as long as the sanitation crew comes by regularly to haul it away. But if the sanitation workers go on strike, the trash will accumulate and eventually build up to levels that will make the neighborhood intolerable and unlivable. This is what happens when too much Aβ builds up in the Alzheimer's brain and isn't cleared away.

If the low levels of Aβ found in healthy brains don't interfere with cognitive function, then something is causing Aβ to build up to dangerous levels in AD patients. There are two possible reasons for this: One is that AD patients are producing more of it; the second is that they are producing normal amounts of it, but it is not being broken down and cleared away as it should be—that is, the sanitation crew is on strike. Research indicates it is the latter.

The main way that Aβ is cleared out is with insulin-degrading enzyme—the same enzyme the body uses to clear away insulin after it has done its job of stopping the liver from releasing stored glucose into the bloodstream (as it does between meals) and helping to move glucose and amino acids out of the bloodstream and into cells. Enzymes are proteins that act as helpers and catalysts to make biochemical reactions happen more quickly and efficiently. I like to think of it this way: Parents of more than one child always claim they don't have a favorite child. Enzymes are not like this; they do choose favorites. In scientific terms, enzymes have higher affinities for certain targets of action (called substrates) than others. Insulin-degrading enzyme has both insulin and Aβ as its targets, but its affinity for insulin is much higher than for Aβ. (Insulin is the "favorite child.") Therefore, when both insulin and Aβ need to be broken down and cleared away, insulin takes precedence. This means that even when just small amounts of insulin are present, insulin-degrading enzyme (the sanitation crew) will focus its attention on clearing away the insulin, leaving the Aβ to accumulate.[14]

So when insulin levels are chronically elevated—as they often are in people consuming a diet high in refined carbohydrates, particularly when this is combined with being sedentary, chronically sleep deficient, and under a lot of stress (all aspects of the modern diet and lifestyle that can contribute to insulin resistance)—the enzyme is occupied with clearing the insulin, thus allowing the Aβ to build up and form plaques. This might be one explanation for why the highest risk for Alzheimer's disease is among people of a certain genetic makeup with type 2 diabetes and who are treated with insulin.[15] The higher the amount of insulin in the bloodstream, the more Aβ will build up, and the more it builds up without being cleared away, the more likely it is to form plaques.

How to Fuel a Struggling Brain

If AD is, at its heart, the result of specific brain regions becoming unable to properly metabolize glucose, coupled with a buildup of amyloid plaques and other neuronal structural changes, secondary to long-term chronically elevated insulin, fatty acid imbalance in the brain, and key micronutrient insufficiencies, then any dietary intervention aimed at improving or preventing this condition should seek to correct the metabolic and structural abnormalities via the following methods: reducing insulin levels; transitioning the body and brain to fuels other than glucose; and providing a rich supply of protective nutrients; in particular, omega-3 fatty acids, vitamin B_{12}, zinc, and other brain-critical vitamins and minerals.

As a model to guide therapeutic intervention, we can look to what happens during fasting or simple carbohydrate restriction to see how the body sustains itself when it is deprived of glucose in the diet. So if Alzheimer's is ultimately the result of neurons that are starving because they can no longer use glucose properly, then the first and most important step is to provide these neurons with a different source of fuel—one they *can* use.

Glucose Versus Ketones as Fuel for the Brain

The major switch that occurs when the body receives very little carbohydrate is that it switches from running on glucose as its primary fuel to instead using fats, another type of fuel called *ketones*, and small amounts of glucose derived from noncarbohydrate sources.[16] (The latter is a process called *gluconeogenesis*, and we will discuss it in detail in chapter 2.) Ketones are produced when insulin levels are very low. They are by-products of the body breaking down fat—from stored body fat as well as dietary fat in the foods we eat. Ketones themselves also serve as fuel, and the brain is particularly well equipped to thrive on ketones. There are a few different ways to elevate ketone levels, which we will explore in chapter 2, but for now it suffices to know that keeping insulin levels low via dramatically reducing carbohydrate intake is effective for most people.

It is often claimed that glucose is the brain's only fuel, or that the brain requires 120–140 grams of glucose per day. This is untrue and oversimplifies human physiology. Glucose is regularly cited as the "preferred" fuel for the body and brain. However, it is only preferred in the sense that it will generally be used first. It is neither more efficient nor physiologically "safer" than two of the other fuels the body and brain can run on: fats and ketones. In the absence of dietary carbohydrates, ketones can provide as much as 40–60 percent of the brain's energy, thus dramatically reducing the amount of glucose required.[17] Moreover, the brain's remaining requirement for glucose does not automatically imply a need for dietary carbohydrate. The human body is the ultimate reuse and recycle machine; it can convert other substances—such as amino acids (from protein) and glycerol (from fats)—into glucose.

Conventional medicine sometimes contends that ketones are harmful, but this is not the case. They are a completely normal part of human metabolism that preferentially fuel the brain and central nervous system while the rest of the body runs on fats during times of very low carbohydrate intake.[18] (The benign state of nutritional ketosis achieved via a very low-carbohydrate diet is not the same thing as the acutely dangerous state known as *diabetic ketoacidosis*. This is further clarified in chapter 2.)

The question you might be asking yourself now is, if ketones are such a useful fuel for the brain, and the Alzheimer's brain is struggling to fuel itself, then why doesn't the brain automatically and immediately shift to using ketones instead of glucose? The answer is: A sufficient supply of ketones isn't available. The body doesn't generate high amounts of ketones on a regular basis. Generally speaking, ketone production only occurs when insulin levels are very low. In fact, levels of ketones sufficient to fuel the brain are generally only produced when carbohydrate intake and resulting insulin levels are low enough to flip the metabolic switch that causes the body to make a wholesale shift away from glucose and toward fats as its primary fuel source. Put very simply, the body only generates high amounts of ketones when it needs to—for example, when carbohydrate intake and glucose availability are low enough that the body *must* shift to using a different source of fuel. Therefore, the most effective way to raise blood ketones and begin providing the brain with a fuel it can use properly is to dramatically reduce dietary carbohydrates. Other dietary and lifestyle factors affect insulin levels, and these will be addressed in subsequent chapters, but greatly reducing carbohydrate intake is among the simplest and easiest strategies to implement right off the bat.

People vary widely with regard to their individual level of carbohydrate tolerance and the precise amount of carbohydrate reduction their bodies require in order to make the transition from running mostly on glucose to running mostly on fat and ketones. However, generally speaking, in order for this to happen, carbohydrate intake needs to be much, much lower than it typically is on the starch- and grain-heavy standard American or Western diet.

A Dietary Path out of the Fog

If Alzheimer's disease is, in fact, another of the modern "diseases of civilization" primarily caused by a diet and lifestyle at odds with human physiology, then returning to a diet more congruent with the one on which our species is believed to have evolved is a reasonable starting point in the battle against this debilitating condition. This might resemble a Paleolithic diet—one made up of relatively high amounts of animal fat and protein; abundant nonstarchy vegetables; and moderate amounts of fruit, nuts, and seeds; and devoid of high-glycemic cereal grains, refined sugars, and chemically manipulated processed foods high in vegetable oils.

This type of diet—combined with appropriate amounts of physical activity, adequate sleep, stress reduction, and exposure to fresh air and daylight in order to support the body's natural circadian rhythm—might help maintain lifelong insulin sensitivity, resulting in vibrant function of the body and brain well into old age. Thus, a physiologically appropriate diet might help to prevent cognitive decline.

However, in order to potentially slow the progression of AD that has already taken hold, or possibly even reverse some of the existing cerebral damage and metabolic derangement observed in AD patients, carbohydrate reduction is a powerful first step. This reduction includes avoiding or greatly limiting otherwise wholesome, unprocessed foods that are high in starch or sugar, such as potatoes, yams, beets, beans, high sugar fruits (such as grapes, bananas, and apples), and other starchy tubers and root vegetables. These foods, which healthy, robust populations have been consuming for millennia, are not detrimental for health, *per se.* I am not suggesting that these foods are not nutritious, nor that they are in any way a cause of disease. Metabolically fit, healthy individuals need not avoid them. But for someone experiencing the ravages of AD or another form of cognitive decline or impairment—someone whose brain has lost the ability to harness sufficient fuel from glucose—providing the body with large amounts of glucose in the form of dietary carbohydrate will likely not be conducive to healing. It is only in the relative absence of dietary carbohydrates—and this includes even the wholesome, nutritious ones—that insulin levels will be low enough for the body to make the shift away from glucose and toward using fats for fuel and will therefore generate enough ketones to provide the brain with nourishment, the severe lack of which is primarily responsible for the signs and symptoms of AD in the first place. The therapeutic and neuroprotective effects of ketones are so impressive, in fact, that one of the premier researchers studying ketones and brain health has suggested that a drawback of the modern, carbohydrate-heavy diet is that it is "keto-deficient."[19]

Very low-carbohydrate ketogenic diets have a long history of efficacy for disorders of the central nervous system, and they seem especially promising for AD and other neurological conditions.[20] If ketones are the brain's primary fuel source under conditions of reduced glucose availability, then AD patients should show improvement in cognitive function on a ketogenic diet or with administration of ketones via an outside source. This has been demonstrated in "gold standard" randomized, double-blind, placebo-controlled studies. Oral administration of ketones has resulted in improved performance on cognition tests compared to placebo.[21]

In a study involving dietary ketosis via a very low-carbohydrate diet (less than 10 percent of total calories coming from carbs) for MCI patients, the low-carbohydrate subjects had better performance on memory tests compared to subjects on a 50 percent carbohydrate diet, with higher scores correlated to higher blood ketone levels.[22] (In other words, the higher the level of ketones in the blood, the better the subjects performed on the tests.) A significant reduction in insulin levels was observed for the low-carb group but not for the higher carb group, meaning that the reduced carbohydrate intake was successful at lowering insulin levels, while there was no significant change in insulin in subjects consuming half their total calories as carbohydrates. The authors speculated that the improved memory might have resulted from a combination of the brain's use of ketones and its improved insulin sensitivity, the latter of which might help it use glucose better.

Classical ketogenic diets have been used for almost a century for epilepsy treatment. These classical ketogenic diets call for upward of 80–90 percent of total calories coming from fat. That's quite a departure from the high-carbohydrate diet that has become the norm in the modern Western world. The good news is, something this drastic and difficult to maintain might not be necessary as a nutritional therapy for AD. Classical ketogenic diets restrict carbohydrates as well as proteins, because high-protein intakes might stimulate insulin secretion, which would undermine the purpose of a diet intended to generate an elevated level of ketones and limit the amount of glucose in the bloodstream. (This restriction on the amount of both carbohydrates and proteins explains why a classical ketogenic diet is so high in fat: there are only three macronutrients, so when we limit intake of two of them, only one is left to fill the gap. Calories and nourishment have to come from somewhere, and on a ketogenic diet, with reductions in carbohydrates and proteins, they come mostly from fat, in the form of stored body fat as well as nourishing fats from wholesome foods, such as grass-fed and pastured meats, wild-caught fish, avocados, nuts, and seeds.)

Rather than a very strict ketogenic diet as a dietary strategy for Alzheimer's, simply lowering carbohydrate intake to a point where some ketones are generated and excessive insulin levels are corrected could potentially have positive effects just by easing the metabolic burden on the brain. Of course, individual insulin sensitivity is a factor, as is an individual's ability to generate elevated levels of ketones. Some people's bodies simply generate higher ketone levels more readily than others', but ketone levels would be expected to rise at least somewhat in anyone following a very low-carbohydrate and higher fat diet.

Moreover, unlike a classical ketogenic diet, a very low-carbohydrate diet (which still generates some ketones) allows for consumption of a wider array of low glycemic load vegetables and fruits, which are typically richer in micronutrients, antioxidants, and phytochemicals than refined grains and sugars, which carry a high glycemic index and load and would be prohibited on such a diet.[23] Therefore, a very low-carb diet as a primary avenue for therapy is more practical, since the difficulty with sticking to classical ketogenic diets is that they're extremely restrictive, and some people might find them unpalatable for the long term. The difficulty of staying on a traditional ketogenic diet for an extended period of time might also explain why much of the research involving ketones as therapy for AD is limited to ketone drink mixtures rather than dietary overhauls. (More on these interesting compounds in chapter 2.) There is also likely trepidation on the part of the medical community regarding such a high fat intake—particularly saturated fat—despite mounting evidence that saturated fat intake is *not* associated with increased risk for cardiovascular disease and that reductions in dietary *carbohydrate*, in fact, can improve multiple markers for heart disease.[24] This wonderfully promising avenue for research in dietary therapy is being hindered by an outdated nutritional school of thought.

Other Factors: Supplements and Lifestyle

The damage observed in the Alzheimer's brain is complex and multifactorial. Therefore, any intervention intended to delay or possibly reverse this damage should be a multifaceted strategy that addresses the root cause as well as ancillary and downstream effects. The majority of these potentially helpful practices are nutritional in nature, but others are alterations in lifestyle practices. Obviously, the foundation of what might be considered an "anti-Alzheimer's strategy" is a diet very low in carbohydrates and high in fats and overall nutrient density. Beyond that, there are nutritional supplements that might be beneficial based on their biochemical effects, and there are also lifestyle interventions that might be effective due to their influence on reducing insulin levels, enhancing overall metabolic efficiency in the body, and directly facilitating better cognitive function by stimulating the brain to form new neuronal connections. We will explore each of these in more detail in parts three and four.

The Takeaway: There Is a Solution

Researchers are beginning to amass evidence that the nutritional and lifestyle strategies introduced here and discussed in more detail throughout this book are, in fact, effective for reversing cognitive impairment and Alzheimer's disease. Dale Bredesen, a researcher and physician at the forefront of this research, has developed a multipronged intervention that has yielded extremely promising results.[26] While the intervention calls for adjusting multiple biochemical and physiological levers via diet and lifestyle, it should come as no surprise that the foundation of this approach is a switch to what Dr. Bredesen calls a *lipid-based metabolism*—that is, following a diet that transitions the body from being fueled primarily by glucose to being fueled primarily by fats and ketones.

> AD is not a mysterious, untreatable brain disease—it is a reversible, metabolic/toxic, usually systemic illness with a relatively large window for treatment.
>
> —*Dale Bredesen*[25]

Some of Dr. Bredesen's patients, whose cognitive function was so severely impaired that they had to leave their professions, are now back at work and leading their normal lives. He has achieved fascinating improvements in patients with mild cognitive impairment as well as full-blown Alzheimer's, and the positive effects were even achieved among individuals who were carriers of the ApoE4 genotype, which is the strongest genetic risk factor for AD. (More on this in chapter 7.)

Dr. Bredesen's program—called MEND, for metabolic enhancement for neurodegeneration—hammers home the point that, with the possible exception of damage caused by physical trauma to the head, skull, or brain, cognitive impairment and dementia are metabolic problems. As such, they require metabolic therapies. There might come a time when pharmaceutical medications help augment these metabolic therapies, but treating the symptoms piecemeal will never be as effective a solution as addressing the root causes.

Other aspects of Dr. Bredesen's program involve just the sort of lifestyle practices we'll explore in part three: good quantity and quality of sleep, brief periods of fasting, stress management, exercise, restoration of vitamin and mineral sufficiency, and more. That these dietary and lifestyle factors are entirely within our control should give us hope that we can have a positive impact on a disease process for which pharmaceutical treatments developed to date have been so disappointing and ineffective.

CHAPTER 2

Brain Fuel Metabolism: Key to Understanding Alzheimer's Disease

I n order for you to understand and appreciate the paramount importance of dietary and lifestyle interventions to reduce insulin levels and generate ketones as a strategy for combating Alzheimer's disease, we will need to dive deeper into the complex world of brain fuel metabolism. Don't be intimidated; I'll keep things simple. These are complicated concepts, but they're not beyond the understanding of nonscientists who simply want to help their loved ones regain healthy cognitive function to whatever extent might be possible, and you certainly don't need a PhD to understand the basics. But understand them you must, for it is only in understanding these fundamentals that the logic behind adopting a low-carbohydrate, high-fat diet and implementing other lifestyle strategies to improve insulin sensitivity and reduce inflammation and oxidative stress will become self-evident and undeniable. With that, let's dive in.

Is Alzheimer's Disease "Type 3 Diabetes"?

In chapter 1, I explained the overlap between metabolic syndrome and Alzheimer's disease, as chronic hyperinsulinemia is one of the primary driving factors behind both conditions. In addition to "type 3 diabetes" and "diabetes of the brain," which are fascinatingly descriptive phrases, researchers have also used the phrase "metabolic cognitive syndrome" to hammer home the point that this particular form of dementia is a *metabolic issue*.[1] Researchers increasingly recognize that cognitive impairment might go hand in hand with MetSy. Metabolic syndrome is a risk factor for Alzheimer's, and while these two conditions have multiple pathological features in common, the most powerful one is insulin resistance.[2]

With all the focus on insulin, carbohydrates, and brain glucose utilization, you might be saying to yourself, "But my loved one isn't diabetic." This might well be true, but it doesn't mean that he has no issues related to disturbed carbohydrate metabolism or dysregulated insulin levels. In order to connect the pathologies of type 2 diabetes, insulin resistance, and cognitive impairment, we will need to explore how type 2 diabetes is currently diagnosed and see why this is problematic.

Type 2 diabetes is typically diagnosed by assessing biomarkers related only to glucose. For example, based on criteria established by the American Diabetes Association, the following represents "increased risk" for diabetes:[3]

- Fasting blood glucose: 100–125 mg/dL (5.6–6.9 mmol/L)
- Hemoglobin A1c: 5.7–6.4% (Hemoglobin A1c [HbA1c] is an approximate average of the blood glucose level during the previous three months or so.)
- Blood glucose measured two hours after a 75-gram liquid glucose load (oral glucose tolerance test): 140–199 mg/dL (7.8–11 mmol/L)

In order to trigger a diagnosis of full-blown type 2 diabetes, measurements need to exceed those ranges:[4]

- Fasting blood glucose: ≥ 126 mg/dL (7.0 mmol/L)
- Hemoglobin A1c: ≥ 6.5%
- Blood glucose response to two-hour oral glucose tolerance test: ≥ 200 mg/dL (11.1 mmol/L)

Notice that none of these diagnostic criteria include anything related to insulin. This is a terribly limited way to look at glycemic control, and by clinging to this myopic vision, thousands—potentially millions—of people with significantly impaired insulin sensitivity remain undiagnosed. Joseph Kraft, MD, who did pioneering work in this area decades ago, uncovered the scope of this underdiagnosis, and frankly, it is shocking. According to Dr. Kraft, "There are far too many who are told, 'Don't worry, your fasting blood sugars are normal.'"[5] What all tests to assess blood glucose fail to do—whether they are measuring fasting values, HbA1c, or response to an oral glucose tolerance test (OGTT)—is provide any data on *insulin* levels. A "normal" blood sugar level, "normal" A1c, and "normal" response to the OGTT might only be normal because pathologically high insulin levels are keeping the blood sugar in check.

With "normal" blood glucose levels, no one could blame an individual for believing they're totally in the clear with regard to their metabolic health. However, as time goes on, and the body is flooded with more and more insulin, the body's cells stop "listening" to insulin's message; that is, they become resistant to it. When cells become resistant to insulin, more insulin is needed to overcome the resistance and force the cells to respond. All the while, as insulin levels rise higher and higher, the blood glucose remains normal. It is only when one of two things (or both) occurs that the blood glucose will rise to the point of alerting a physician that the patient is prediabetic or diabetic: (1) the body's cells become so resistant to insulin that they no longer take up glucose from the bloodstream in a timely fashion; or (2) the cells that secrete insulin from the pancreas (called *beta cells*) can no longer keep up with the extreme demand for insulin (sometimes called *beta cell burnout*). Both of these have the same result: a sustained elevation of blood glucose.

So you can see that blood glucose might be the last thing to rise in individuals with impaired insulin sensitivity. Insulin levels might have been damagingly high for years—decades, in some people—before glucose rises to the point of triggering a type 2 diabetes diagnosis. For this reason, Dr. Kraft began administering his patients an OGTT that extended the standard two hours to five hours, and even more importantly, included insulin measurements. (During a typical OGTT, a patient drinks 50–75 grams of glucose in liquid form, and their blood glucose is measured at thirty-minute intervals for two hours.) This is how he discovered that thousands of people with seemingly normal glucose levels were maintaining those levels only as a result of dangerously high insulin, leading him to write that OGTTs without insulin assays have

> Insulin resistance is usually at or near the top of the list of known lifestyle-related factors heightening the risk of declining cognition in the elderly.
>
> —*Stephen Cunnane and colleagues*[7]

"awesome shortcomings."[6] To describe the state of hyperinsulinemia with normal blood glucose, Dr. Kraft coined the phrase "diabetes in-situ," or "occult diabetes." (Occult meaning *hidden*—the diabetes [high glucose] is hidden by the high insulin.)

An emerging body of evidence suggests that an increased prevalence of insulin abnormalities and insulin resistance in Alzheimer's disease may contribute to the disease pathophysiology and clinical symptoms.

— *G. Stennis Watson and Suzanne Craft*[8]

If a hyperinsulinemic Alzheimer's patient is not a diagnosed diabetic, this is simply the artifact of type 2 diabetes being diagnosed solely via glucose measurements with no concern whatsoever for insulin levels. But make no mistake: These individuals are in serious metabolic trouble. With sky-high insulin levels, all that remains is for enough time to pass that the regulatory mechanisms begin to derail and blood glucose does rise to the point of a diabetes diagnosis. Very high insulin levels are a common finding among AD patients, and hyperinsulinemia is an independent risk factor for developing cognitive decline and dementia.[9] (Meaning, regardless of genetics, for someone diagnosed as diabetic or who has other risk factors, chronically elevated insulin alone is a significant risk factor.) In fact, one study concluded that people with hyperinsulinemia had double the risk for developing AD compared to those with normal insulin levels—and these individuals were not diabetic.[10] At least, not by conventional standards. Dr. Kraft—and I—would disagree.

Aside from elevated blood glucose, you might also be thinking that you or your loved one doesn't exhibit one of the other common comorbidities of type 2 diabetes: excess body fat or obesity. But even if you have a "healthy" body weight or body mass index (BMI), this does not at all preclude MetSy or type 2 diabetes—or cognitive impairment. In fact, many older individuals with Alzheimer's disease are underweight. But being underweight or at a healthy weight is not indicative that they have a healthy metabolism. While many people accumulate excess body fat as a result of chronically high insulin levels, many others do not. According to Dr. Kraft, "Not everyone with type 2 diabetes is obese. . . . Normal weight, normal BMI, normal fasting blood sugar, and normal fasting insulins do not exclude hyperinsulinemia, type 2 diabetes."[11]

There is growing awareness in the medical community that looks can be deceiving and that what we consider a "healthy" body weight really says very little about what's going on inside someone's body. It's entirely possible—and increasingly common—for people to have multiple features of MetSy and insulin resistance while still remaining lean. Excess body weight (particularly around the midsection) is only one indicator of metabolic derailment. Its absence does not imply that no other indicators are present. (Other factors that would suggest MetSy include hypertension [high blood pressure], elevated triglycerides, low HDL cholesterol, elevated fasting insulin, and high fasting glucose or high HbA1c.) Researchers call these individuals the "normal weight obese," or, more informally, TOFI—thin outside, fat inside.[12] It should come as no surprise that these individuals—people who appear healthy on the outside but who have metabolic profiles that indicate extreme damage and dysregulation internally—are at greater risk for cardiometabolic disease and overall mortality and compromised health than are healthy people, as well as overweight individuals with biomarkers within the normal ranges (called the "metabolically healthy obese").[13] One study found that between 7 percent and 36 percent of obese people are metabolically healthy, while between 21 percent and 87 percent of nonobese people are metabolically unhealthy.[14] So it might sound strange, but the fact is, being at a "healthy" body weight and having "normal" blood sugar levels don't give anyone a free pass with regard to MetSy or chronically elevated insulin. If anything, they provide a false sense of security and might mask underlying metabolic problems.

Dr. Kraft's extended OGTT with insulin assays revealed that the incidence of hyperinsulinemia is wildly underestimated and underappreciated. The scope of the problem with chronically elevated insulin is difficult to quantify, but for certain, the millions of people diagnosed with type 2 diabetes and MetSy are just the tip of the iceberg. There are strong physiological and biochemical mechanisms now linking chronic hyperinsulinemia to the vast majority of modern illnesses afflicting millions around the world, including conditions that have historically been deemed idiopathic—meaning no one knows what causes them—such as vertigo, tinnitus, and Ménière's disease.[15]

There is no question that people with type 2 diabetes have an increased risk for cognitive impairment and Alzheimer's disease.[16] But we must not let the term *type 3 diabetes* mislead us into thinking that type 2 diabetes is required for the development of Alzheimer's disease or MCI. Many Alzheimer's patients have absolutely normal glucose levels and therefore are not diagnosed diabetics. Remember, the problem isn't glucose; it's insulin. Or rather, it is insulin resistance, either in the brain or in the rest of the body—or both.[17] Alzheimer's patients frequently exhibit high levels of insulin in their blood but low levels in the brain and cerebrospinal fluid, which helps explain some of the pathological features of AD that we'll explore later.

Type 2 and type 3 diabetes are not the same illness, and certainly one need not be a diagnosed diabetic to develop Alzheimer's disease, and many Alzheimer's patients are not diagnosed diabetics. As we established previously, while they're not the same conditions, they likely have the same primary underlying causes. It's simply the ultimate manifestation of the underlying insulin resistance that differs. People with type 2 diabetes have a higher risk for cognitive decline than people without diabetes, but as some researchers have done, it seems more accurate to say that "patients with Alzheimer's disease may have a greater risk for glucoregulatory impairments than do healthy older adults."[18] And it might be more accurate still to say that patients with glucoregulatory impairments have a greater risk for Alzheimer's disease than do healthy older adults.

With body weight often remaining normal, and fasting glucose and A1c being the *last* things to rise, I'll co-opt a famous expression from a political campaign years ago: "It's the insulin, stupid." (Fasting insulin levels are easily measured in a physician-ordered blood test. However, even if the fasting insulin level is normal, this doesn't preclude problems with insulin remaining elevated for a prolonged period after meals and, therefore, most of the day. The five-hour OGTT with insulin assay can provide an eye-opening look at your body's handling of carbohydrates. Drinking 50 or 75 grams of glucose in liquid form is not something I recommend, and it doesn't much mimic the way we eat "in the real world," but it will give you a good look at your or your loved one's insulin levels in response to a large amount of simple sugar. This is not a common test to have run, but your doctor should be able to locate a laboratory that can perform it.)

Brain Fuel Metabolism: Getting Energy from Glucose and Ketones

As I discussed in chapter 1, the reduced use of glucose in brain regions involved in memory and other processes that are compromised in MCI and

AD is one of the invariant signatures of these conditions. In fact, the extent of the reduction is tied to disease severity—meaning, the lower the cerebral metabolic rate of glucose (CMRglu), the more severe the condition. To give you a sense of the numbers here, a longitudinal study using PET scans to measure CMRglu in people aged fifty to eighty showed that a reduced hippocampal metabolic rate of glucose at baseline (meaning the start of the study) strongly predicted progression from normal cognitive function to AD, with the greatest reductions at baseline correlating with the quickest development of overt AD.[19] In other words, the more compromised someone's CMRglu was when it was measured at the beginning of the study, the more quickly they progressed to full-blown Alzheimer's. (Think of it like buying a brand-new car that's never been driven before versus purchasing a used car that already has some mileage on it, as well as a few dents and dings. The used car, with its preexisting damage, is likely to develop additional problems more quickly than the new one in pristine condition.) At baseline, in people who progressed from normal cognition to MCI, hippocampal glucose metabolism was 15 percent reduced, with an annual rate of decline of 2.4 percent. In individuals who progressed from normal cognition to AD, baseline CMRglu was 26 percent below that of people who did not develop AD, and the annual rate of decline was 4.4 percent—almost twice as high as that of those who developed the less severe MCI, and more than five times higher than the mere 0.8 percent annual rate of decline measured in subjects who had normal CMRglu at baseline and did not develop AD.[20] (A slight and gradual decline in cognitive function with advanced age is to be expected and might even be inevitable; it is a relatively drastic and more rapid decline that leads to MCI and AD.) Assuming the rates of decline were somewhat constant, extrapolating backward indicates that the decline might have started several years before baseline testing, perhaps decades before overt signs of AD began to manifest.

At baseline, despite the already decreased CMRglu in some subjects, all subjects were cognitively normal, which suggests that the brain is able to compensate for quite some time before its compromised energy generation becomes insurmountable and symptoms start showing themselves. This starting point of reduced glucose utilization in the brain and a stronger rate of continued decline might be one of the earliest triggering events leading to an ultimate end point of AD. In fact, in this longitudinal study, the risk for future cognitive decline was twofold greater and the time of survival twofold less per one-unit reduction in hippocampal metabolic rate of glucose.[21] (The larger the reduction in the metabolic rate of glucose, the higher the risk for cognitive decline, and the shorter the person's life span.) Other studies support these findings. Compared to healthy controls (people with normal cognition), AD patients have shown up to a staggering 45 percent reduction in CMRglu, with one study's authors claiming that this is the "predominant abnormality" and "primary pathophysiological mechanism" in AD.[22] It is particularly insidious that the disease process might have its origins so many years before noticeable signs and symptoms are present, because in the absence of overt symptoms, there is no reason to suspect metabolic derangement is brewing that might ultimately lead to severely compromised cognitive function. For this reason, potential prevention strategies and reduction of risk should be lifelong concerns. Although it might well be possible to reverse some of the impaired cognition in those with Alzheimer's and MCI, it is far easier to take control of matters long before the horse has gotten out of the barn. As they say, an ounce of prevention is worth a pound of cure. (We'll address potential prevention in chapter 24.)

Since this reduction in glucose usage in specific brain regions is one of the things that happens earliest in MCI and AD—long before the formation of beta-amyloid plaques and before any noticeable decline in cognition—it is likely one of the primary causal factors. Also recall that this reduction is observable via PET scan in people in their thirties and forties, long before signs of dementia begin to appear. The question researchers long sought to answer was, if neurons involved in learning and memory processing were not metabolizing glucose at the normal rate, was this because they weren't taking up enough glucose, or because though they were taking it up just fine, they were not using it effectively? In other words, was the problem one of supply or of demand? It was a bit of a chicken-and-egg question, but researchers now believe that the problem begins with demand. Brain uptake of glucose appears normal in many cases of MCI and even in the early stages of AD. It's the metabolism of the glucose that's reduced. After this goes on for a while, the cells then take up less glucose: If there's little demand, then there's no need for a large supply.

Since compromised fuel metabolism in regions of the brain involved in memory processing, learning, and some aspects of behavior seems to be the driving factor behind cognitive impairment, let's explore how the brain gets its energy.

How the Brain Gets Its Energy

The brain is an energy hog; it requires a great deal of fuel. Under "normal" dietary conditions—that is, when someone consumes a diet with a significant amount of carbohydrates—the brain's primary fuel is glucose. However, as we know, the brain is somewhat adaptable and can run on another type of fuel, too: ketones. The brain's flexibility in the kinds of fuel it is able to use was essential to our survival throughout evolutionary history. During times of famine, food scarcity, or even just a long winter when there might not have been significant amounts of carbohydrate-rich plant foods available, if we'd had no ability to use fuels other than glucose, we would have been in serious trouble.

Fortunately, when glucose is in short supply, the brain is more than happy to run on ketones—provided they are available. However, as mentioned previously, ketones are only produced in the body when insulin levels are low, typically as a result of restricting dietary carbohydrates. (Many other factors affect insulin levels and insulin sensitivity, but for most people, carbohydrate intake has the largest impact. We'll look at other relevant factors in part three.) For this reason, among people consuming a typical modern Western diet—which is high in carbohydrates—ketone levels are almost always very low. They might rise a little bit overnight—several hours pass since the last meal was eaten and insulin presumably comes back to its low baseline level, so ketone levels might be very slightly elevated first thing in the morning—but this is almost insignificant compared to the levels that are generated around the clock when someone eats very little carbohydrate.

Textbooks and scientific papers cite different estimates for the brain's daily requirement for glucose, but they typically range from 110–145 grams per day.[23] However, being that glucose is not the brain's only viable fuel source, when ketone levels are elevated, ketones can provide as much as 60 percent of the brain's energy requirements, which would leave the brain needing far less than 110–145 grams of glucose.[24] Not only that, but compared to when glucose is burned for fuel, ketones actually help to generate more energy while inducing less damage, making the fueling system more efficient overall. (Think of ketones as a "clean energy" source compared to glucose.) The ability of ketones to supercharge the body and brain has led one prominent ketone researcher to say, "Ketone bodies deserve the designation of a 'superfuel.'"[25]

We've established that the Alzheimer's brain is struggling because critical regions have lost the ability to harness energy from glucose. And even though a logical and obvious solution to this problem would be for the brain to simply switch over to using ketones instead of glucose, recall that the brain can't use ketones if a steady supply of them isn't available. And as long as there are large amounts of insulin in the bloodstream, the body has no reason to generate ketones. In fact, high levels of insulin directly inhibit the formation of ketones. So for someone who wants to generate enough ketones to provide a significant amount of fuel to neurons that are starving, high insulin levels are a nearly insurmountable roadblock. (At the risk of complicating matters, there are ways to raise ketone levels when insulin is high. We'll get to those in a bit. For now, let's stick with how the body generates ketones under normal circumstances.)

We know that glucose uptake and utilization are impaired in the Alzheimer's brain. Do we know for sure that the AD brain is able to take up and use ketones? Yes, we do. A Canadian research team led by Stephen Cunnane, PhD, has proven that brain ketone uptake and metabolism are not impaired in AD.[26] In general, the higher the ketone levels in the blood (within safe limits), the more ketones the brain takes in. According to Dr. Cunnane and colleagues:

> Results suggest that ketones are actually the preferred energy substrate for the brain because they enter the brain in proportion to their plasma concentration irrespective of glucose availability; if the energy needs of the brain are being increasingly met by ketones, glucose uptake decreases accordingly. This decrease in brain glucose uptake when both ketones and glucose are available supports the notion that ketones are the brain's preferred fuel. Nevertheless, it is uncommon for both ketones and glucose to be available; normally, when one is increased in the blood the other is decreased. Under conditions of normal energy sufficiency and three meals per day, ketogenesis is supressed [sic] and glucose supplies >95% of the brain's energy requirements; hence, glucose . . . is the brain's dominant but not actually its preferred fuel.[27]

The fact that the brain can fuel itself with ketones—even an aged, Alzheimer's-ravaged brain—should point us immediately toward dietary and lifestyle strategies that reduce insulin levels and elevate ketones, such as a very low-carbohydrate diet and the other interventions we'll explore. That elevation of ketones improves cognitive function in individuals with MCI and Alzheimer's has been shown time and time again, including in "gold standard" randomized, double-blind, placebo-controlled studies.[28] Ketones are a premier fuel source for the brain that—albeit unintentionally, via our carbohydrate-dense diet—we are preventing our bodies from generating in amounts significant enough to serve this critical purpose.

However—and I cannot emphasize this enough—it is only the brain's *glucose* energy supply that is insufficient. If we can elevate ketones—and we can—then we can provide a significant amount of alternative fuel to power these struggling neurons. As if that weren't enough, studies show that mice put on a diet designed to generate ketones not only have an increased brain utilization of ketones but also have an increase in the cerebral metabolic rate of glucose, as well—a win-win![30] Granted, this was shown in mice, not humans, but it's still promising.

> When the brain's energy supply is insufficient to meet its metabolic needs, the neurons that work hardest, especially those concerned with memory and cognition, are among the first to exhibit functional incapacity (for example, impairment of memory and cognitive performance).
>
> —*Sami Hashim and Theodore VanItallie*[29]

Moreover, when MCI and AD patients show markedly improved cognitive function when their ketone levels are elevated, it suggests that the affected areas of the brain are not "dead," but rather are dormant, perhaps just waiting to receive adequate nourishment before springing back into action. According to Dr. Cunnane's group, the brain-energy deficit "can at least in part be bypassed by ketogenic treatments. A core element of this interpretation is that brain cells and/or networks that were previously dysfunctional can start to function more normally again once they are provided with more fuel, that is, they were starving or exhausting but not dead; otherwise this cognitive improvement would not be possible."[31]

I hope you're as fascinated and excited as I am! This is cutting-edge research, and it's a therapeutic avenue far more promising than any pharmaceutical drug developed to date. Yet, sadly, it's a strategy you're unlikely to hear about from your family physician, and indeed, even from most neurologists. This information is readily available in the scientific and medical literature. But it does no good languishing in journals that loved ones and caregivers of AD and MCI patients are unlikely to read. No one has been bringing this critical information to the people who need it most—until now.

Why are you unlikely to hear about these fascinating—and potentially life-altering—strategies from your medical teams? There are several reasons: (1) Physicians don't always have time to keep up with the latest developments in their own specialties, let alone come across research on ketones and brain fuel metabolism in esoteric journals that might be targeted toward other fields. (2) Understandably, it's nearly impossible to wrap one's head around the possibility—the mere possibility—that something as seemingly complex and intractable as Alzheimer's disease can be improved with a special diet. (3) Despite a plethora of journal articles, books, websites, podcasts, social media campaigns, and professional conferences highlighting the astounding therapeutic potential of ketogenic diets as therapy for a wide array of chronic illnesses, there is still a great deal of ignorance and confusion surrounding what, exactly, ketones are, what they do, and whether they're safe.

I cannot do anything about the first issue. My goal in writing this book is to change your mind about the second. Regarding the third, we've got some work to do.

Two points are clear—(i) AD is at least in part exacerbated by (if not actually caused by) chronic, progressive brain fuel starvation due specifically to brain glucose deficit, and (ii) attempting to treat the cognitive deficit early in AD using ketogenic interventions in clinical trials is safe, ethical, and scientifically well-founded. —*Stephen Cunnane and colleagues*[32]

Ketosis Versus Ketoacidosis

Ketones, as I've outlined, are produced as a by-product of the breakdown of fats. Let's go a bit deeper. Consider the human body as being like a hybrid car: It can run on several different types of fuel. In fact, we run on multiple types of fuel concurrently, depending on the activity we're engaged in and which organ or type of cell we're looking at. For example, red blood cells must run on glucose; they lack the "machinery" to use fats or ketones. Most cells in the brain use glucose or ketones; they don't fuel themselves on fats. When we consume a diet very low in carbohydrate, there isn't enough glucose to fuel the body, so the body is forced to transition to fueling itself primarily with fat, thus "sparing" what little glucose is available for the tissues that absolutely require it. (I might start to sound repetitive here, but it's so important to understand this fact, it's worth repeating.) Humans generally don't use protein as an energy source. We might break down small amounts of protein to use amino acids for fuel, but the fuel the body likes to use best is fat—that's why we store so much of it. (Some of us more easily than others!)

Researchers often claim that ketones are a kind of "backup" fuel, turned to only during fasting or times of food scarcity. However, this is based on the assumption that glucose is the preferred fuel for the body. In order to show that glucose is likely not the body's preferred fuel, and that, in fact, it might be fat that we are better suited to run on, let's take a quick detour into fuel storage in the human body. I promise, there's a method to the madness: Understanding these basic concepts will give you or your loved one the confidence to adopt a very low-carbohydrate, high-fat diet. This isn't a fringe idea, or some off-the-wall approach being peddled by the latest TV snake oil salesman; it is a nutritional therapy rooted in the fundamentals of human physiology.

Let's start at the top of table 2.1 and work our way down. Our bodies have three compartments to hold carbohydrate (abbreviated CHO)—specifically,

Table 2.1. Energy Reserves in Humans

Stored Fuel	Type of Tissue It's Stored in	Fuel Reserves (grams)	Fuel Reserves (kcal—"calories")
Glucose (CHO)	Body fluids	20	80
Glycogen (CHO)	Liver	70	280
Glycogen (CHO)	Muscle	120	480
Protein	Muscle	6,000	24,000
Fat	Adipose (body fat)	15,000	135,000

Source: Thomas M. Devlin, ed. *Textbook of Biochemistry With Clinical Correlations.* 7th Edition. (Hoboken, NJ: John Wiley & Sons, Inc., 2011): 849.
Note: Based on an adult weighing -155 pounds (70 kg)

glucose. The first is in body fluids—mostly blood but also cerebrospinal fluid, the vitreous humor surrounding the eyeballs, and other body fluids. This is 20 grams—80 calories—of fuel. (One gram of carbohydrate provides 4 calories of energy.) That's not much. Eighty calories isn't anything to write home about when we're talking about supplying fuel to the whole body and brain, so let's move on to the other form of stored glucose in our bodies: glycogen.

Glycogen is to human beings what starch is to plants: It's the form in which we store carbohydrate. (We store it as glycogen, while a potato, for example, stores it as starch.) Since our blood can only hold so much glucose at any given time (even for a type 2 diabetic with sky-high blood sugar), our bodies have to find somewhere else to put it. "Somewhere else" is in our liver and in our muscles. The liver can only hold about 70 grams of carbohydrate as glycogen, or about 280 calories' worth. That's still not much. As a native New Yorker, I can tell you that just one of those classic New York bagels nearly the size of your head can pack close to a 70-gram wallop of carbohydrate all by itself. So this liver glycogen, like the glucose in the blood, doesn't seem like such a great fuel for the body to rely on.

But the muscles—now we're getting somewhere. Even a relatively nonmuscular person still has a fair bit of muscle mass. The hypothetical 155-pound person represented in table 2.1 stores about 120 grams of carbohydrate in their muscle glycogen, for around 480 calories. Not too shabby, but still nothing to brag about. (If you've ever been to an Italian or Chinese restaurant, you've likely consumed more than 120 grams of carbohydrate in a single meal, courtesy of fresh bread, pasta, dessert, and wine, or rice, noodles, wonton and dumpling wrappers, and sugary sauces thickened with cornstarch.) One hundred twenty grams of carbohydrate from muscle glycogen is not a reliable fuel source. And, the more important factor working against muscle glycogen as a fuel for the whole body (or brain) is that it can only be used to power activity in the muscles in which it's stored. It does the rest of the body no good. Glycogen stored in, say, your biceps, can't be released into the bloodstream when your blood sugar gets low. Only liver glycogen can do that, so muscle glycogen can't serve as fuel for the rest of the body.

Moving down to protein, we have about 6,000 grams of body protein, for 24,000 calories of stored fuel. (One gram of protein provides 4 calories.) Now that is a lot of stored energy! But where is that protein stored? In our muscles. And also in our organs, glands, bones, tendons, ligaments, and other precious tissues that we would not want to break down (catabolize) for fuel. Protein is far too valuable for these other purposes to be siphoned off and used as an energy source. So those 24,000 calories are awfully tempting, but as a fuel source, they're out.

There's one more potential fuel source remaining: fat. And look at that: 15,000 grams of fat stored in the adipose tissue (body fat), for a whopping 135,000 calories! (One gram of fat provides 9 calories of energy.) Now we're talking!

The human body has an almost unlimited capacity to accumulate adipose tissue—that is, to store fat. (Many of us know this only too well!) Taking this into account, it almost seems as if nature, evolution, the big voice in the sky, or whatever you choose to believe in, evolved, created, or designed our bodies to run on fat, because fat is the fuel the "gas tank" of the human body is equipped to hold the most of. Plus, if 1 gram of carbohydrate provides only 4 calories of fuel, and fat provides 9, then gram for gram, fat gives us more than twice as much energy. Remember this the next time you hear someone say that carbohydrates are the body's "preferred fuel source."

Many clinicians and researchers alike—particularly physicians who encounter daily the devastating effects of the modern, high-carbohydrate, high-insulin-inducing diet—now believe that fat is the body's preferred and premier fuel source, and that fat and ketones are not the "backup" or emergency fuels but, rather, the ones we're supposed to be running on most of the time. This helps explain why a low-carbohydrate diet must also be high in fat. If we're getting very little fuel from carbohydrate, and we don't want to use protein as a main fuel source, then the only thing left is fat—both our stored body fat and the fat in our food. To be clear, the body does require glucose, but it doesn't require it in anywhere near the levels we force it to handle from constant infusions of breakfast cereal, crackers, granola bars, pasta, bread, cookies, juice, and soda.

Okay, fine . . . fats, proteins, carbohydrates. Where do ketones fit in?

A side benefit to fueling the body primarily with fats, rather than carbohydrates, is that when the breakdown of fats exceeds the body's capacity to utilize all of that fuel, some of the fats are converted into ketones, and the ketones themselves are an additional fuel source. This is a normal, healthy metabolic process, called "nutritional ketosis" or what Dr. Robert Atkins (yes, *that* Dr. Atkins) called "benign dietary ketosis."

Nutritional ketosis—a perfectly normal physiological response to the body's need for a fuel other than glucose—is a completely different metabolic state from *diabetic ketoacidosis*. Confusion regarding beneficial nutritional ketosis and harmful and pathological diabetic ketoacidosis—even among educated medical professionals, who ought to know better—is what so often prevents doctors and nutritionists from recommending low-carbohydrate and ketogenic diets for their patients. Just because they both have "keto" in their names doesn't mean they're the same thing. As longtime low-carb researchers Jeff Volek, PhD, RD, and Stephen Phinney, MD, PhD, have said, "Suggesting these two states are similar is like equating a gentle rain with a flood because they both involve water."[33] The water analogy is a good one: The difference between benign dietary ketosis and diabetic ketoacidosis is like a spring shower versus a catastrophic tidal wave or monsoon.

Diabetic ketoacidosis is a pathological and potentially life-threatening condition that might occur in type 1 diabetes and sometimes in type 2. Recall that I said insulin directly inhibits the formation of ketones. Well, people with type 1 diabetes produce little to no insulin. Therefore, unless they take an adequate dose of injected insulin, they run the risk of having too little insulin in their bloodstream. And with insufficient insulin in the body, blood glucose rises to very high levels, and there is also nothing stopping the production of ketones. So diabetic ketoacidosis results in simultaneously sky-high blood glucose and ketones. The problem with very high ketone levels is that ketone molecules are acidic. A buildup of very high ketones will overwhelm the body's capacity to buffer this acidity in the blood, and this is a truly dangerous situation.

However, benign dietary ketosis is completely different. During nutritional ketosis, blood glucose is relatively low. Ketone levels stay well below the harmful threshold and blood pH remains in a perfectly normal, healthy, and safe range. So while the gentle rain/monsoon analogy is illustrative, one I prefer even more is related to drinking alcoholic beverages: Nutritional ketosis is like having a glass of wine or two and being a little more relaxed and mellow than usual but still in full control of your faculties, whereas ketoacidosis is like being falling-down drunk. They both involve alcohol, but they're completely different states of being. Table 2.2 provides the ranges of ketone levels (in this case, beta-hydroxybutyrate [βOHB], a ketone measured in the blood) that typically occur under a variety of metabolic conditions.

Table 2.2. Ketone Levels in Different Metabolic States

Metabolic State	Blood Ketones (βOHB, mmol/L)
Mixed (high-carb) diet[34]	0.1-0.2
Overnight fast on mixed diet[35]	<0.5
Nutritional ketosis[36]	0.5-5.0
Medically therapeutic ketosis[37]	2.0-7.0
Total starvation[38]	5.0-8.0
Diabetic ketoacidosis[39]	15-25

As you can see, diabetic ketoacidosis generates ketones in much higher concentrations than would be generated via nutritional ketosis from a low-carbohydrate diet or, indeed, even under conditions of total starvation. In healthy individuals who produce adequate insulin, relatively small amounts of insulin are enough to suppress the formation of excessive ketones, so there is no need to worry about ketoacidosis. Moreover, ketones themselves actually stimulate insulin secretion. In a properly regulated body, when ketone levels start creeping up too high, they induce insulin secretion, which then inhibits ketone formation, thereby keeping their own production in check. Healthy amounts of insulin will not allow ketones to reach dangerous levels. However, let me repeat that this is what occurs in a properly regulated body. People with type 1 diabetes or insulin-dependent type 2 diabetes need to be much more careful. Even so, ketogenic diets have been used safely and effectively in both conditions.[40] In fact, Keith Runyan, MD, a physician in Florida, has type 1 diabetes, and he uses a ketogenic diet to manage his condition and keep his blood glucose and ketones at safe levels.[41]

Doctors who warn people with diabetes—both type 1 and type 2—about "the dangers of ketosis" are confusing nutritional ketosis with ketoacidosis. It is a sad state of affairs when "ketones and nutritional ketosis continue to be casually discounted by both dietetic and medical educators, many of whom lack a basic understanding of the role ketones play in human energy metabolism."[42] I am not a physician (nor do I play one on TV), but if I were one, for doctors and nutritionists mired in this quagmire of physiological and metabolic ignorance, I would prescribe rereading a biochemistry textbook, where the following gems can be found: "Many tissues prefer to use fatty acids and ketone bodies as oxidizable fuels in place of glucose. Most such tissues can use glucose but prefer to oxidize fatty acids and ketone bodies."[43] And, "During prolonged starvation acetoacetate and β-hydroxybutyrate replaced glucose as the predominant fuel for the brain. Muscle avidly consumes ketone bodies early in starvation but switches to fatty acid oxidation as starvation progresses, thereby sparing ketone bodies for metabolism by the brain. Thus, ketone bodies are a normal fuel for a variety of tissues and are part of a complex pattern of fuel metabolism."[44]

Let's keep in mind what Samuel Henderson, PhD, a leading researcher into the use of ketones for Alzheimer's disease, wrote:

> In a normal Western diet, rich in carbohydrates (>50% of total calories consumed), significant ketogenesis is inhibited the vast majority of the time. . . . Throughout much of human evolution, ketosis likely served as a valuable survival mechanism to fuel brain metabolism during times of food scarcity. Hence, in some ways, the modern diet can be considered "keto-deficient."[46]

Obviously, as an alternative fuel for the brain—one that has been proven effective—ketones hold incredible promise for improving cognitive impairment and Alzheimer's disease. However, the brain cannot run exclusively on ketones, and as I mentioned earlier, some cells in the body cannot run on fats or ketones and therefore must use glucose. So even on a very low-carbohydrate diet, there's still a requirement for some glucose in the body and the brain. On a low-carb diet, small amounts of glucose come from the carbohydrates in vegetables, fruits, nuts, seeds, and dairy products. But a human can survive for quite some time, even during a period of total starvation, with no food intake whatsoever—and, therefore, zero dietary glucose. (We must have water within two to three days, but we can survive without food for significantly

---

By far, the greatest criticism of ketogenic diets is that ketosis is unhealthy, dangerous, and can even cause death. But where are the bodies? If it's so dangerous, why aren't the casualties piling up? More to the point, why does it keep saving so many lives?

—John Kiefer[45]

longer.) With no glucose whatsoever coming into the body, from where does the body get this absolutely necessary glucose?

Gluconeogenesis: Making Glucose from Other Compounds

Recall what I said earlier about the human body being a master at reusing and recycling. We are excellent at converting things into other things. To suggest that because the brain requires glucose we all must consume plentiful carbohydrate is as narrow-minded and incorrect as saying that because oranges are a good source of vitamin C, we all must consume oranges. Indeed, oranges are a good source of vitamin C, but they're not the only source. We can get ample vitamin C from broccoli, bell peppers, and spinach, for example. In the same way, dietary carbohydrates are the most obvious source of glucose, but we can also make glucose from several other molecules.

There are essential amino acids (from proteins) and essential fatty acids (from fats). There are no essential carbohydrates. This is not to say that the body has no requirement for glucose, only that the requirement for glucose does not automatically imply a requirement for dietary carbohydrate. According to Jeff Volek and Stephen Phinney in their book, *The Art and Science of Low Carbohydrate Performance*, "Within the class of nutrients called 'carbohydrates,' there is no molecule that is essential for human health or well-being. This does not mean that blood sugar is completely unimportant, but rather that blood sugar can be well-maintained via metabolic processes such as gluconeogenesis without dietary carbohydrates in the keto-adapted human."[47]

According to the Food and Nutrition Board of the Institute of Medicine of the US National Academy of Sciences, "The lower limit of dietary carbohydrate compatible with life apparently is zero, provided that adequate amounts of protein and fat are consumed."[48] I am not suggesting that consuming no carbohydrate whatsoever is optimal or advised; I am simply noting that, due to the body's capacity to produce glucose from other substances, it is *possible*. How? Through a process called *gluconeogenesis*.

Don't be put off by the technical-sounding word. It's just science-speak for "making new glucose," and it's the biochemical process by which the body creates glucose out of other molecules in order to supply the brain and other tissues that must have it. In this sense, rather than forcing the body to use glucose for fuel, such as after eating a bagel, the glucose supply in the body is demand-driven: the body will generate the required glucose as needed. And remember, when the body and brain run on fats and ketones, the total demand for glucose is reduced.

Gluconeogenesis goes on in the body all the time. We run on different kinds of fuels simultaneously, while the body performs its reuse and recycle acrobatics. But in general, gluconeogenesis really ramps up when it has to—such as when we eat very little carbohydrate but we still have to get glucose from somewhere. As mentioned earlier, we first get glucose from glycogen stored in the liver. Glycogen gets broken down into individual glucose molecules that can be used for fuel. But remember, the liver stores only a small amount of glycogen. Once those reserves start running low (they're never completely depleted), we tap into other sources.

One of the other sources we tap into is protein. Many of the amino acids that make up proteins can be converted into glucose. At first, before the body has made the transition to running mostly on fats and ketones, it's still looking for its typical large amount of glucose. It will get this glucose by breaking down small amounts of body proteins in order to get these glucogenic amino acids. This only goes on for a short time, though. Once the body is adapted to using fats and ketones, the overall glucose demand drops, and it's no longer necessary to break down body proteins to fill that glucose gap. (Also, amino acids we consume in dietary protein can be converted to glucose, so the body has no reason to break down its hard-earned and valuable muscle tissue.)

Another source of the small amount of required glucose is fat. When we break down fat to use for fuel, some parts are burned for energy and other parts are converted into glucose (which subsequently becomes a fuel source as well). Fats are stored as triglycerides in the body, and for the sake of simplicity, we can think of them as looking like the letter *E*. The backbone of the triglyceride molecule, from which three fatty acids extend (the "tri" in *triglyceride* indicates that *three* fatty acids are joined together), is called *glycerol*. Two glycerol molecules can be combined to form one molecule of glucose. So you see, when carbohydrate intake is very low—or even completely absent—the body can internally generate the glucose it needs. No pasta or apple juice required! Even so, as you'll see, the diet recommended in this book is a *low*-carbohydrate diet, not a *no*-carbohydrate diet. Not all carbohydrates are starchy. We tend to think of potatoes, rice, and bread when we hear the word "carbohydrate," but lettuce, broccoli, zucchini, asparagus, and cauliflower are a few examples of nonstarchy, lower-carbohydrate vegetables, all of which are permitted in this nutritional strategy. So right off the bat, this diet does provide some glucose.

Raising Ketone Levels

We've covered a great deal of groundwork and laid a solid foundation for understanding how we can use a dietary strategy to induce whole-body biochemical changes in order to nourish parts of the brain that have lost the ability to harness sufficient energy from glucose. We know that the glucose required for certain tissues can be provided by small amounts of dietary carbohydrate as well as via gluconeogenesis. And we also know that we want to raise ketone levels, because the core of this strategy is that ketones will feed those struggling neurons!

If you're thinking now that there's no way—*no way*—your loved one will commit to a very low-carbohydrate, high-fat diet, you might be feeling discouraged and wondering if there's anything you can do—anything at all—to somehow elevate their ketone levels. Is there some kind of sneaky, backdoor way to raise ketones even when someone has high insulin levels or consumes a lot of carbohydrate? There is!

High insulin levels (driven mostly, but not entirely, by a high carbohydrate intake) prevent the formation of significant amounts of ketones. But there are ways around this, ways to get ketones to the brain even when the metabolic state should preclude this. One way is to provide the body with large amounts of substances that it will readily turn into ketones, and another is to give the body ketones directly. Let's start with the first.

The simplest and most cost-effective way to raise ketones in the body is by consuming medium-chain triglycerides (MCTs). MCTs are a special type of fat that is not digested and absorbed in the same way as other fats. Instead of going through the same route that fats like olive oil or sesame oil take within the human body, MCTs are delivered directly to the liver, which converts them into ketones and releases them into the bloodstream, where they can travel to other tissue to serve as fuel. (The liver generates the vast majority of ketones in the body, but it does not use them. It exports them to be used elsewhere.)

MCTs occur naturally in some fats and oils. Coconut oil and palm kernel oil are the richest sources. However, MCTs make up only a small percentage of the total fatty acids in these oils. There are now purified MCT oils available at health food stores and online, and these are 100 percent MCT, compared to approximately 15 percent for coconut oil. (Depending on the source cited, coconut oil might consist of as much as 57 percent MCTs. There's a bit of debate over the precise definition of a medium-chain triglyceride, but regardless, coconut oil is still a good source, though even at 57 percent MCT, it is lower than pure MCT oil.) Studies in animals and humans confirm that intake of MCTs elevates blood ketone levels. In fact, a physician whose husband was afflicted with AD witnessed a noticeable improvement in his cognition upon making no other changes to his diet or lifestyle other than feeding him coconut oil.[49]

The fascinating thing about the potential of MCT-rich oils to improve cognitive function is that ingestion of MCTs will elevate ketones regardless of insulin and blood glucose levels. Moreover, the brain's uptake and use of ketones is supply driven: The higher the ketones, the more the brain will take them in and use them, both for healthy people and those with MCI and AD.[50] (We'll discuss coconut and MCT oils in greater detail in chapter 13.)

The second way to raise ketones even when insulin levels are high is with exogenous ketones. *Exogenous* means "from the outside." This is in contrast to when the body produces ketones internally, either from taking in MCT-rich fats or from being adapted to a very low-carb diet. Think of exogenous ketones as a kind of "ketone supplement." They're available online and typically come either as a beverage or in powder form that you can add to your beverage of choice. Compared to coconut or MCT oils, however, these are not cost-effective for most people.

People with MCI and AD show improved cognition with higher ketone levels, whether these are achieved via a very low-carb diet or via ingestion of MCT oils or exogenous ketones.[51] They show marked improvements in standard assessments of cognitive function, as well as in other, less formal measurements, such as word recall and other tasks to test memory. This finding alone should point us toward the use of ketones and ketogenic diets as at least part of a therapy for cognitive impairment. However, exogenous ketones don't automatically help everyone with AD. For example, individuals with the ApoE4 genotype—the strongest genetic risk factor for AD—often don't experience results as promising as people with other genetic profiles.

As promising as MCT-rich oils and exogenous ketones are for improving cognition, they are by no means a panacea. They're akin to putting a drugstore Band-Aid on a sucking chest wound: It's better than nothing, but it's not exactly going to do a whole lot to improve the situation. Or think of it like bailing water out of a leaky boat without first stopping to patch the hole: Raising ketone levels via MCTs and exogenous ketones merely improves the symptoms of cognitive impairment, but it does nothing to correct the underlying causes and therefore does nothing to delay, halt, or possibly even reverse disease progression. So while I absolutely believe raising ketones by any means possible can be helpful in the short term, the real benefit—the wham-bam, one-two punch, if you will—comes from a *combination* of carbohydrate reduction and liberal use of MCT products or exogenous ketones.

We owe a debt of gratitude to universities and private companies that are developing ketogenic supplements that might eventually be readily available for the public. I do believe they have an important place in this nutrition and lifestyle strategy, but the fact is, providing ketones from an outside source without addressing the root causes of cognitive dysfunction will allow this internal root cause to keep getting worse. The same can be said of insulin. Although Alzheimer's disease and MCI typically go hand in hand with elevated insulin in the blood, levels in the brain might actually be *low*. (And this contributes to some of the structural alterations seen in the brains of affected individuals.) This being the case, if there were a way to administer insulin directly to the central nervous system, then patients might show some improvement. Such experiments have been conducted, and they reflect the same obstacle as exogenous ketones: Insulin infusion into the central nervous system helps in the short term, but it might actually make things worse in the long run. Additionally, not all individuals respond positively to insulin in the central nervous system; cognition in some people gets worse.[52]

Individual and genetic variations might explain, at least in part, why ApoE4 gene carriers don't improve as much as other people after taking exogenous ketones. It might be that, for some individuals, simply supplying ketones isn't sufficient to have a noticeable impact. These people would likely still improve to some degree, but not as dramatically as others. For reasons we'll explore in chapter 7, people with the ApoE4 gene might suffer the ravages of the modern diet and lifestyle more severely than others, and it might be that having elevated blood ketones, by itself, just isn't enough to overcome whatever damage has taken hold. In order to experience a significant benefit from these elevated ketones, perhaps they would have to adopt some of the additional strategies we'll explore. Remember, both MCI and AD are the result of a lifetime of accumulated metabolic and physiological insults. It shouldn't surprise us that some people don't experience marked improvements with nothing more than exogenous ketones. What should surprise us is that so many people *do*.

Exogenous Ketones and Measuring Ketones at Home

There are two important questions to consider: (1) Should you or your loved one use exogenous ketones? and (2) Can you measure ketone levels at home, and should you? The answer to both is yes, but . . .

To address the first: As I've said, MCT-rich oils and exogenous ketones quite impressively improve the signs and symptoms of impaired cognitive function—in the short term. They are a quick fix, the effects of which might wear off as soon as the ketones are no longer available in the body. Moreover, without any other dietary or lifestyle changes, nothing is being done to address the fundamental causative factors, so over time, affected individuals will need to take higher and more frequent doses of MCTs or ketones, as the underlying issues will only have gotten worse, and more ketones will be needed to overcome this. (The half-life of elevated βOHB in the blood induced by exogenous ketones is only about one to one-and-a-half hours, so their effects are fleeting.)[53] Contrast this with strategies that do correct the underlying hyperinsulinemia, inflammation, and oxidative stress—most powerfully, a very low-carbohydrate diet. Both of these strategies—a ketogenic diet and exogenous ketones—are likely to help independently, and combining the two might be a way to get truly astounding results. Moreover, diligently following a low-carbohydrate diet will keep at least a low level of endogenous (internal) ketone production going nearly all the time.

This sounds impressive, but let's take things back to reality for a moment. Individuals of very advanced age or very severe disease progression are unlikely to give up their morning toast and orange juice in favor of eggs cooked in coconut oil. And for loved ones and caregivers, even attempting to implement this change can be extremely frustrating and add to the stress of what is already an emotionally overwhelming situation. In these cases, I absolutely encourage the use of large amounts of coconut or MCT oil, or outside ketones. We are trying to feed neurons that are starving to death, and elevated ketones—however they are achieved—will do this.

Even though the disease process will continue unabated, the short-term, temporary improvements these people might experience could allow them to live their final few years with slightly better control of their faculties, and perhaps just as importantly, it might ease some of the burden and improve quality of life for their loved ones and caregivers.

On the other hand, AD and MCI are striking people ever younger. For individuals experiencing cognitive impairment in their fifties or sixties—who might have twenty-five to thirty more years of life ahead of them, I would recommend using MCT-rich oils, but I would place far more emphasis on implementing as many of the other dietary and lifestyle changes as they are willing and able to pursue. Giving high doses of ketones is like applying a tourniquet to a profusely bleeding wound: This immediate step is necessary to manage the acute crisis, but you wouldn't quit after the tourniquet and provide no other treatment. You would get the injured person to a hospital, where they can actually fix the problem. So yes, raising ketone levels is key, *while also addressing the underlying issues.* The younger someone is, the more likely their body will be able to adapt and respond to these changes. The human is body is remarkably resilient—when we allow it to be.

To address the second question: Yes, you can measure ketone levels at home, but it is not strictly necessary. There's a lot of controversy surrounding measuring ketones. Most of this comes from people using ketogenic diets for weight loss or optimizing athletic performance, and their concerns do not necessarily apply to people using nutritional ketosis for the goal of improving cognitive function.

Let's get one thing out of the way: Due to the exploding incidence of type 2 diabetes, blood glucose meters are ubiquitous at supermarkets and corner drugstores these days. And even though many people with type 2 diabetes use low-carb diets to manage their blood sugar, there isn't much point in an MCI or AD patient measuring blood glucose levels. After all, remember, it's the insulin, not the glucose, and at the time of this writing, there are no home meters for measuring insulin. (Measuring glucose is not entirely useless, though. It will still give you some insight into how your loved one is responding to certain foods; just keep in mind that blood glucose might be "normal" because of high insulin.)

It is possible to measure ketones at home, but the best measure of whether this strategy is working is how the affected individual is faring. Due to genetics and other factors, people vary widely in their ability to generate ketones; some people's bodies just make higher levels of ketones more read-ily than others', even upon consuming the same foods or supplements and doing the same types of physical activity. And as of yet, there's no firmly established ketone "threshold" above which someone would be guaranteed to experience improvements in cognition and below which there would be no effect. Just as people vary in their ability to generate ketones, they also vary in their response to ketones. So all measuring ketones does is show you a number; it doesn't tell you whether or not your loved one is deriving a benefit. Some people might experience improvement with mild ketone elevation, while others would need to sustain higher levels.

Nevertheless, measuring ketones has its place. Since there is not neces-sarily an automatic correlation between higher ketone levels and better cognition in everyone (although most studies support a relationship), the best purpose measuring ketones can be put to is encouragement. Seeing concrete proof that you or your loved one has achieved nutritional ketosis can be a huge source of motivation to continue sticking with a diet that isn't always easy to adhere to. Moreover, if your loved one does not exhibit improvement after several weeks on a very low-carbohydrate diet (or from taking exogenous ketones), it's possible this is because they never actually achieved a state of nutritional ketosis. Measuring ketones will show you whether this is the case.

There are three ways to measure ketones at home. Each measures a different type of ketone. A molecule called *acetone* is measured in the breath. (This is responsible for the "keto breath" many people experience when adopting this diet. More on this in chapter 20.) Breath testing can tell you whether or not you've achieved ketosis, but I prefer the other ways of measuring: blood and urine.

Blood ketone meters measure levels of β-hydroxybutyrate, and they require no more than a single drop of blood from a finger prick. (These meters operate the same way standard blood glucose meters do.) The meters are inexpensive, but the test strips are pricey. Depending on your budget, blood ketone testing might not be a realistic option for you. And again, while some people might show nice improvements in cognition with blood ketones at 1.0 or 1.5 mmol/L, others might not exhibit improvements unless they're higher. It's not the numbers, but the effects. (As seen in table 2.2, the range for nutritional ketosis is βOHB at 0.5–5.0 mmol/L. Noticeable responses might occur anywhere in between.)

Urine test strips (sometimes called *ketostix*) measure another type of ketone, called *acetoacetate*. These strips are available in drugstores and online, and they're a far more economical way to test for ketosis. Unlike blood testing, urine testing doesn't give a precise reading but rather gives an indicator of the general level of ketosis. (The reagent section of the test strip will turn from beige to pink or purple within about fifteen seconds. The darker the color, the greater the concentration of acetoacetate. But just like the blood ketones, higher acetoacetate in the urine doesn't automatically mean your loved one will have better cognition. After all, this acetoacetate is being excreted, so it's not fueling the brain. Seeing the strip change color is really just a morale boost—but don't discount the importance of this.)

Should you choose to use urine test strips, keep the following in mind.

- Darker purple does not indicate a state of "deeper ketosis." If the color shows very dark purple, it might be a sign that the person is not drinking enough water and the urine is strongly concentrated due to dehydration. Any noticeable color change is a good sign, even light pink. Darker isn't necessarily better, and you shouldn't feel discouraged if you only see pink. Pink is still indicative of ketosis.
- If you have steady hands, cut the test strips in half the long way— you'll get double the amount of test strips for the same price! (*Note*: this works only for the urine test strips, not the blood test strips.)
- As time goes on, the strips might show less change, and you might think you're not producing ketones anymore. But less change can also mean that the body is becoming more efficient at using the ketones for fuel and is therefore having to "waste" less of them by passing them out in the urine. So don't become discouraged if you see less of a color change over time, but do keep an eye on diet: Perhaps too many carbohydrates have been trickling back in.

Another point against obsessing over ketone measurements is that some ketone generation happens within the brain itself and is therefore not measureable with a blood meter. Researchers have shown that cultured astrocytes (a type of brain cell important for the "care and feeding" of neurons) metabolize MCTs into ketones.[54] In a living animal or human, nearby neurons take up these ketones for fuel.[55] All of this happens in the brain, hidden from view, and is undetectable with a blood meter. So even if measurements of blood ketones are low, that doesn't mean neurons are not being nourished by clinically relevant amounts of ketones.

There are additional complicating factors when measuring for blood or urine ketones. For some people, βOHB levels might be higher in the evening than in the morning or vice versa. And when you test for ketones—particularly in the blood—you are really just taking a snapshot in time: one moment of recorded data. Levels might have been different had you tested just an hour earlier or later, and considering the price of the test strips, testing multiple times a day might not be realistic for everyone.

You can see now why I support measuring ketones as a source of motivation and encouragement, but I don't think it's required, nor do I think it's worth chasing high ketones for the sake of a high reading. The real proof of whether ketones are fueling the brain is the degree of improvement in cognitive function. The results are more important than the numbers. Blood levels of βOHB or urinary acetoacetate really only provide surrogate indicators. The guiding factor should not necessarily be high levels of βOHB, but rather, how the affected person is faring. You don't need ketone measurements to tell you that your loved one's memory is working better or that they're more like their "old self" when interacting with people and that they've had fewer uncharacteristic behavioral outbursts. Numbers are a guide. Trust your instincts; you'll know if your loved one is improving.

If you choose not to use a blood ketone meter or urine test strips, there are other, more subjective ways to gauge whether you or your loved one have made the transition to running on fat and are producing elevated ketones. Some of the signs to look for include:

- Bad breath (keto breath from acetone)—sometimes described as "metallic" or "fruity"
- Reduced appetite (ability to go many hours between meals without feeling overly hungry or irritable)
- Increased energy levels
- Positive mood; optimistic outlook
- Relatively low blood glucose (among people who measure glucose), but no physical or psychological signs of hypoglycemia
- Sharper thinking; less brain fog

Now that we've laid the groundwork establishing why keeping insulin levels low and allowing the body to become a ketone-producing machine are so critical for people with AD and cognitive impairment, in the next few chapters we'll explore some of the physical and biochemical changes that occur in the disease process, with a focus on why nutrition and lifestyle interventions that lower insulin and blood glucose, raise ketones, and provide specific nutrients for brain health might be the most promising weapons we have in our arsenal to fight cognitive decline.

CHAPTER 3

The Shape and Structure of Neurons and Their Role in Alzheimer's Disease

I n order to understand how the specific nutritional recommendations in this book are connected to reducing and possibly even preventing and reversing the physiological damage driving Alzheimer's disease, it is important to have a basic understanding of the structure and function of neurons—the main types of cells in the brain that are responsible for normal cognitive function, including things like memory processing, emotional behavior, and impulse control. Let's start with the structure of a neuron.

Figure 3.1 shows the basic structure of a neuron.

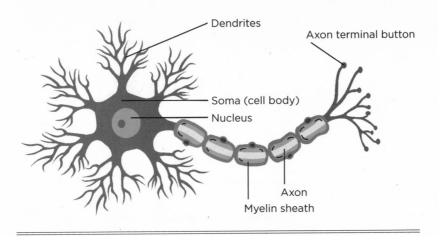

Figure 3.1 Basic neuron structure. Image by Jacky Co/Shutterstock.com.

The main part of the neuron is the *cell body*. The long, thin projection extending out from the cell body is called the *axon*, and it ends in *axon terminals*, where the axon branches off into several end points. Branching out from the cell body at the other end of the neuron are smaller projections, called *dendrites*. Think of axons and dendrites as "senders" and "receivers," respectively. The way neurons communicate with each other is by sending signals from one to the next. The axon of one neuron sends a signal out, and the dendrites of the next one receive it. The very small spaces between the axon terminals and the dendrites are called *synapses*. There are literally trillions of synapses in the brain.

Figure 3.2 depicts a nerve impulse traveling down through an axon.

It is critical that neurons and neuronal synapses have the correct shape (structure), without damage or distortion. If the shape of a synapse is altered,

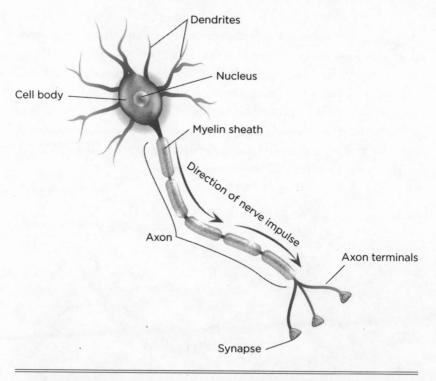

Figure 3.2 Nerve impulse transmission. Cellular communication occurs via electrical impulses traveling from the cell body down through the axon (protected and insulated by the myelin sheath) and out through the axon terminals. Image by Tefi/Shutterstock.com.

it will not function properly, and if synapse function has been compromised, communication between neurons breaks down. The result of a breakdown in neuronal communication is impairment of cognitive function.

Now that we have a very basic overview of how the connections between neurons work, let's delve a little deeper into what is happening in the brain of someone with Alzheimer's, and why their cognitive function has been impaired.

We have established that the fundamental cause of Alzheimer's is the death or deterioration of brain cells resulting from their inability to metabolize glucose. This seems to be the malfunction with the biggest impact underlying the condition, but it is not the only contributing factor. When coupled with long-standing recommendations for all population groups to limit cholesterol intake, as well as the exponential explosion in prescriptions for antacids and statin drugs (to fight indigestion and acid reflux and to lower cholesterol, respectively), brain cells don't stand a chance.

Deformed Synapses: How Shrinking Axons and Dendrites Result in Impaired Cognition

As discussed earlier, the synapse is the space between axons and dendrites. It is the connection between neurons—the place where communication in the form of nerve impulse transmission occurs. Therefore, if the shape of the synapse has been compromised, proper communication cannot happen inside the brain. Many things can compromise the shape of synapses. Let's explore some of them.

Beta-amyloid (Aβ) plaques, which I've mentioned briefly already and which we'll cover in detail in chapter 6, are one of the classic hallmarks of Alzheimer's disease. Recall that these are insoluble protein fragments that accumulate inside the brain. Some researchers think that Aβ plaques *cause* Alzheimer's, but an understanding of the biochemical processes involved in creating and clearing Aβ plaques suggests that they are more likely a *result* of the condition and are intimately related to chronically high insulin levels.

Regardless of whether they are a cause or an effect of the underlying metabolic disturbances in AD, one thing that these amyloid protein fragments do is compromise synapse function. When these protein fragments start to accumulate, they join together and aggregate into insoluble plaques. Over time, these plaques get larger and larger, forming cross-linkages between each other, until they begin to block the synapse and impede or "get in the way of" nerve impulse transmission. Think of this like an emergency exit in a crowded building. If there are boxes and other things being stored in front of the fire door, then the exit is blocked and no one can get out. This creates an extremely dangerous situation in a crisis. Consider what happens inside the brain when the exit (synapse) is blocked and nerve impulses cannot get through. The implications for cognitive function are obvious—and frightening.

A second change to the shape of neurons and synapses that negatively affects cognitive function is the shrinking of axons and dendrites. Let's take a closer look at a synapse (figure 3.3). There is a small amount of space between the axon terminal that sends the nerve impulse and the dendrites that receive it.

The electrical impulses (as well as nutrients and other materials) have to travel across this small space in order to be passed from one neuron and received by the next one. Think of it like jumping across a hole in the ground. If the hole—the distance between the axons and dendrites—gets larger, it will be harder for the nerve impulse to travel across that space.

In Alzheimer's disease, the space—the synapse—actually does get larger, thereby reducing communication between neurons. Here's how it

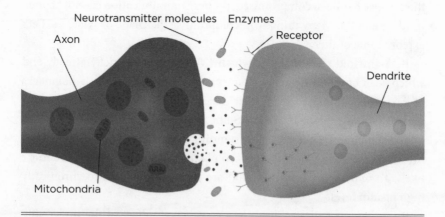

Figure 3.3 Close-up of a neuronal synapse. Electrical impulses and chemical messengers (neurotransmitters) travel across the space between neurons, exiting from the axon terminal of one neuron and being received by receptors on the dendrites of another. In order for neuronal communication to happen properly, the axons, dendrites, and the synapse itself must have the correct structure. Image by joshya/Shutterstock.com.

works: Recall that the primary issue in Alzheimer's is the degeneration and death of neurons, essentially by starvation. However, neurons don't die right away. Our cells are powerful, robust entities. They want to stay alive. One way by which neurons protect their survival when they're struggling for fuel is by making their axons and dendrites smaller in order to conserve energy for the cell body. If they don't have to expend energy maintaining a nice, long axon and many branches of dendrites, then they stand a better chance of staying alive. So the axons and dendrites recede, or become shorter, as the cell shrinks. Picture a vacuum cleaner with a retractable cord and you'll have a good visual for how this works: The long, thin cord gets reeled back into the main part of the machine for storage. The cell body of the neuron sucks the axon back in, just like a vacuum cord being retracted. If the axons and dendrites have receded into the cell body, then the synapse is no longer viable. It is too far a distance for the nerve impulse to travel—if the neuron even has enough energy to create that impulse at all.

Neurofibrillary Tangles: Malformed Cells, Malfunctioning Brain

The deleterious alterations to neuron structure we've covered so far would be more than sufficient to result in impaired cognition. But there's even more. The primary metabolic hallmark of AD is the reduced cerebral metabolic rate of glucose. The primary physical hallmark is the amyloid plaques. A second physical hallmark consists of neurofibrillary tangles (NFTs) made up of hyperphosphorylated tau proteins. (How's that for a mouthful?!) Tau proteins are part of what make up cell cytoskeletons. Think of cytoskeletons as internal scaffolding that gives cells their proper shape. ("Cyto" means *cell*.) They're like the foundation and load-bearing walls of a building: Without these, the building would collapse. If cytoskeletons are malformed or become weakened or damaged, then cells themselves will become malformed, leading to a collapse in cellular function.

Owing to their unique shape, neurons must have properly constructed cytoskeletons; otherwise axons and dendrites will not function properly. As we have been exploring the role of insulin resistance in driving cognitive impairment, it should come as no surprise that problems with insulin sensitivity and signaling are intimately involved in interfering with the assembly of tau proteins and the formation of viable cytoskeletons. An enzyme called glycogen synthase kinase-3β (GSK3β) plays a role in several cellular processes, one of which is influencing the trafficking of tau proteins and their assembly into the cytoskeleton.

Overactivity of GSK3β causes tau proteins to fold in on themselves, forming "tangles," rather than constructing a proper cytoskeleton. Activity of GSK3β is regulated in part by insulin. Insulin inhibits this enzyme, thereby preventing overactivity and limiting the formation of NFTs. And while many AD patients are hyperinsulinemic—that is, they have too much insulin in the bloodstream—they have too little insulin in the brain and central nervous system. This "deficit" of insulin in the brain allows GSK3β activity to proceed unabated, resulting in increased formation of NFTs, increased malformation of cell cytoskeletons, and increased neuronal dysfunction. Moreover, GSK3β might also be directly involved in promoting the formation of beta-amyloid plaques.[1] For these reasons, inhibition of GSK3β has been a target for pharmaceutical drugs for AD.[2]

To tackle the problem head-on, as discussed in chapter 2, direct infusion of insulin into the central nervous system seems to help in the short term, but it does nothing to correct the underlying problems of either why sufficient amounts of insulin aren't getting to the brain or why neurons aren't responding to it once it arrives. Pharmaceutical drugs that target individual symptoms—such as beta-amyloid plaques or NFTs—might provide temporary improvement for an AD patient, but they fail to address the ultimate causal factors, which is why nearly all Alzheimer's drugs developed to date have been disappointing.

The Myelin Sheath and the Crucial Role of Vitamin B$_{12}$

Think of neurons as live wires. This analogy isn't too far off the mark; neurons really do carry and transmit electrical impulses, just like power lines do. And just like electrical wires and power cords, neurons need to be insulated so they don't short out or shock anybody. The substance that insulates neurons is called *myelin*, and because it surrounds and encases axons and nerve cords the way a sheath encases and protects a sword, it is often referred to as a *myelin sheath*.

One of the primary building blocks of myelin is cholesterol. Despite what you are used to hearing about cholesterol "clogging the arteries," cholesterol is one of the most crucial substances for building cells and tissues throughout the human body. And because there is a multitude of brain cells forming trillions of synapses, and axons are covered in myelin, the brain is loaded with nourishing cholesterol. In a typical human being, the brain accounts for just 2 percent of total body weight, but it holds 25 percent of the body's cholesterol—that is how important cholesterol is for brain function.[3] (If you are old enough to remember a time before we were cautioned against consuming dietary cholesterol, eggs were once considered "brain food" specifically because of their cholesterol and nutrient content!) Imagine now what might result from a long-term avoidance of dietary cholesterol or from years of taking medication designed to disrupt the body's internal synthesis of this life-sustaining substance. We'll cover cholesterol in detail in chapter 9, but to give you a preview of how important cholesterol is for brain health and cognitive function, consider what lipid researchers Roger Lane and Martin Farlow wrote about this fascinating molecule: "Approximately 25% of the total amount of cholesterol in the human body is found in the brain, mostly in the specialized membranes of myelin and in the membranes of neuronal and glial cells."[4]

Cholesterol is not technically an "essential" nutrient, because the human body can and does manufacture cholesterol for itself. We can synthesize it from fatty acids and other nutrients, but because cholesterol is such an integral part of so many physical structures and biochemical processes in the body, sometimes our bodies can't produce enough to meet our needs. There isn't always enough to go around, so to speak. This is why, regardless of the fact that we do produce some cholesterol "from scratch," we would still do well to consume some in our foods, and this might be especially true for people who are trying to restore healthy cognitive function.

A low cholesterol supply for the brain is made much worse when coupled with statin drugs or other pharmacological agents designed to lower cholesterol levels. Statin drugs work by blocking endogenous production of cholesterol. This means they block the internal manufacturing of choles-terol, which is so critical for our health far beyond just the structure of myelin. If you or your loved one are taking a drug designed to prevent your body from making cholesterol, and you are combining it with a diet low in cholesterol-rich foods (such as butter, egg yolks, red meat, shellfish, and pork fat), this creates the absolute worst possible nutritional environment for a struggling brain.

Another factor complicating the synthesis of healthy myelin is vitamin B_{12} deficiency. Vitamin B_{12} is required for proper formation and functioning of myelin, and as a population, older people tend to have low levels of B_{12}.[5] There are several reasons older people are frequently deficient in B_{12}. One is that robust levels of stomach acid are required for absorption of B_{12} from foods, and stomach acid levels naturally decline with age. To make matters worse, many older people have been taking antacids for years, some for decades. Whether these are over-the-counter antacids (like Tums or Rolaids) or prescription medications (called "proton pump inhibitors" or PPIs, such as Prilosec and Nexium), they have the same end result: lower levels of stomach acid. And low levels of stomach acid will prevent the digestive tract from being able to liberate B_{12} from food. (See chapter 21 for more on digestive function.)

The influence of low stomach acid on B_{12} absorption is exacerbated by the tendency of older people to consume fewer foods that are rich in B_{12} to begin with. The foods highest in B_{12} are animal proteins; specifically, red meat and organ meats (especially liver), and shellfish (such as oysters, mussels, and clams). We have been cautioned against consuming organ meats and shellfish due to their cholesterol content.

In addition to avoiding B_{12}-rich foods due to concerns about fat and cholesterol, older people—particularly ones who live on their own—are less likely to go to the effort of grilling a steak or braising liver and onions for dinner when it is easier to simply pour themselves a bowl of oatmeal or toast up a slice of bread. Unfortunately, for older people who might have limited mobility, the easiest foods to prepare are the exact starchy carbohydrates that are likely contributing to incapacity of the brain. Elderly people who live on their own are more likely to consume these convenient carbohydrates rather than preparing a meal of good quality fat and protein for themselves. So in yet another nutritional double-whammy for proper myelin formation, we have reduced intake of B_{12}-rich foods coupled with a reduced capacity to digest and absorb what little is consumed in the diet.

Moreover, many B_{12}-rich foods are harder to chew than starchy carbohydrates. If your loved one has ill-fitting dentures, weak teeth, or some other problem in the mouth that prevents adequate chewing of meat, then they are more likely to gravitate toward foods that are easy to chew, such as noodles, spaghetti, and muffins—precisely the things they should be avoiding.

Something important to note is that severe B_{12} deficiency (known as *pernicious anemia*) is occasionally misdiagnosed as dementia. Some of the most insidious signs of long-term B_{12} depletion are depression, peripheral neuropathy (numbness, pain, tingling, or feelings of coldness in the extremities), memory loss, and changes to cognitive function. I recommend that you work with a licensed physician to have your loved one's B_{12} levels assessed and start supplementation as soon as possible if they are low. If the deficiency is sufficiently deep and longstanding, some of the neurological damage might be irreversible, but you might be able to prevent or at least slow further decline by replenishing B_{12} levels.

Low B_{12} levels are absolutely a hindrance to strong cognitive function and brain health. In a study examining vitamin B_{12} status in the elderly, the authors concluded, "Low vitamin B_{12} status should be further investigated as a modifiable cause of brain atrophy and of likely subsequent cognitive impairment in the elderly."[6] They went on to say:

> *Our data suggest that subclinical low vitamin B_{12} status, within what is usually considered to be the normal range, can affect brain volume even in the early stages of cognitive decline, possibly by disturbing the integrity of brain myelin or through inflammation. Thus, early treatment of low vitamin B_{12} status may prevent further brain volume loss.*

Please note that they said "subclinical low vitamin B_{12} status, within what is usually considered to be the normal range." This means that even if your B_{12} levels are within the "normal range," you might still benefit from supplementation. Depending on the laboratory, the "normal range" can vary, but a typical range is 260–935 pg/mL. That's a large range! Think about it: Your B_{12} levels could be 930 pg/mL, and you would be considered "normal," or they could be at 260 pg/mL—three and a half times lower—and you'd still be considered "normal." But if your loved one's levels are at the very low end of the normal range, perhaps they would benefit from raising them to the middle or high end. Please be aware: Just because levels of certain nutrients are "normal" doesn't mean they're optimal, particularly when the range of what is considered "normal" is so wide.

The same study authors wrote, "Our study shows that low vitamin B_{12} status . . . is an important risk factor for loss of brain volume in older community-dwelling adults. These findings suggest that plasma vitamin B₁₂ status may be an early marker of brain atrophy and thus a potentially important modifiable risk factor for cognitive decline in the elderly."[7]

If digestive function is compromised, then oral B₁₂ supplementation might be effective. Absorption of B₁₂ from supplements doesn't require the same degree of stomach acid and digestive fire as the B₁₂ bound up in food. It is available in tablets and capsules, but another effective delivery strategy for B₁₂ is a sublingual lozenge that dissolves under the tongue. (It can also be used as a kind of hard candy and allowed to dissolve elsewhere in the mouth.) According to David Brownstein, MD, author of *Vitamin B-12 for Health*, the methyl or hydroxyl/hydroxy forms of B₁₂ seem to be more effective than the "cyanocobalamin" form found in most common multivitamins.[8] Look for "methylcobalamin" or "hydroxycobalamin" on the label, rather than cyanocobalamin. Methylcobalamin or methyl B₁₂ lozenges are available at most health food stores and online.

When B₁₂ levels are especially low, B₁₂ injections might be the most effective way to raise them. Injections bypass all compromises in digestive function that might interfere with B₁₂ absorption. As always, work with a physician or other qualified health care practitioner to assess vitamin and mineral status and decide on an appropriate course of action to address any insufficiencies.

You can now understand why the last several decades of advice that have guided supposedly "healthy diets" have been a disaster for brain health. We have been told to limit cholesterol as much as possible, even though cholesterol is the brain's number one nutrient. We have been told to base our diet (literally base our diet—remember the old food pyramid?) on starchy carbohydrates—specifically, grains, the high glycemic load of which, in many people, leads to chronically elevated blood glucose or insulin levels and might induce insulin resistance. We have also been cautioned against consuming natural, stable, saturated fats in favor of "heart-healthy" polyunsaturated vegetable oils. These new man-made fats alter the structure and function of cell membranes not just in the brain, but throughout the entire body. (More on this in chapter 4.) And last, but not least, as a side effect of having been advised to avoid foods that are high in cholesterol and fat, we have unintentionally also avoided foods that are rich in vitamin B₁₂.

To return to robust cognitive health, return to a robust, nutrient-dense diet, low in carbohydrates and high in the nutrients the struggling brain needs most: cholesterol, natural fats, omega-3 polyunsaturated fats, antioxidants, and micronutrients (vitamins and minerals).

CHAPTER 4

Cell Membranes:
The Bouncers of the Body

I hope by this time you aren't having flashbacks to high school biology class. Don't be intimidated; I'll keep things simple. It is extremely important that you understand the structure and function of cell membranes and other membranes in the body—what they're made of and what they do. Keeping your cell membranes healthy is critical for brain health.

Cells are the teeny-tiny, itty-bitty things that make up our bodies. Every part of us, from our eyeballs to our pinkie toes, is made of cells. We have erythrocytes (red blood cells); hepatocytes (liver cells); enterocytes (small intestine cells); myocytes (muscle cells); adipocytes (fat cells); astrocytes, glial cells, and neurons (brain cells); and cells in every other type of tissue and organ. We are made up of trillions of these things. Basically, we're just walking, talking sacks of cells. (Or if you're a Carl Sagan fan, we're actually recycled stardust, but for the purpose of our discussion here, we'll call ourselves big sacks of cells, and it's "trillions and trillions," rather than Mr. Sagan's catchphrase, "billions and billions.")

Everything that happens inside our bodies happens because of actions at the cellular level. When you touch a hot pan and pull your hand away as fast as you can, that movement happens because sensory cells in your hand felt something hot, transmitted that to your brain, and your brain told the motor cells to move—in this case, to move your hand away from the pan. It is not an exaggeration to say that everything that happens inside our bodies happens because of activity inside or right outside these trillions of cells. We can digest food because cells lining our stomach and gastrointestinal tract secrete hydrochloric acid and digestive enzymes. We can breathe because cells in our lungs exchange oxygen and carbon dioxide in our blood.

Regardless of the kinds of cell we're talking about, all cells have membranes. To be specific, I'm talking about plasma membranes, which surround the miniorgans inside our cells (called organelles) and also surround the whole cell itself. They separate the inside of the cell from whatever's outside. Think of cell membranes like bouncers at a club: They decide who's allowed to come in and who has to be kicked out. If the bouncers are going to do their job well, they need to look a certain way, right? You wouldn't want scrawny, timid, weak people at the club's entrance, would you? Of course not. These are the security guards; you'd want bouncers who are broad, strong, tough, and brawny.

The same is true of our cell membranes: They have to be built a certain way in order to function properly. When cell membranes don't function properly, all kinds of things can go wrong. If the membrane is like a bouncer, then when it doesn't work correctly, good things (like vitamins, minerals, amino acids, and glucose) can't get into the cells, and bad things (like toxins and normal metabolic waste products) can't get out. This is a recipe for disaster.

So what does any of this have to do with how the modern diet can influence the pathology of Alzheimer's disease? Cell membranes are made of fatty acids. (They are composed of phospholipids, glycoproteins, cholesterol, and other substances, but the major components are phospholipids, and the major components of those are fats.) And they're made from all three kinds of fatty acids: saturated, monounsaturated, and polyunsaturated. All three kinds of fatty acids are required for proper cell membrane structure and function. The membranes for different types of cells have different requirements for the particular proportion of saturated versus unsaturated fats in them, so there isn't an exact formula for the cell membrane of, say, a neuron versus a cardiac muscle cell versus a pancreatic beta cell. For our purposes here, it's enough to know that we need all three types of fat to some extent. For this to make sense, we'll need to see what a cell membrane actually looks like (figure 4.1).

The cell membrane is a *phospholipid bilayer*. (Don't worry; it sounds much more technical than it is. All this means is that the membrane is like a double door—it has two layers.) The "phospho" is for the phosphate groups, which are depicted as the spheres at the top and bottom of the membrane

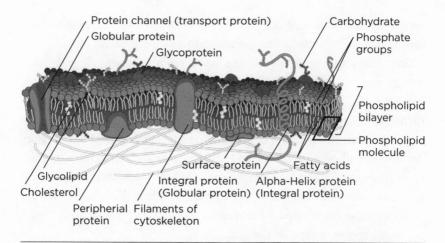

Figure 4.1 Cell membrane structure. The double-layered cell membrane consists mainly of fatty acids, phosphate molecules, and cholesterol. Various structural proteins and carbohydrates, plus receptors, pores, and channels, are anchored to or embedded within the membrane, allowing important substances to get into and out of the cell.

in figure 4.1. The "lipid" portion—the "tails" extending from the spherical phosphate groups—is the one we are more concerned with. Each of those tails is a fatty acid. Some are saturated, some are monounsaturated, and some are polyunsaturated. The cell membrane can only do its job effectively when it has the right mix of these fats and the fats have not been damaged. When the membrane has the right building blocks and is structurally sound, it can perform well, just like a bouncer who has the right build.

But membranes aren't made only of fatty acids. There are many other molecules embedded in the membrane that also help it do its job. Think of it like an impressive, sprawling estate—the home of someone extremely wealthy (the kind of residence that has a name, not an address—like Chateau de la Mer, instead of 319 Old Dirt Road). There are a lot of different ways to get into and out of an estate like that: There's a front door, a back door, windows, the servants' entrance, balcony doors, the ballroom entrance, the underground driveway for deliveries, and so on. And in order for these entrances to let people in and out, the house itself has to be built correctly, right? If the house were constructed poorly, perhaps the doorways and windows wouldn't be the right shape or size, or if the house started sinking into its foundation, the underground entrance would become inaccessible.

The cell membrane works the same way. As depicted in figure 4.1, embedded on and within the membrane itself—like doors and windows—are ion channels, transporters, and other things that are designed to bring certain things into the cell and send other things out—things that can't just slip through the membrane without help. Cell membranes are *semipermeable*. This means some molecules can pass right through very easily, while others only gain access to the inside of the cell via a special route or by having another molecule escort them through, like security guards who stand outside the mansion and only let in people they recognize. For example, specialized receptors on cell membranes recognize things like thyroid hormone, insulin, testosterone, and the neurotransmitters serotonin and dopamine.

It should be obvious now what could happen if the cell membrane isn't built properly. Things that are supposed to get in are blocked from doing so, and things that are supposed to get out can't. And it doesn't end there. If the membrane itself is shoddy, then some of those transporters, channels, and receptors aren't going to work correctly, just like a house with doors and windows that aren't the right shape or size. To give us some idea of what this means in a practical sense, if our cellular LDL receptors aren't working right, we'll have more LDL particles floating around in our bloodstream because they can't get into the cells. (If you're thinking LDL is known as the "bad cholesterol," you're right, but that is a major oversimplification of the facts. You will learn more about cholesterol in chapter 9.) If your insulin receptors and glucose transporters aren't doing their jobs because the cell membrane is poorly constructed, your blood glucose levels will be higher than they should be because insulin can't help get the glucose into the cells. The right building blocks mean the difference between cell membranes that are able to perform their physiological function and cell membranes that malfunction, causing havoc throughout the body and brain.

So what does it mean when we talk about the cell membrane not being built correctly? Remember that fatty acids give the membrane its basic structure. And we need all three kinds of fatty acids—saturated, monounsaturated, and polyunsaturated. But for over half a century, we've been told to avoid saturated fats. We've been told to limit our intake of saturated fats and emphasize the unsaturated ones. Ditch the butter, cheese, bacon fat, beef tallow, egg yolks, and fatty cuts of meat, and use olive oil, soybean oil, corn, canola, sunflower, and safflower oils instead.

These dietary imbalances affect the structure of our cell membranes. Too many polyunsaturated fats in the diet will mean too many get incorporated into the membranes. And when there are too many polyunsaturates, the membrane becomes weak and unstable. In order to improve the structural stability of these weakened membranes, the body sends in reinforcements—kind of like load-bearing walls or studs—something that keeps the rest of the house (or membrane) from collapsing. What do these reinforcements consist of? Cholesterol!

This might be one reason that diets high in polyunsaturated fats have sometimes been shown to lower serum cholesterol: Cholesterol is removed from the bloodstream and inserted into the membranes, because too many polyunsaturated fats make for poorly constructed membranes, and they need cholesterol to reinforce and stabilize them. The human body can manufacture saturated fats, just as it does cholesterol. So saturated fat is not an essential nutrient, but there might be individuals whose internal synthesis of saturated fatty acids is unable to keep up with demand, and certain disease or trauma states might require a larger supply of saturated fat and cholesterol for repair purposes.

The perimeter of cells is not the only place where there are membranes in our bodies. The subcellular structures inside of cells are also surrounded by membranes. The ones we are most concerned with as they relate to brain function and Alzheimer's disease are the mitochondria, and we will look at them in detail in the next chapter.

— CHAPTER 5 —

Mitochondrial Function and Dysfunction

As explained in the previous chapter, membranes do not only appear at the outside border of cells. They surround the mini structures called *organelles* inside the cell as well. The structures we are especially concerned with are the mitochondria (singular = mitochondrion). The mitochondria are the "powerhouses" or energy factories of our cells. They are the sites where energy is produced. Figure 5.1 provides an illustration of basic mitochondrial structure.

As you can see, mito-chondria have both an outer membrane and an inner membrane. And the process of energy production takes place along a system embedded within the inner mitochondrial membrane. The final stop is an enzyme called ATP synthase. There are thousands of ATP synthases studded along the inner mitochondrial membrane, as represented in figure 5.2.)

> Accumulating evidence suggests that mitochondrial dysfunction is intimately associated with AD pathophysiology. . . . Mitochondrial dysfunction and the resulting energy deficit trigger the onset of neuronal degeneration and death.
>
> —*Paula I. Moreira and colleagues*[1]

ATP is the "energy currency" of the human body: In order to conduct economic business in the United States, we use dollars; in order to conduct physiological and biochemical business, the cells in our bodies use ATP. And if ATP is our energy currency, then think of mitochondria as the mints where the currency is manufactured.

The term *mitochondrial dysfunction* is being used more and more to describe what underlies neurological degeneration—including Alzheimer's disease, Parkinson's disease, amyotrophic lateral sclerosis (ALS, also known as "Lou Gehrig's disease"), multiple sclerosis, and more.[2] If mitochondria are what literally create energy, then damage to them will result in a cellular energy crisis. And by now, you are coming to understand that Alzheimer's disease is a cellular energy crisis in the brain.

Mitochondria might malfunction for many reasons, including inborn genetic errors and mutations. In this chapter, we will explore glycation and oxidation, two of the most prominent causes of mitochondrial dysfunction over which we can exert an influence. They are both largely

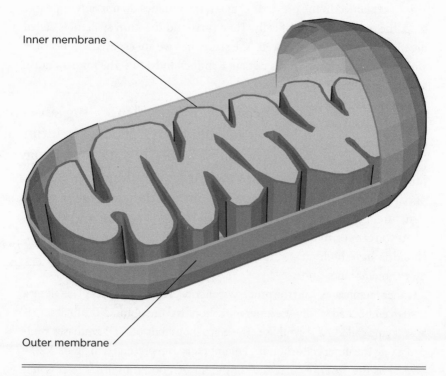

Inner membrane

Outer membrane

Figure 5.1 Basic mitochondrial structure. Each mitochondrion is a double-layered entity. An inner membrane surrounds the inside portion, and an outer membrane encapsulates the mitochondrion as a whole. Image by Yurii Andreichyn/Shutterstock.com.

the consequences of excessive consumption of the refined carbohydrates and isolated vegetable and seed oils that make up such a large part of the modern diet. You will see that you can keep your mitochondria healthy by adopting a nutrient-dense, reduced-carbohydrate diet, getting adequate sleep, and managing your stress levels. Your mitochondria will also benefit from regular physical activity, whether this means walking, biking, gardening, weightlifting, golf, yoga, pilates, swimming, senior aerobics—whatever you can handle and enjoy. You will see this again when we discuss exercise in chapter 17, but it's important enough to say twice: When it comes to your mitochondria, think of the phrase, "Use 'em or lose 'em." Staying active gives the body a reason to generate new, healthy mitochondria. Physical

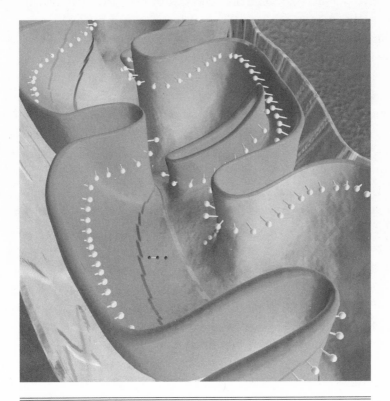

Figure 5.2 Close-up of the inner membrane of a mitochondrion. The enzymes that produce ATP are embedded within this inner membrane. Many cells in the body contain thousands of mitochondria, and each individual mitochondrion contains thousands of these energy-generating enzymes. Image by sciencepics/Shutterstock.com.

movement—especially higher intensity movement—provides the stimulus the body needs to create more mitochondria, and combined with regular dedication to low-intensity activity (such as walking or gardening), it can keep the ones it has in good working order. Give the body a reason to make and maintain healthy, well-functioning mitochondria, and it will.

In order to more fully understand the nutritional strategy outlined in this book—in particular, the importance of improving insulin sensitivity and blood glucose control and the emphasis on including certain types of dietary fats and avoiding others—it will be helpful for you to become familiar with the terms *glycation* and *oxidation*.

Glycation and oxidation are processes that occur in the human body as the result of normal, healthy metabolism. They are consequences of simply being alive, breathing, metabolizing food, and physically moving our bodies. However, glycation and oxidation are supposed to happen at low levels, very slowly, over a long period of time. When they happen more quickly and to a greater degree than normal, they overwhelm the body's capacity to repair the cells and tissues these processes can damage. Out-of-control glycation and oxidative stress are associated with (and might also directly or indirectly cause) many chronic illnesses of our time, including Alzheimer's disease.

Uncontrolled glycation and oxidation in the brain can be thought of as two types of "brain damage" that are part of the vicious cycle of Alzheimer's. This cycle is initiated by glucose- and insulin-handling problems, as well as by an imbalance of fatty acids in the diet. Glycation and oxidation are part of the vicious cycle because metabolic problems with carbohydrate intolerance come first, but once rampant glycation and oxidative stress take hold, they make it even more difficult for neurons to function properly and for communication to occur smoothly between brain cells. Below we will discuss these in more detail, beginning with glycation.

Glycation

Have you ever left a lollipop or hard candy on the dashboard of a car on a hot summer day? What happens? The sugar melts, spreads all over the nearby surface, and makes everything sticky and almost impossible to clean. And when the sugar hardens and dries, it solidifies and becomes almost as brittle as glass.

Something similar happens inside the body when we have a large amount of sugar (glucose) in our blood for extended periods of time. The medical term "hemoglobin A1c," which we've already discussed, refers to hemoglobin (the protein that carries oxygen in the blood) that has become sticky with sugar. It is *glycated* hemoglobin. Glycation is a function of glucose exposure and time—that is, the greater the amount of glucose in the blood, and the longer the high blood sugar is sustained, the more glycation will occur throughout the body. Diabetics with poorly controlled blood glucose typically have elevated A1c values because their blood sugar is almost always a little higher than is healthy. (You might recall from chapter 2 that hemoglobin A1c is an approximate average of the blood glucose level during the previous three months or so.) And when A1c is elevated, think of it like the blood being sticky and gunky. Its consistency or viscosity has gone from watery to more like maple syrup or molasses, and when the blood is thicker, it doesn't flow as smoothly as healthy blood. This can lead to a number of problems resulting from poor delivery of oxygen and nutrients from the blood to the tissues that need it.

Hemoglobin isn't the only thing in the body that can become glycated. Almost any structure inside us can suffer this fate of getting mucked up and sticky with sugar, including the structural proteins that make up the arteries, capillaries, and other blood vessels. Healthy blood vessels are like soft rubber hoses that are very accommodating—meaning, they can readily dilate and expand in order to easily accommodate blood flow. In contrast, blood vessels that are glycated become hard and unyielding, acting more like glass tubes—brittle and fragile. So when blood glucose is chronically high, instead of water flowing through a nice rubbery hose, we have something akin to thick, dense molasses being forced through a brittle glass tube that is less able to expand and accommodate the volume of blood. Think how much harder the heart needs to work in order to pump blood through this smaller space, and how much harder the blood will press up against the blood vessel walls. This might contribute to high blood pressure (hypertension), which is very common in individuals with type 2 diabetes and insulin resistance. Hypertension is one of the defining diagnostic criteria for metabolic syndrome, and chronically high insulin levels are a likely culprit behind essential and idiopathic hypertension.[3] (It is also why high blood pressure very often resolves upon adopting a low-carb diet.)

The logical and almost inevitable outcome of compromised blood vessel health and vessel dysfunction secondary to chronically high blood glucose and insulin is the high incidence of the various cardiovascular complications many people with diabetes experience that go far beyond hypertension: heart attack, burst blood vessels in the eyes, poor circulation, kidney failure (due to damage to the tiny blood vessels involved in filtering blood), loss of feeling in the extremities (diabetic neuropathy), and more.[4]

The consequences of blood sugar and insulin dysregulation on the cardiovascular system are devastating. Now consider the effects that might take place in the brain. Brain cells can become glycated (just like the car dashboard), and if they become covered in sticky sugar or sugar that is hardened and fragile like glass, these cells will cease to function properly. Glycation is one of the connections between abnormal blood glucose and insulin levels and damage to the brain.

But the damage glycation causes doesn't stop there. Sometimes, glycated structures connect (or bond) with each other, forming larger groups of harder and stickier cells and tissues, called advanced glycation end-products, commonly referred to by the not-ironic acronym "AGEs." In fact, glycation of proteins in the skin might contribute, in part, to the visible signs of aging, such as dry and brittle skin, sagging skin, and lines and wrinkles. But what happens to the skin on the outside is nothing compared to what happens to the brain on the inside. According to researcher Stephanie Seneff and colleagues, "With increased exposure to glucose, multiple proteins in both astrocytes and neurons are susceptible to glycation damage. A glycated protein suffers from a loss of function, increased susceptibility to oxidative damage, and increased resistance to degradation and disposal."[5]

Another way to think of AGEs is like charred or blackened meat. Think of the dark crust that forms on the surface of meat when you grill or sear it—that is also an advanced glycation end-product. The health consequences of consuming AGEs in our foods are quite different from when they form inside our bodies, but it is still a helpful image for us to use to think about the damage or "burning" that occurs when AGEs form inside the brain:

- Sticky, damaged cells
- Cells that are no longer capable of transmitting nerve impulses
- Cells whose damage prevents access to long- and short-term memory
- Cells whose damage interferes with proper behavior and impulse control
- Cells whose damage results in the signs of Alzheimer's disease

Oxidative Damage

The other major form of what we can think of as "brain damage" in the Alzheimer's sufferer is oxidative damage, also called oxidative stress, or simply oxidation. Like glycation, a low level of oxidation is a normal, unavoidable consequence of healthy human metabolic processes. It is only uncontrolled, chronic, overwhelming, and unrelenting oxidation that contributes to cognitive decline in the Alzheimer's brain, and there are many different things that can lead to this uncontrolled oxidative stress. The two most relevant and most easily modifiable factors are poor diet and chronic stress (including insufficient sleep).

If you read health publications or follow health stories on the TV news, you have probably heard the term *free radicals*. It is beyond the scope of this book to delve deeply into the science of what these are; for our purposes, we can think of free radicals as being pinballs inside our cells: They bang around and crash into things. What are these "pinballs" inside us? Technically speaking, these free radicals are "reactive oxygen species," or ROS. Biochemically, they are molecules with unpaired electrons. Molecules with unpaired electrons are unstable, so they will "steal" electrons from somewhere else in order to remedy this unpaired situation. This leaves another molecule with an unpaired electron, and on and on, in a kind of chain reaction. Among the places ROS steal electrons from are the fatty acids that make up cell membranes. When a molecule loses an electron, it is said to be oxidized. And when fatty acids experience this, the damage is called oxidation. In looking to repair this damage, whatever was oxidized (hit by the pinball) tries to steal resources from some other place, resulting in the aforementioned chain reaction of oxidation. The nutrients called *antioxidants* are helpful for limiting this damage and sometimes preventing it from occurring at all.

So where do the free radical pinballs that wreak havoc as they knock around from cell to cell and structure to structure come from? One source of them is vegetable oils, which are rich in polyunsaturated fatty acids. (Examples include soybean, corn, cottonseed, and safflower oils.) When exposed to heat, light, or air, polyunsaturated fats oxidize, creating ROS that we then consume upon eating foods that contain these oils or were cooked in them. (We'll explore this in more detail in chapter 12.)

Another source of ROS is everyday human metabolism. At a cellular level, the mitochondria (remember, these are the mini furnaces that create energy inside our cells) create ROS. We have natural, "in house" antioxidants generated by our own bodies (most notably glutathione and superoxide dismutase) that are designed to limit the damage caused by these ROS, but when too many ROS leak out, they can overwhelm the body's natural antioxidant capacity, leading to greater amounts of oxidative damage. The creation of ROS during energy production is a normal and unavoidable occurrence, but it happens to a larger and more overwhelming degree when the body is trying to create energy from glucose than when producing it from fat. As alluded to earlier, fats are a more efficient and "cleaner burning" fuel than glucose. The generation of energy (ATP) from glucose and fatty acids is slightly different on a molecular level, and this slight difference is enough to account for a greater amount of damaging free radicals generated by the metabolism of glucose. As for how this affects cognitive function, according to researcher Paula Moreira and colleagues, "If the amount of free radical species produced overwhelms the neuronal capacity to neutralize them, oxidative stress occurs, followed by mitochondrial dysfunction and neuronal damage."[6] Transitioning the body from the constant burning of carbohydrate to a fat-based metabolism instead is one way to reduce the oxidative burden in the body and brain.

Considering the important role of antioxidants in limiting the extent of oxidative stress, you might be thinking that high doses of antioxidant nutrients would be beneficial. Indeed, there might be a role for increasing the antioxidant pool in the body, but supraphysiologic doses of antioxidants are not recommended. Oxidation isn't all bad; it's a normal and necessary part of human physiology. In fact, oxidation is one of the tools the immune system uses to neutralize invading pathogens: Cells involved in the immune response oxidize pathogens, thereby killing them or tagging them for removal or excretion. Oxidation is also involved in a process called *apoptosis*, which is a kind of programmed "cell suicide" or cellular self-destruct mode. This is one way the body has of dismantling and disassembling old, worn out, or malfunctioning cells that are supposed to be gotten rid of. (Cancer cells evade apoptosis, which is why they continue to grow and spread, even though they are not functioning properly.) So while it's important to have an adequate pool of antioxidants to keep oxidative damage from overwhelming the body's tissues, inundating the body with massive doses of antioxidants might actually be detrimental because it could interfere with this critical balancing act. A sensible way to introduce more antioxidants into the body is by consuming foods that are rich in antioxidant nutrients. Many of the vegetables and low-glycemic fruits permitted on a very low-carbohydrate diet fit this bill, as do most herbs and spices, such as turmeric, rosemary, basil, garlic, oregano, allspice, and thyme. Liberal use of these in cooking is encouraged; it is highly unlikely that you would "overdo" antioxidants from food sources.

The brain is more susceptible to oxidative damage than any other major organ because of its high oxygen consumption. Neurons are particularly vulnerable to oxidative stress because their metabolic rate is about five times that of other brain cells. In addition, neurons contain a high proportion of polyunsaturated fatty acids that can interact with ROS to set off a self-propagating chain of lipid peroxidation and molecular breakdown.   —*Mortimer Mamelak*[7]

Mitochondrial Mayhem

Being the powerhouses that generate energy for us, mitochondria are both a source and a target for free radicals. In fact, owing to the fragile polyunsaturated fatty acids that are such a large part of the structure of the inner and outer mitochondrial membranes, these tiny generators are especially susceptible to oxidative stress. Just think of the burden they face in light of our modern diet: high in refined sugars and grains, and high in ROS-forming vegetable oils. They become glycated and also suffer constant blows from oxidation. They get a double whammy.

Mitochondrial dysfunction is a major problem in Alzheimer's disease. Mitochondria quite literally produce most of our energy. If they are damaged or reduced in number, it will clearly result in less energy produced in the whole body and, obviously, in the brain. Alzheimer's is a sort of "perfect storm" situation in which brain mitochondrial glycation and oxidation have combined to do serious damage to neuronal health and cognitive function.

It is crucial to protect the mitochondria by limiting the amount of damage that occurs in the first place and also by providing helpful nutrients to clean up and clear away the normal amount of damage that is unavoidable, inevitable, and natural. This is true for healthy people, but it is even more imperative for the Alzheimer's sufferer. The Alzheimer's brain has been suffering the effects of rampant oxidation and glycation for years, sometimes decades. The more quickly and effectively the damage is cleared away, the more quickly the Alzheimer's patient's cognitive function might improve. This is why the powerful nutritional strategy in this book is advised and also why specific supplements are suggested as adjuncts to the diet. This is no time for half-measures. This is the time for a drastic intervention in a race against time. We are trying to preserve and possibly restore healthy cognitive function, in part by restoring mitochondrial health.

One way oxidative damage causes a breakdown in healthy cognition is by changing the shape of the neurons themselves. As discussed in chapter 3, neurons are covered in myelin, which is primarily made up of cholesterol and fatty acids. If we consume too much of the wrong types of fat, these oxidized fats will be incorporated into the myelin structure, and the myelin will not function properly—leading to a breakdown in cellular communication and transmission of nerve impulses between neurons, which is one of the causes of memory loss and poor cognitive function in Alzheimer's. Simply put, the brain cells go "on the fritz," and the logical results are cognitive impairment, memory loss, and behavioral changes.

The same is true for cell membranes: They are made up of fatty acids, cholesterol, and other materials. If we eat an improper balance of fats in our diet, then too many of the wrong types of fat might be inserted into the cell membranes, which will become oxidized, and again, cellular function will be compromised.

To get a true appreciation for why this is so important and for why an alteration in the structure and function of something as seemingly inconsequential as cell membranes holds so much influence over all aspects of health—including cognitive function—let's keep in mind what cell membranes do. Remember, cell membranes are the bouncers of the cell: They allow the good things in and send the bad things out, and they also help cells retain their proper shape. Alter the shape of a neuron, alter its function.

Now that we've explored some of the cellular and subcellular damage that contributes to memory loss, behavioral changes, and other characteristics of Alzheimer's disease, there's another important biochemical factor to address: beta-amyloid plaques. These plaques, and the debate surrounding their role in disease progression, are the subject of the next chapter.

—CHAPTER 6—

Beta-Amyloid as a Cause of Alzheimer's: Guilty Party or Wrongly Accused?

I f you or your loved ones have done research into the causes of Alzheimer's disease, you have no doubt come across the term *beta-amyloid (Aβ)*. Beta-amyloid plaques, which I discussed briefly in chapter 1, figure prominently in almost all scientific papers related to Alzheimer's, but there is no consensus as to the exact role these plaques play in the condition. Many researchers contend that Aβ is a primary cause of AD, while others hold that it is an effect. Based on the etiology of AD as outlined in this book, and as is the case with so many nuances of human physiology, it is a little bit of both.

Aβ plaques can be likened to a fever: Fever is a natural protective mechanism the body employs to kill and neutralize invading pathogens. (The goal is to raise the body's core temperature to a level that is fatal to the bugs and viruses that cause illness.) However, even though it is a protective mechanism, if a fever goes too high, it can have disastrous effects for other parts of human physiology. The same can be said for Aβ. It might start out as a defensive step in the brain, but it progresses to a point where, rather than being helpful, it becomes harmful.

We can speculate with some degree of certainty that the accu-

> The production of the amyloid is a protective response. . . . The idea of just getting rid of the amyloid without understanding why it's there actually makes very little biological sense. —*Dale Bredesen*[1]

mulation of Aβ and its formation into widespread plaques is not a *cause* of AD, because the property that is an even greater hallmark of the condition— the reduced use of glucose in the brain—happens years, and sometimes decades, prior to the appearance of Aβ plaques. The formation of Aβ plaques is not the first step in AD pathology and is therefore not the most likely triggering factor.

A prominent and well-characterized feature of AD is progressive, region-specific declines in the cerebral metabolic rate of glucose (CMRglc). . . . Carriers of a common Alzheimer's susceptibility gene [APOE Ɛ4] have functional brain abnormalities in young adulthood, several decades before possible onset of dementia. Therefore, low regional CMRglc appears to be a very early event in the disease process, well before any clinical signs of dementia are evident, and well before cell loss or plaque deposition is predicted to have occurred.

—*Samuel Henderson*[2]

Furthermore, there is no evidence that Alzheimer's sufferers overproduce Aβ. It seems that the accumulation of these protein remnants and their formation into insoluble plaques is not the result of excess accumulation but rather of impaired clearance. That is, as explained in chapter 1, the reason Aβ builds up in the Alzheimer's brain is that it is not being effectively broken down and removed. A key factor preventing the efficient removal of Aβ is chronically elevated insulin. According to researcher Sónia Correia and colleagues, "Under hyperinsulinemic condi-

---

Insulin-degrading enzyme (IDE), a major Aβ-degrading enzyme, might be competitively inhibited by insulin, resulting in decreased Aβ degradation. It was shown that elevated insulin levels in type 2 diabetes induce Aβ accumulation through competition between insulin and Aβ for IDE.

—*Sónia Correia and colleagues*[4]

tions, insulin competes with amyloid β (Aβ) for insulin-degrading enzyme, leading to the accumulation of Aβ and senile plaque formation."[3]

Recall again that insulin and Aβ are both degraded and cleared away by insulin-degrading enzyme (IDE), but insulin is IDE's "favorite child." This means that as long as insulin levels are elevated, IDE will prioritize clearing the insulin, thus allowing the beta-amyloid to accumulate. Only when insulin levels are low—such as on a low-carbohydrate diet and with other lifestyle modifications—will IDE be able to focus on going after the amyloid proteins.

Beta-Amyloid as a Protective Factor

As discussed in the preceding sections, long-term overconsumption of refined carbohydrates and damaged polyunsaturated vegetable oils is a primary driver of rampant glycation and oxidation throughout the body and also in the brain. In order to prevent more of this kind of "brain damage" from occurring, the brain might be employing Aβ as a tool to shut off the glucose spigot. If the amount of glucose being metabolized in the brain is reduced, then glycation and oxidative stress will be reduced as well.

One way by which Aβ proteins aid in limiting glucose metabolism is by inhibiting some of the enzymes involved in converting glucose into energy. It is understandable why some researchers see this as a causative step in Alzheimer's pathology. If we know that Aβ reduces glucose usage in the brain—in part by interfering with the activity of relevant enzymes—and reduced brain glucose metabolism is one of the key hallmarks of AD, then it is reasonable to speculate that the accumulation of Aβ is causing the lowered use of glucose. But research suggests the reduction in brain glucose metabolism occurs long before the accumulation of Aβ plaques. Moreover, if neurons are damaged from long-term metabolic derangement, Aβ proteins might indeed be playing a protective role by interfering with the continued influx of glucose, the overabundance of which was likely a key contributing factor to the metabolic derangement in

The formation of Aβ may actually be an element in the brain's defense against oxidative stress. . . . Oxidative stress may then provoke the protective release of Aβ.

—*Mortimer Mamelak*[5]

the first place. From this perspective, at a cellular level, Aβ is actually doing the brain a favor.

Unfortunately, in the context of the high-carbohydrate modern Western diet, putting the brakes on the brain's use of glucose is an absolute disaster, because glucose serves as the primary fuel for the brain. And because glucose is the primary fuel for the brain when carbohydrate intake is high, the reason neurons deteriorate from a reduced ability to use glucose is because no alternative fuel is available. Remember, the other fuels that can feed the brain—ketones—are only generated in sufficient supply when insulin levels are very low (or MCT oils or exogenous ketones are ingested). There are several ways to reduce insulin levels, but one of the most effective is via a very low-carbohydrate diet. In the context of the starch and grain-based American diet, there is no elevation of ketones; therefore, brain cells struggle for fuel and ultimately degenerate. This occurs over a long period of time. (It is important to remember that Alzheimer's disease doesn't develop overnight. In the early stages, the brain might be able to compensate for the reduction in energy, but eventually, the signs and symptoms start appearing. This might lead to a diagnosis of mild cognitive impairment, but if nothing is done to reverse the metabolic derailment driving this, the end stage will be full-blown Alzheimer's disease.)

Continuing with the perspective of Aβ as an initially protective mechanism—but one that eventually gets out of hand and becomes harmful—how does this occur? One way is that large amounts of Aβ plaques alter the shape of the synapse between neurons. (Think of it as the plaques "getting in the way" and blocking nerve impulse transmission.) If axons and dendrites are like transmitters and receivers, imagine if someone jammed those transmitters and receivers. Messages would be garbled or lost altogether, and communication between neurons would break down, resulting in the observable outcomes of memory loss, foggy thinking, behavioral changes, emotional outbursts, and the other effects associated with Alzheimer's disease. In addition to altering the shape of the synapse, Aβ plaques themselves are subject to glycation and making cross-linkages between each other, forming advanced glycation end products, which compromise structure and function in the brain even further.

Since Aβ is likely not a main causal factor in AD, it's not surprising that pharmaceutical drugs developed to specifically target the secretion of these proteins and their formation into plaques have had little impact on disease progression.[6] The approach that is known as the "amyloid hypothesis" or "amyloid cascade hypothesis" has many shortcomings and fails to account for many of the metabolic and physiologic abnormalities in AD and MCI. Continuing to funnel research dollars toward this failed trajectory will only delay research into avenues that are far more promising.[7] Researchers are slowly beginning to realize this, and some are shifting from the amyloid focus to a mitochondrial hypothesis, wherein mitochondrial dysfunction— and the resulting disruption of cellular energy production—is believed to be a driving factor of cognitive decline.[8] Understanding AD as a systemic metabolic disturbance involving abnormal insulin signaling, glucose usage, inflammation, and oxidative stress, rather than something exclusively localized to the brain, suggests novel therapeutic avenues that are likely to be far more effective than what has been attempted to date. We will only begin to make real progress in the fight against this condition when we focus therapeutic efforts on the underlying causes of AD, rather than on managing individual symptoms.

CHAPTER 7

ApoE4:
Is There an Alzheimer's Gene?

I n learning about your or your loved one's diagnosis of MCI or Alzheimer's disease, you have likely come across the term *ApoE4*. ApoE4 is shorthand for the Ɛ-4 allele of the gene that encodes for the apolipoprotein E molecule. Don't be intimidated by the science-speak. All this means is that ApoE4 is a variant of a gene that expresses itself in some way in the body. Just as some people have genes for blue eyes and others have genes for brown eyes, some people have genes for ApoE4, and others have genes for ApoE2 or ApoE3. These genes create apolipoprotein E particles.

So what is this apolipoprotein molecule the ApoE gene creates?

Substances that are not water-soluble cannot travel through the bloodstream on their own. There are several critical nutrients and structural components for the body that are not water-soluble, so in order to be transported to where they are needed, they must be packaged inside molecules that can travel in the bloodstream. These molecules are called lipoproteins, and we can think of them like cargo ships on the ocean. We can't very well send all our cargo out on the ocean in cardboard boxes; the boxes would never survive and make it to their destination. So we put them on ships, which can deliver the precious items safely. Things like vitamins A, D, E, and K; cholesterol; and fatty acids—which are required for good health and proper functioning of the body and brain—are the non-water-soluble cargo inside our bodies, and they need to be protected inside these lipoproteins. And just as cargo ships have special equipment to help them dock in a port, lipoproteins have special molecules on their outsides to help them "dock," or attach to places inside our body where the cargo is needed. These special molecules that aid in the delivery of precious nutritional and biochemical cargo are the apolipoproteins.

Continuing a little further with our cargo ship analogy, if a ship were left unprotected during a hurricane, a great deal of damage could happen to the docking equipment. Similarly, in the face of the nutritional hurricane that is the modern diet—high in sugar, refined carbohydrates, and vegetable oils—the apolipoprotein molecules suffer damage. The apoE4 molecules seem to accrue more damage than the apoE2 and apoE3 molecules, which is one of the reasons why the ApoE4 gene is associated with greater risk for Alzheimer's disease than the other variants, and greater disease severity if and when the condition takes hold.

Why is damage to apolipoproteins a problem? Neurons in the brain have apoE receptors (places for these particles to dock), which suggests that apoE plays a role in the delivery and clearance of crucial fatty acids, cholesterol, and phospholipids to and from the brain. (Apolipoprotein E does a great deal more than this. It's a signaling molecule for as many as 1,700 genes, many of which directly influence cellular processes involved in the pathogenesis of Alzheimer's disease.[1] However, for our purposes at this point, we'll focus on its role in lipid transport and delivery.) Delivery and recycling of cholesterol in the brain is essential because the brain contains 25 percent of the body's total cholesterol—used as an antioxidant, electrical insulator, and key structural component of cell and plasma membranes. Despite its unfortunate reputation as a dangerous substance, cholesterol is, in fact, an absolutely integral contributor to structure and function throughout the entire body, but perhaps especially in the brain, and any interruption in its supply is likely to have dire consequences for cognitive function. (We'll discuss cholesterol in detail in chapter 9.)

Cholesterol is delivered throughout the body primarily by low-density lipoproteins. The ApoE4 gene is associated with less-effective LDL uptake than the other ApoE variants; therefore, ApoE4 carriers experience the consequences that result from this more frequently and to a greater extent than people with other genotypes. One of these consequences is reduced delivery of cholesterol and fatty acids to astrocytes, which are specialized brain cells whose primary role is to receive these critical substances and "feed" them to nearby cells.[2]

The reason the apoE2, E3, and E4 molecules function differently and influence disease risk in different ways is because they have different shapes.

Like all proteins, these apolipoproteins are made from long chains of amino acids, like words placed in a certain order to form a sentence. Change the word order, and you change the meaning of the sentence. (Think of "Man bites dog" versus "Dog bites man.") Changes in just one or two of the amino acids affect the shape of the protein. The proteins that make up the apoE2, E3, and E4 particles differ in just a few amino acids, but seemingly tiny changes at this biochemical level can have extraordinary consequences for an organism—a human being—as a whole. The different shapes of these apolipoproteins means they differ in the way they bind to other molecules and structures in the body and brain, which explains why they're associated with different trends in lipid (cholesterol) processing. (For example, E4 carriers seem to be at greater risk for cardiovascular disease. However, this might not be the result of the E4 genotype, *per se*, but rather, the mismatch between E4 and the modern diet.) *Change the structure, change the function* is a principle often taught on the first day of a biochemistry class in order to hammer home the powerful role of the order of amino acids in determining protein structure and the ultimate actions of those proteins.

The ApoE4 Genotype and Risk for Alzheimer's: Hunter-Gatherers in a Modern Supermarket World

The ApoE4 gene has become important in Alzheimer's disease research because people with one copy of it are at greater risk for developing AD than those without one, and people with two copies are at even greater risk.[3] (We have two copies of each gene in our body; one from our mother and one from our father.) The risk for developing Alzheimer's among carriers of the ApoE4 gene is so significant that one study's authors called it "the susceptibility gene."[4] People with one copy of the ApoE4 gene have a fivefold increased risk of developing AD, while people with two copies are estimated to have a staggering lifetime risk between 50 percent and 90 percent.[5] However, the ApoE4 gene does not *cause* AD. What it does is make a person more susceptible to the metabolic damage inflicted by the modern Western diet and lifestyle. As many researchers are fond of saying, "Genetics loads the gun, but diet and lifestyle pull the trigger."

Despite this seemingly damning genetic heritage, the ApoE4 allele is neither required nor sufficient for development of AD, as 50 percent of people with AD are not E4 carriers, and some E4 homozygotes (two gene copies) never develop the disease.[6] On the other hand, the other known risk factor—chronic hyperinsulinemia—elevates risk independently of ApoE status. And since chronic hyperinsulinemia occurs in approximately 40 percent of people over age sixty, it's not surprising to find a correlation between it and a condition that preferentially strikes the aging, such as AD.[7] In fact, evidence indicates that the risk for AD attributable solely to hyperinsulinemia is as high as 39 percent.[8]

So if you have one or two copies of the ApoE4 gene, this does not mean it is inevitable and unavoidable that you will develop dementia. It simply means that you must be especially careful about what you eat and how you live so that you do not tempt fate and trigger your increased susceptibility. ApoE4 is considered a *risk gene*, and according to the Alzheimer's Association in the United States, "Risk genes increase the likelihood of developing a disease, but do not guarantee it will happen."[9]

The APOE Ɛ4 allele may not be inherently damaging but only in combination with a high-carbohydrate diet, which is damaging in itself and is likely to be a major contributor to the high risk of CAD [coronary artery disease], and possibly AD, in modern populations with or without the APOE Ɛ4 allele. . . . AD may be similar to obesity, coronary artery disease, and type II diabetes mellitus in being a consequence of the conflict between our Paleolithic genetic constitution and our current Neolithic diet.

—Roger Lane and Martin Farlow[10]

It should be noted that Ɛ4 is not an inherently damaging allele; it is only deleterious in combination with a HC [high-carb] diet (which is deleterious on its own).

—Samuel Henderson[11]

In the world population, the frequencies of the E2, E3, and E4 genotypes are approximately 8 percent, 77 percent, and 15 percent, respectively.[12] The different versions of the ApoE gene are hypothesized to stem from human evolutionary migration patterns and the historic adoption of grain-based agriculture.[13] Groups with the longest exposure to grain consumption have a lower E4 frequency, which suggests that high carbohydrate intakes might have selected against this genotype.[14] That is, ApoE4 might have persisted among ancestral populations that were hunter-gatherers, who presumably consumed far fewer grains (carbohydrates) than their pastoral farming contemporaries. Populations with the lowest E4 frequencies include Arabs living in Northern Israel (4 percent), Greeks (6.8 percent), and Mayans (8.9 percent), while E4 is vastly more common in traditional hunter-gatherer groups such as African Pygmies (40 percent) and the North American Inuit (21 percent).[15] Arabs and Greeks might have had a higher grain intake via wheat than their hunter-gatherer contemporaries, and Mayans might have consumed more grain via corn.

This suggests that people with the ApoE4 genotype might be biologically better suited to a diet lower in carbohydrates—or, at least, lower in grain-based carbohydrates. (Perhaps their denser carbohydrate sources would have been roots and tubers, such as potatoes, beets, yams, yucca, and taro.) This theory makes sense in light of what we know about the damaging effects of the refined carbohydrate load of the modern Western diet. It seems that certain population groups are simply better suited for a higher intake of fat and protein, with a lower intake of carbohydrates, particularly from cereal grains.

By itself, having the ApoE4 genotype is not sufficient to cause Alzheimer's disease.[17] We know this because many people with the ApoE4 genotype do not develop AD. In fact, only about half of people homozygous for ApoE4 develop the disease by age ninety.[18] This is, of course, an extraordinarily high incidence, but we should note that it also means about half of E4 homozygotes *don't* develop AD. So by itself, having these genes is not sufficient to cause AD. When AD develops in an E4 carrier, it is more likely a result of the combination of a diet high in carbohydrates and low in micronutrients and essential fatty acids with the increased susceptibility this genotype confers, rather than possession of the E4 alleles, *per se*. AD is estimated to affect approximately 47 percent of people over eighty-five years of age, but the incidence of ApoE4 worldwide is far lower than 47 percent, so there are clearly other factors contributing to AD risk besides one single genetic trait.[19]

People with any and all combinations of ApoE2, E3, and E4 gene alleles are susceptible to AD. No genotype confers immunity; there are no genetic "get out of jail free" cards. Among patients diagnosed with AD, estimates put the prevalence of the E4 genotype as greatest in Northern Europe and lowest in Asia and Southern Europe.[20] This seems to support the hypothesis that populations with a longer exposure to higher carbohydrate intakes from grains (presumably from rice in Asia and wheat in Southern Europe) would have a lower prevalence of E4, while those from colder climates— such as Northern Europe—might have genetic constitutions better suited to diets higher in animal fat and protein.

A modified "Paleolithic prescription" may prevent AD. The Paleolithic prescription proposes a change in diet and activity to a level more similar to our Late Paleolithic ancestors. . . . Therefore, reducing dietary intake of high-glycemic carbohydrates and increasing protein, fiber and fat would be preferred. Similar diets appear to reduce the risk of AD. Since HC [high carb] diets are proposed to be the primary cause of AD regardless of apoE genotype, such a diet would generally reduce the risk of AD. However, this diet is predicted to be particularly beneficial to carriers of apoE4.

—Samuel Henderson[16]

We also know that it is possible to develop AD without the ApoE4 gene—that is, this genotype is not required to induce AD. We know this because many Alzheimer's patients are *not* carriers of the E4 gene. In fact, the majority of AD patients are not E4 carriers. So while ApoE4 gets a lot of attention in AD research, it is a side issue that distracts us from the real root cause: chronic hyperinsulinemia, driven by excessive carbohydrate intake and other factors of modern life that are believed to contribute to insulin resistance, inflammation, and uncontrolled oxidative stress.

ApoE4 has garnered attention because apoE4 molecules are the ones most heavily damaged by the modern diet that is so far removed from the hunter-gatherer lifestyle under which it is believed to have been conditioned. I emphasize again: The ApoE4 genotype does not cause Alzheimer's.

It increases susceptibility under certain dietary and lifestyle conditions, in the same way that specific genes are associated with certain types of cancer but do not necessarily cause the cancer to develop in the absence of other contributing factors.

If the ApoE4 genotype makes someone more susceptible to the metabolic insults of a modern diet heavy in refined carbohydrates and damaged fats and oils, then it is critical that people with this genotype return to the types of foods for which their individual physiology might be better suited: abundant nonstarchy vegetables, seafood, poultry, meats, nuts and seeds, and seasonal low glycemic fruits, with little to no cereal grains or dairy.

Research is emerging that suggests people with the ApoE4 genotype might respond negatively to larger amounts of saturated fat in their diet. Specifically, they might see unfavorable changes to their blood lipids (cholesterol) as reflected in laboratory tests. The ApoE4 genotype is associated with elevated LDL in the blood as well as elevated triglycerides. The only way to know whether a low-carbohydrate, high-fat diet is affecting you this way is to get tested regularly, perhaps every few months. However, I must caution here that what some practitioners in the modern conventional medical establishment consider an "unfavorable" or "at risk" cholesterol profile has been called into question by many cardiologists and lipid experts, and that neither a high total cholesterol level nor a high level of LDL cholesterol, by itself, is necessarily harmful, particularly in older people.[21] (More on this in chapter 9.) In fact, higher cholesterol later in life is associated with reduced risk for all-cause mortality, and among elderly individuals without dementia, low cholesterol is a strong predictor of mortality.[22]

If your genetic constitution leads you to believe you or your loved one should err on the side of limiting intake of saturated fat, you can most certainly still follow a diet low in carbohydrate and high in fat. The main modification you might look to make is emphasizing monounsaturated and polyunsaturated fats rather than saturated fats—for example, doing most of your cooking with olive or avocado oil, rather than tallow, lard, or ghee; and consuming polyunsaturated fats as they occur naturally in whole foods, such as in nuts and seeds, rather than vegetable oils such as soybean and corn oil. Regarding animal protein, poultry and seafood are higher in mono- and polyunsaturated fats than beef and pork, but please note that beef and pork both also contain substantial amounts of monounsaturated fat. One more category you might wish to moderate your intake of, or eliminate altogether, is dairy (butter, cheese, sour cream, yogurt), as dairy fat is predominantly saturated. (If the E4 genotype is more closely associated with hunter-gatherer populations rather than agriculturalists, then individuals with this genotype in the modern world might be as unsuited to dairy as they are to grains.)

This is similar to the recommendations of Steven Gundry, MD, an expert in nutrition for the ApoE4 genotype. Dr. Gundry has pointed out that Nigerians have a high incidence of the ApoE4 genotype, yet they experience extraordinarily low rates of dementia.[23] According to Dr. Dale Bredesen, whose groundbreaking work in reversing Alzheimer's disease and MCI I mentioned in chapter 1, ApoE4 is the oldest genotype, with the other variants having first appeared more recently in evolutionary history.[24] With this in mind, E4 carriers might do well to avoid the majority of foods that would not have been consumed in great quantities in many parts of the world several millennia ago—namely, grains and dairy products. Dr. Gundry recommends a diet free of grains and dairy, with a modest amount of animal protein coming primarily from shellfish and seafood, with small amounts of high-quality grass-fed and grass-finished beef and lamb, and pastured poultry. The long-chain omega-3 fats found predominantly in marine foods and in smaller amounts in land animals are especially beneficial for E4s. (We'll discuss omega-3s in more detail in chapter 13.) The vegetables recommended for ApoE4 carriers include nonstarchy items, with emphasis on leafy greens (for example, spinach, dandelion, collards), cruciferous vegetables (broccoli, cauliflower, brussels sprouts, cabbages), and alliums (onions, garlic, leeks, chives, scallions, shallots). Dr. Gundry advises against "seeded vegetables" (tomatoes, eggplant, peppers, squash), as these might act more like fruits in E4 carriers, which might increase triglycerides. He encourages liberal consumption of monounsaturated fats—as much as one liter of olive oil per week—with very little saturated fat, including from coconut oil.[25] (Dr. Gundry encourages the use of MCT oil in lieu of coconut oil.) Other wonderful sources of unsaturated fats are olives, avocados, and nuts and seeds: macadamias, almonds, walnuts, hazelnuts (filberts), pecans, Brazil nuts, and pistachios.

We've covered a lot of ground so far! From the fundamental issue of Alzheimer's disease as an energy crisis in the brain to the role of glucose and ketones as fuel, from how changes in the shape of neurons and damage to the energy-generating mitochondria influence disease progression to genetic factors that influence risk for developing dementia, we've laid the foundation upon which to construct a diet to reduce and possibly even reverse and prevent the neuronal injuries that underlie Alzheimer's. Part two will walk you through the details on how to do just that.

A Nutritional Strategy for Restoring Healthy Cognitive Function

This section presents a low-carbohydrate, higher fat diet to nourish the struggling brain. We'll do some myth busting regarding cholesterol and saturated fat so you'll feel confident embarking on this nutritional journey. Here you'll find everything you need to guide you through the dietary change: what to eat, what to avoid, and how to navigate your new food landscape when grocery shopping, cooking, and dining out.

CHAPTER 8

Low-Carbohydrate Diet Basics

B ased on what you have read so far, it should be obvious that the underlying tenet of this nutritional strategy to fight Alzheimer's disease and
cognitive impairment is a dramatic reduction in dietary carbohydrate.
This is a low-carbohydrate diet. It is not a no-carbohydrate diet, but it does
require consuming far less carbohydrate than you or the person you care
for are probably accustomed to. The focus of the diet is fat and protein,
with a small amount of carbohydrate (but little to none from grains). The
majority of your calories will come from fat, a moderate amount from
protein, and very little from carbohydrate. This is likely the opposite of what
you're accustomed to hearing from the conventional medical world as what
constitutes a "healthy diet," but remember, we are intentionally inducing a
metabolic shift in the body away from carbohydrates and toward fats. If we
think of the body like a car, if we want our engine (the brain) to be fueled
by ketones—which come from breaking down fats—then it does no good
to keep filling the gas tank with carbohydrates.

As I've described in part one, by using this nutritional strategy, we are
moving the body and brain away from using glucose as their primary fuel.
It is important to note that "glucose" is not just what we think of as sugar.
This diet requires limiting refined sugar, of course, but it also requires limiting all starchy carbohydrates, because these are broken down into glucose
inside the body. So it's not just obvious forms of sugar—candy, cakes, cookies, soda, juice—that we need to limit; it's all high-carbohydrate foods that
end up as glucose inside us. This makes the diet a little more nuanced.

The degree of carbohydrate restriction required to make the metabolic
shift differs from person to person. Most people will experience the metabolic and cognitive effects of carbohydrate reduction if they consume fewer
than 50 grams of carbohydrate per day. Some people will be able to be

The primary event leading to the development of AD is consumption of an evolutionarily discordant high carbohydrate diet. This hypothesis predicts that relatively simple preventative measures, such as lowering the consumption of starchy carbohydrates and increasing essential fatty acids in the diet will be effective.

—*Samuel Henderson*[1]

more liberal with their carbohydrate intake, but others might need to go even lower than that, particularly if the cognitive impairment or dementia is severe and has been present for a long time. As they say, drastic times call for drastic measures.

Compared to the standard American diet (not ironically referred to as the *SAD*), 50 grams of carbohydrate might not sound like much. It's not unusual for people to consume 250 grams of carbohydrate per day—and sometimes more! Fifty grams is not a lot when you consume starchy, carbohydrate-dense foods like bread, bagels, pasta, rice, corn, potatoes, crackers, breakfast cereal, fiber bars, and the like. (A large bowl of pasta can be over 50 grams all by itself!) But 50 grams allows for consumption of a substantial amount and a wide variety of nonstarchy vegetables, such as leafy greens, summer squash, eggplant, bell peppers, asparagus, cauliflower, and low-glycemic fruits, like berries.

While this way of eating might seem like a radical departure from what you're accustomed to, rest assured, it's not that radical at all. It's not difficult, just different (see table 8.1).

The Body's Big Three Macronutrients: Protein, Fat, Carbohydrate

There are three main macronutrients that the body recognizes as sources of energy (calories): protein, fat, and carbohydrate. All foods fall into one or more of these categories. (Alcohol is sometimes considered a macronutrient because it provides energy—7 calories per gram—but alcohol is not a prime source of calories on this plan.) Some foods are almost entirely (or predominantly) one macronutrient, while others are combinations. For example, olive oil and coconut oil are pure fats, but a rib eye steak is both protein and fat. Egg whites are nearly all protein, but almonds are fat and

Table 8.1. The Ground Rules

What this diet is:	What this diet is not:
• A dietary strategy based on the facts of human physiology and biochemistry • A way to restore metabolic balance and promote healing **Above all:** • A safe, nontoxic, drug-free, nutritional therapy	• An overnight miracle cure for Alzheimer's disease

What this diet requires:	What this diet does NOT require:
• An open mind • A willingness to let go of longstanding and deeply held beliefs about what a "healthy diet" looks like • A willingness to buy, prepare, and cook more food at home and abandon packaged, processed "convenience foods" • A willingness to try new foods and abandon old favorites that are interfering with cognitive function • A commitment to spending (just a little) more time in the kitchen	• Hunger and deprivation • Shakes, bars, and "meal replacement" products • A second mortgage to afford only organic foods • Fancy foods available only at specialty stores • Trips to four different grocery stores to hunt down uncommon ingredients • Specialized kitchen equipment • Being a professional chef

protein (with a small amount of carbohydrate in the form of fiber). Beans and pulses—black beans, lentils, chickpeas—are carbohydrate and protein.

The proportions of the three main macronutrients in the diet you will follow depend on how sensitive you are to carbohydrates. As mentioned above, everyone has a unique threshold or tolerance for carbohydrate consumption, below which they can switch their metabolism to running on fat and generating significant amounts of ketones to fuel the brain. Some people can consume as much as 60–80 grams of carbs per day and still reap the metabolic and cognitive benefits, while others will need to restrict much further, for example, to under 30 grams per day.

(continued on page 93)

A Four-Tiered Approach to a Low-Carb, High-Fat Dietary Plan

Macronutrient Ratio = Fat 65%: Protein 20%: Carbohydrate 15%

Figure 8.1 represents a good general place to start.
On 2,000 calories per day, this works out to:

- Fat—1,300 calories (144 grams)
- Protein—400 calories (100 grams)
- Carbohydrate—300 calories (75 grams)

On 1,700 calories per day, this works out to:

- Fat—1,105 calories (123 grams)
- Protein—340 calories (85 grams)
- Carbohydrate—255 calories (64 grams)

Macronutrient Ratio = Fat 70%: Protein 20%: Carbohydrate 10%

Figure 8.2 is the next step, incorporating more fat and restricting carbohydrates even further.
On 2,000 calories per day, this works out to:

- Fat—1,400 calories (156 grams)
- Protein—400 calories (100 grams)
- Carbohydrate—200 calories (50 grams)

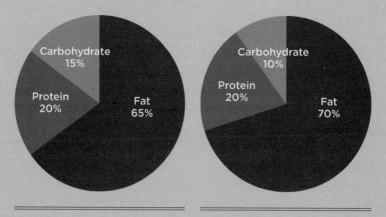

Figure 8.1   Figure 8.2

On 1,700 calories/day:
- Fat—1,190 calories (132 grams)
- Protein—340 calories (85 grams)
- Carbohydrate—170 calories (42 grams)

If your body seems especially resistant to generating enough ketones to deliver a good, steady supply of fuel to your brain, you can increase fat, decrease carbs, and also decrease protein slightly. This might be helpful because protein raises insulin levels, although not to the degree that carbohydrates do. The level of protein intake that might be considered "too much" is completely individual. You will have to experiment and see where you feel best, and how your body and brain respond.

A higher fat and lower protein intake would look like the following:

Macronutrient Ratio = Fat 75%: Protein 15%: Carbohydrate 10%

Figure 8.3 is the next step.

On 2,000 calories per day, this works out to:
- Fat—1,500 calories (167 grams)
- Protein—300 calories (75 grams)
- Carbohydrate—200 calories (50 grams)

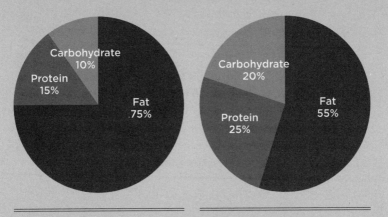

Figure 8.3   **Figure 8.4**

On 1,700 calories per day:
- Fat—1,275 calories (142 grams)
- Protein—255 calories (64 grams)
- Carbohydrate—170 calories (42 grams)

If you are very physically active and think you can tolerate a higher carbohydrate intake while still experiencing the benefits of lower insulin, lower glucose, and elevated ketones, experiment with a slightly higher carbohydrate intake, with slightly less fat and perhaps more protein. Others who might be successful with a higher carbohydrate intake include individuals whose cognitive impairment is very mild and of recent onset. In these cases, a very low-carbohydrate diet might not be necessary. Some people might experience benefits from a somewhat moderate carbohydrate intake—higher than the other approaches shown here, but still significantly lower than typical carbohydrate intakes in the modern industrialized world, perhaps in the range of 25 percent to 30 percent of total calories, with those additional carbohydrates coming predominantly in the form of more vegetables and perhaps small amounts of fruit, beans, or starchy tubers, rather than from refined sugars and grains. Most people will find it difficult to produce significant ketones at this level of combined carbohydrate and protein intake, but again, there might be some people with relatively mild cognitive issues who don't need to follow a very strict low-carb diet to reap some of the benefits. (Some individuals who are especially physically active might do well in this range, but overall, this is likely too much for the average individual, especially if they are of advanced age or have very severe Alzheimer's.)

Macronutrient Ratio = Fat 55%: Protein 25%: Carbohydrate 20%

Figure 8.4 is the next step.
On 2,000 calories per day, this works out to:
- Fat—1,100 calories (122 grams)
- Protein—500 calories (125 grams)
- Carbohydrate—400 calories (100 grams)

On 1,700 calories per day:
- Fat—935 calories (104 grams)
- Protein—425 calories (106 grams)
- Carbohydrate—340 calories (85 grams)

One thing is certain: The majority of your caloric intake will come from fat. Fat will make up at least 55 percent of your total calories, and likely closer to 65 percent or even 70 percent or more. Depending on your individual carbohydrate sensitivity and ability to generate sufficient ketones, your macronutrient breakdown could resemble one of the scenarios presented in this chapter. Please keep in mind that these are just examples. Ideally you will work with a qualified health care practitioner familiar with these types of diets in order to determine the macronutrient ratios and specific amounts of food that are right for you. Also, please note that, depending on your gender, body size, and activity level, your daily caloric needs might be different from the examples provided. As a general rule, men need more total calories than women, larger people need more calories than small-framed people, and more active people need higher calories than those who are sedentary.

The specific foods that are and are not suitable for this dietary strategy are discussed in the next few chapters. The truth is, there are no foods that are entirely "off limits." However, if you are looking to make the metabolic shift to fuel the brain as quickly, efficiently, and effectively as possible, you would do well to avoid certain foods entirely, while emphasizing others. It's not that bread, pasta, rice, and other starchy grains are prohibited outright. They are simply best avoided because even very small amounts of these foods will put most people's total carbohydrate intake over the limit, and it's just not worth it. To reach your carbohydrate quota for the day, you could have one medium serving of starch or grain, or several generous servings of cauliflower, spinach, zucchini, and other low-carbohydrate vegetables. We will address the types of carbohydrates to eat on your new nutritional plan in chapter 10.

Before that, though, there's something even more pressing we need to cover. Many of the foods recommended in this strategy are high in cholesterol. In dutifully following dietary advice from the government or likely even your own doctors or dietitians, you might have banished these foods from your diet for years. In order to add these foods back into your life without trepidation, we need to set the record straight about cholesterol—what it is, what it does, why you don't need to be afraid to eat cholesterol-rich foods, and most of all, why cholesterol is king of all nutrients when it comes to restoring healthy cognitive function.

—CHAPTER 9—

Cholesterol:
The Brain's Best Friend

If you are going to proceed with confidence in adopting a low-carbohydrate, high-fat diet or guiding your loved one through it, it is imperative that you understand some basic facts about cholesterol. Many of the foods emphasized in this nutritional strategy—eggs, butter, fatty cuts of animal protein—are high in cholesterol, and it is important that you let go of your fear of bringing these formerly taboo foods back into your diet. You do not need to fear these foods; in fact, they should be welcomed with open arms and given a place of honor. There is almost

> Lack of cholesterol supply to neurons impairs neurotransmission and synaptic plasticity, inducing neurodegeneration and tau pathology.
>
> —*Roger Lane and Martin Farlow*[1]

nothing more nourishing to a struggling brain than cholesterol. I can't stress it enough. Cholesterol is the single most misunderstood, maligned, and wrongfully vilified nutrient in all of health science.

Functions of Cholesterol in the Body

I cannot emphasize this point enough: Cholesterol is not the dangerous substance we've been led to believe it is. Just the opposite, in fact. Cholesterol is absolutely one of the most critical and essential factors for overall good health, and it is especially critical for brain health and cognitive function.

Before we get into the specifics of cholesterol's role in the brain, let's explore a few of the wonderful things cholesterol does for us throughout the body:

- Serves as an essential structural component for cell membranes and plasma membranes
- Serves as an essential structural component of the myelin sheath, which insulates and protects neurons and facilitates communication between them
- Is required for synthesis of all steroid hormones, including testosterone, estrogen, progesterone, aldosterone, cortisol, and more
- Serves as a raw material for endogenous (internal) production of vitamin D, via the interaction of sunlight with our skin
- Is required for proper function of serotonin receptors in the brain
- Serves as an essential component of bile salts, which are required for the digestion of fats and fat-soluble vitamins and phytonutrients
- Serves as a repair substance, needed for repair and regeneration of damaged tissue

With cholesterol serving so many vital functions in our bodies—and in the brain, in particular—imagine what would happen under a long-term deficiency, such as might be induced by a very low-cholesterol diet or statin drugs or other cholesterol-lowering medication. As Jimmy Moore and Eric Westman, MD, authors of the book *Cholesterol Clarity*, put it, "The knee-jerk reaction to push a statin medication to lower your cholesterol as the first line of defense without looking further into the cause is one of the most foolish things your doctor could ever do."[3]

> There is no evidence that cholesterol—by itself—blocks coronary or cerebral arteries, causing heart attacks or strokes. Cholesterol is a co-participant in lipid deposition into the endothelium of arterial vessels damaged by hyperinsulinemia.
>
> —*Joseph Kraft*[2]

As it relates to brain function, recall the discussion of myelin in chapter 3. Myelin is made largely out of cholesterol. If there isn't enough cholesterol in the body to create and maintain this myelin, then neurons will "short out," like ungrounded electrical wires. The natural outcome of neurons misfiring and failing to communicate with each other would be the exact kind of memory loss, confusion, and behavioral changes that characterize MCI and Alzheimer's disease.

Going beyond that, as cholesterol is an essential component of all cell and plasma membranes, we can easily see what would happen to health at a cellular and subcellular level if the body's supply of cholesterol were limited. Recall the analogy of the cell membrane as a kind of security guard: In order for good things (nutrients, fuel, antioxidants) to get into the cell, and for bad things (toxins and normal metabolic waste products) to get out of the cell, they have to pass through the membrane. If the body doesn't have enough cholesterol to construct well-formed cell membranes, it's a recipe for disaster. The good stuff can't get in, and the bad stuff can't get out.

All cells in the body are largely made out of membranes. The cellular wall, the walls of organelles inside the cells and the walls that separate different compartments in each cell from each other are all membranes.... Our bodies are made out of cells; every organ, every tissue, every little speck of us is made out of cells. It has been estimated that from 40 to 80% of our body cells are membranes.... Well, what are the membranes made of? The answer is this: all membranes are made out of fats and cholesterol, which means that our bodies are largely made out of fats and cholesterol!

—*Natasha Campbell-McBride*[4]

Taking this one step further, let's consider the mitochondria. Recall that the mitochondria are our cells' energy generators. The structure of the mitochondria is such that they are loaded with cholesterol. Mitochondria have two sections, both of which are surrounded by cholesterol-rich membranes. The actual "pumps" that generate energy (ATP) inside the mitochondria are embedded within the inner membrane. So if these membranes are malformed or malfunctioning due to insufficient cholesterol, it is obvious that there will be devastating effects on a cell's ability to generate energy. And remember: Alzheimer's disease is largely the result of brain cells that are no longer able to generate sufficient energy. They shrivel up and eventually starve to death. Want to make well-built and well-functioning membranes? Be sure to provide your body with enough cholesterol to do so.

What about "High" Cholesterol Levels?

Just as is happening with fats overall, and saturated fat in particular, mainstream medicine is slowly—very slowly—coming around to the idea that we have been wrong about the "dangers" of cholesterol. Dead wrong. (Pun absolutely intended.) The truth is, studies of older people have shown that higher levels of cholesterol later in life are associated with a *reduced* risk for dementia.[8] The cerebrospinal fluid of people with Alzheimer's is lower in cholesterol than that of healthy, nondemented people of the same ages.[9] Higher cholesterol levels are associated with *better* cognitive function in older individuals.[10]

Having too low cholesterol is actually much worse than having too high cholesterol. Cholesterol is part of every cell in the body and plays a role in keeping those cells healthy. So to think that you need to reduce cholesterol and cut down on the amount of it that you eat is just absurd.

—*Fred Pescatore*[5]

Study after study has shown that people with a normal level of cholesterol die from heart disease just as often as people with a high cholesterol, and that blood cholesterol level cannot predict a heart attack. At least 60% of the people who have heart attacks have normal levels of blood cholesterol.

—*Natasha Campbell-McBride*[6]

Dietary cholesterol is not the problem. . . . You don't induce heart disease by consuming dietary cholesterol.

—*Fred Kummerow*[7]

We might have gotten the story wrong on cholesterol for people of all ages, but particularly for older people, who are obviously the population most afflicted with cognitive impairment not resulting from physical trauma. Regarding cardiovascular health, among older people, high total cholesterol and even high LDL are not risk factors for increased all-cause mortality or death from coronary heart disease. As a matter of fact, some researchers suggest *low* cholesterol is more indicative of underlying health problems and is a stronger predictor of increased mortality risk than high cholesterol.[11] Study after study confirms that in older people high LDL cholesterol is associated with lower risk for all-cause mortality, leading researchers to say that it's time to reevaluate what we consider a "healthy" or "optimal" cholesterol level in the elderly.[12] Authors of a large data analysis that looked at cholesterol levels among people sixty years of age or older uncovered an inverse relationship between all-cause mortality and LDL cholesterol—meaning, the higher the LDL cholesterol, the *lower* the risk for mortality.[13] (Granted, the risk for mortality for all humans alive is 100 percent. We're all going to die sometime, from something. Stated simply, a reduction in risk for all-cause mortality means a lower chance of dying from any particular illness or chronic condition than from simply old age.)

Because it contradicts so strongly with what we've been led to believe about how dangerous cholesterol is, some researchers have written that the seemingly protective role of higher total cholesterol—as well as higher LDL—is a "paradox."[14] Let's dive a little more deeply into cholesterol, and we'll see that this is not a paradox at all but, in fact, makes perfect sense.

Cholesterol in Our Food Versus Cholesterol in Our Bodies

Dietary cholesterol—that is, the cholesterol we get from food—has very little effect on our *serum* cholesterol (the levels measured in our blood). It is not the case that when you eat foods that contain cholesterol, the cholesterol lodges itself in your arteries like when you pour bacon grease down the drain of your kitchen sink and it clogs up the pipes. The human body doesn't work this simplistically. When you eat broccoli, do you turn green? Of course not. That's not how the body works. So when you consume egg yolks or butter, the cholesterol doesn't automatically get stuck in your blood vessels. Please give your body—your complex, strong, fascinating, wondrous body—more credit than that.

The vast majority of the cholesterol inside us comes from inside us. We make it ourselves. Cholesterol is such an important substance for the human body that when we consume less cholesterol, our bodies make more, and when we consume more of it, our bodies make less. Ultimately, the amount of cholesterol in our bodies is the amount of cholesterol our bodies need at that particular point in time. And sometimes, such as when we are under a great deal of stress, have suffered a physical trauma, or are trying to restore healthy cognitive function, we might benefit from even more cholesterol in our diets, because during these times, our bodies have a very high demand for this nourishing substance, and we might not be able to produce enough of it to meet our needs. We can give our damaged bodies and brains a leg up by getting more cholesterol from our foods.

Since we know that cholesterol is one of the body's most important repair substances, instead of a knee-jerk reaction to lower cholesterol levels at all costs, we should be digging deeper and asking why cholesterol levels are high in the first place. What is causing cholesterol to build up in the blood? Why is someone's body, in its beautiful, innate wisdom, generating a large amount of cholesterol?

> The statement "even if you didn't eat any cholesterol, your liver would manufacture enough for your body's needs" has been made so frequently it is often believed. But in fact, there is evidence that for some people cholesterol is an absolute dietary essential because their own synthesis is not adequate. —*Mary Enig*[15]

Looking at it from another angle, why is the body not able to clear away the cholesterol it produces, such that it is building up to "high" levels in the blood? There are reasons we might produce "excessive" amounts of cholesterol, and there are reasons we might not dispose of it in a timely manner. This "elevated" cholesterol level is the result of whatever these underlying factors are. Therefore, we should stop targeting cholesterol itself and probe further to find out why the cholesterol level is elevated, and address *that*. Like so much of modern conventional medical care, prescribing statins and other cholesterol-reducing medication is treating a symptom, not the root cause. And when we only treat the symptom, the root cause continues unabated. (To use a helpful analogy, taking a statin drug to lower cholesterol is like putting electrical tape over the "check engine" light in your car. Just because you can't see the check engine light anymore doesn't mean you've actually fixed the problem. You've merely masked the sign that was alerting you to the fact that something was wrong. If anything, the problem is likely to get worse, because it's going to be ignored, rather than corrected. We could say the same thing about administering insulin to reduce blood sugar in people who have type 2 diabetes, most of whom are hyperinsulinemic or insulin resistant—meaning they already produce too much insulin. Giving insulin masks the symptom of elevated blood sugar but does nothing to address why the tissues are responding poorly to the insulin that's already there.) Jimmy Moore and Eric Westman said it well: "Conventional medicine immediately advises taking a statin drug to lower the cholesterol when it is higher than what is considered normal, but that ignores what has caused the cholesterol to go up in the first place."[16]

Cholesterol might be elevated for many reasons. When you have blood drawn for a cholesterol test, it's just one snapshot in time. It's the level of cholesterol in your blood at that moment. It could be significantly higher or lower the next day, the next week, the next month. Moreover, because it's such an essential structural component of all cells, cholesterol will be elevated when repair is happening to a greater extent than usual, such as after a physical trauma (accident, surgery), dental work, or during an acute illness or infection. As for cholesterol being elevated because of impaired clearance from the blood, low thyroid function is just one possible factor, as thyroid hormone is required for proper functioning of the LDL receptor.

Just because cholesterol is found in the plaques implicated in heart disease (atherosclerosis) doesn't mean cholesterol is *causing* atherosclerosis. This is guilt by association. Think of it this way: Just because we see firefighters every time there's a building on fire doesn't mean the firefighters are causing the fires. Just the opposite! They are there to stop the fire, right? The same is true of cholesterol. The fact is, there are many things that can damage the linings of arteries. Among the most common irritants to these blood vessels are high levels of blood glucose and insulin, and a high intake of unstable, easily oxidized polyunsaturated fats. (More on this in chapter 12.) So you can see that the modern American diet—rich in refined carbohydrates and unsaturated vegetable oils—provides huge amounts of arterial irritants, and it might be that elevated cholesterol levels are the body's way of protecting us. The body generates more cholesterol to repair the arterial damage inflicted by these harmful foods.

Recall that cell membranes are made of different types of fatty acids: saturated, monounsaturated, and polyunsaturated. When we consume too many polyunsaturated fats—as is very common in the modern American diet, which is high in soybean, corn, canola, and cottonseed oils—too much of this type of fat gets incorporated into the membranes, and the membranes don't work properly. In order to restore the correct shape and fluidity to the membranes, cholesterol gets incorporated as well. Cholesterol stabilizes these otherwise malformed membranes, so it might be that the body produces more cholesterol because more cholesterol is needed. According to the late Mary Enig, PhD, a prominent lipid researcher, "Cholesterol molecules give the proper amount of rigidity to the membranes. In other words, cholesterol helps a membrane keep its proper shape. . . . How much cholesterol a membrane has depends on how unsaturated the fatty acids of the phospholipids are; the more unsaturated they are, the more cholesterol is needed to provide the membrane with just the right amount of stiffness or flexibility."[17]

More research is coming out every day about how wrong we've been about the connections between cholesterol and heart disease. Think about it logically: The treasured, most commonly used fats of yesteryear—the fats our grandparents and great-grandparents used for cooking and eating— were largely the naturally occurring animal fats, which are rich in saturated fat and cholesterol: lard, beef and lamb tallow, butter, ghee, and schmaltz (chicken fat). And yet, heart disease was not a major medical epidemic until the mid- to late-1900s. So how is it that healthy, robust people were regularly consuming these fats but didn't suffer from heart disease at the rates we do today? The answer is that these types of fats do not cause heart disease. As British naval surgeon T. L. Cleave wisely noted, "For a modern disease to be related to an old-fashioned food is one of the most ludicrous things I ever heard in my life."[18]

What does contribute to heart disease—at least on some level—is the huge amount of vegetable oil we consume these days—oils that are only available in significant quantities thanks to mind-boggling feats of modern processing technology (more on this in chapter 12). These oils are especially damaging when combined with chronically high blood glucose levels induced by excess refined carbohydrate consumption.

Cholesterol Synthesis and the Consequences of Cholesterol Fearmongering

As if all that wasn't eye-opening enough, the decades-long fearmongering regarding cholesterol has had unintended—but devastating—consequences. Here are just two examples:

1. Fear of cholesterol has kept people from consuming cholesterol-rich foods that are also rich in choline. Choline is a nutrient that is required for production of acetylcholine, a neurotransmitter (brain chemical) involved in memory processing and learning. Alzheimer's patients have reduced levels of acetylcholine in the brain. Some of the best dietary sources of choline are egg yolks, liver, and shrimp—precisely the kinds of foods we have been cautioned against consuming due to their cholesterol content. On the contrary, egg yolks, liver, and cholesterol-rich shrimp should be considered superfoods for the brain. (Choline is present in some plant foods, but the richest sources are high-cholesterol animal foods.) Choline is also necessary for creating phosphatidylcholine and sphingomyelin, two compounds that are part of most cell membranes and widely needed in neurons. Moreover, liver and egg yolks are also high in vitamin B_{12}, which you'll recall is critical for healthy myelin. We couldn't have gotten our dietary recommendations more backward for brain health if we'd tried!

2. The metabolic pathway by which cholesterol is synthesized internally also creates a compound called *coenzyme Q_{10}* (CoQ_{10}). CoQ_{10} is an integral part of the process by which energy is created inside mitochondria. Moreover, CoQ_{10} is also a crucial antioxidant in the brain. Statin drugs target this pathway in order to block cholesterol production, but in so doing, they also block production of CoQ_{10}.

With that in mind, anything that interferes with the production of CoQ_{10}—such as certain cholesterol-lowering drugs—could have severe implications for healthy mitochondrial function and cellular energy generation. In reducing production of both cholesterol and CoQ_{10}, statin drugs are the worst kind of double-whammy for a brain that is struggling to protect itself and use fuel efficiently.

Figure 9.1 is a simplified look at the cholesterol synthesis pathway.

As you can see, even this condensed and simplified version is quite complex, and cholesterol isn't the only thing created along the way. In fact, it is only one of the very end products. Many other helpful compounds are made as well, including CoQ_{10}, and statin drugs reduce synthesis of all of them. This is because these drugs target a chemical reaction that occurs very high up in the pathway, thereby interfering with everything that comes later, not just cholesterol production. (You can see the point at which statins exert their effects, highlighted near the top of figure 9.1.)

> CoQ may function as an antioxidant, protecting membrane phospholipids and serum low-density lipoprotein from lipid peroxidation by quenching lipid radicals or lipid peroxidation initiating species and, it also protects mitochondrial membrane proteins and DNA from free radical-induced oxidative damage.
>
> —*Paula Moreira and colleagues*[19]

Toward the bottom of the image, you will see three things circled. The first is cholesterol, reinforcing the fact that cholesterol truly is at the end of a very long pathway that statins inhibit far upstream. The next is ubiquinones. Ubiquinone is another way of saying CoQ_{10}. And at the bottom right, you will see prenylated proteins. These are specialized proteins that have several functions in the body, among which are proper secretion of insulin from the pancreas and proper insulin-mediated glucose transport.[20] That is, they contribute to one of the biological mechanisms by which glucose is taken out of the bloodstream and brought into cells. This is why some statin drugs have been associated with an increased risk for type 2 diabetes.[21] Statins affect both insulin secretion and sensitivity, with one study showing as much as a 46 percent increased risk for developing diabetes among statin users compared to those not taking statins.[22] For two popular types of statins—simvastatin and atorvastatin—this effect is dose-dependent, which means the higher the dose of the drug, the greater the chance of developing diabetes. If these drugs interfere with proper insulin secretion, insulin sensitivity, and transport of glucose into cells, then it's perfectly logical that they're a risk factor for diabetes. Glucose will remain in the bloodstream for a longer period of time, ultimately

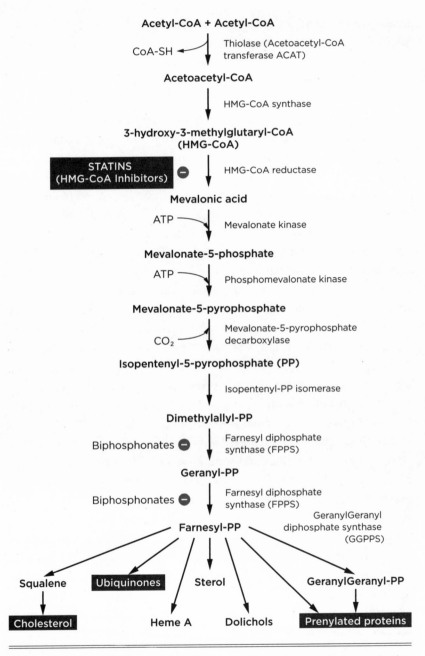

Figure 9.1 The biochemical pathway that produces cholesterol also produces an array of other important molecules. Note that statin drugs interfere with this pathway relatively early, thus inhibiting synthesis of all molecules that come later.

leading to the myriad downstream complications that result from blood sugar abnormalities—potentially including Alzheimer's disease. Moreover, according to Dominic D'Agostino, PhD, a researcher who specializes in the therapeutic applications of ketones, "The up-regulation of proinflammatory pathways associated with high blood sugar and insulin is going to be more detrimental to your cardiovascular health than elevated cholesterol."[23]

The interrelationships between statin drugs, disturbed blood glucose management, and cognitive impairment are well known. According to the Mayo Clinic, one of the most highly respected medical institutions in the United States, side effects of statin drugs include "increased blood sugar or type 2 diabetes" and neurological side effects, including confusion and memory loss.[24] (Moreover, the Mayo Clinic informs that individuals aged sixty-five or older are among the people at higher risk than the general population for experiencing side effects from statins. It's no coincidence that these older individuals are also at greater risk for dementia.) Now that you know the crucial roles of cholesterol in the body and especially the brain, these side effects should come as no surprise. The US Food and Drug Administration (FDA) has also acknowledged that statin users have reported "cognitive (brain-related) impairment, such as memory loss, forgetfulness and confusion" and "people being treated with statins may have an increased risk of raised blood sugar levels and the development of Type 2 diabetes."[25] Additionally, according to the FDA, "Memory loss and confusion have been reported with statin use. These reported events were generally not serious and went away once the drug was no longer being taken."[26] But how often do you think doctors advise patients to *stop* taking statins? If the medication is causing these effects (most likely due to a disruption in the synthesis of cholesterol and CoQ_{10}), then as long as someone is taking the medication, the memory loss and confusion will continue.

Knowing what we do about the role of insulin and glucose in the etiology of Alzheimer's disease, the critical need for sufficient cholesterol for healthy neuron structure and function, and the role of CoQ_{10} in cellular energy generation, statin drugs present a damning triple threat for cognitive function and the development and worsening of dementia.

The Dangers of Low Cholesterol

Now that you know some of the valuable things cholesterol does for us, let's look at just a handful of the health problems that can result from cholesterol levels that are too low. The following are all linked to low cholesterol—and are also well-documented side effects of statin drugs. (Though I hesitate to call them "side effects." They are not side effects. Because of the mechanism by which statin drugs inhibit internal cholesterol production, these are direct effects of the drugs. They aren't incidental, bystander-type effects but, rather, are unavoidable and obvious consequences of what happens when we deprive our bodies of something as essential and important as cholesterol.)

- **Depression:** Cholesterol is required for proper functioning of serotonin receptors. Serotonin is one of the "feel good" neurotransmitters that helps promote positive moods. Low serotonin has been linked to depression, "winter blues," and an overall negative outlook.
- **Fatigue, muscle pain, and weakness:** Recall that statin drugs block production of CoQ_{10}, the molecule that is part of the mitochondrial energy generators. The thing to note here is that CoQ_{10} isn't just required for energy production in neurons; it is required in almost every cell in the body! It doesn't take a PhD to hazard a guess as to what might happen if muscle cells can't generate energy. Fatigue, muscle pain, and muscle weakness are completely logical and utterly predictable consequences of CoQ_{10} depletion driven by statin drugs.
- **Hormonal imbalances and infertility:** Because cholesterol is the raw material from which testosterone, progesterone, and estrogen are produced, insufficient cholesterol can lead to hormonal problems and infertility in both women and men.
- **Loss of libido:** For the very clear reason stated above—we need cholesterol to synthesize the "sex hormones." Now you can see why so many older men—who have been advised for decades to decrease consumption of foods rich in cholesterol and are likely also taking statins—require pharmaceutical drugs to get or maintain an erection and boost their sex drive, which has been killed by a lack of cholesterol. (Sex drive can be affected in women, as well.)
- **Poor digestion of fats and fat-soluble nutrients:** Cholesterol is necessary to produce bile, which helps us break down fats in order to digest and absorb not only the energy in them, but also other compounds that are best absorbed along with fats. These include (among other things) fat-soluble vitamins (A, D, E, K) and

carotenoids, such as beta-carotene—the orange/yellow pigment in carrots, sweet potatoes, and other similarly colored foods. (So put butter on your sweet potato! Or drizzle olive oil on your roasted carrots! Nutrients in these foods are absorbed better when they're eaten with fat.) Long-term poor digestion and malabsorption of these nutrients can lead to a number of health problems. The old adage "you are what you eat" doesn't tell the whole story. You're not what you eat, but rather, what you digest and absorb.

- **Memory loss and poor cognitive function:** It should be obvious by now that any disruption in cholesterol or CoQ_{10} synthesis will have dire consequences for cognitive function, to say nothing of the role of statins in inducing blood sugar abnormalities and problems with insulin signaling. The brain cannot work without cholesterol and CoQ_{10}. Let me say that again: The brain cannot work without cholesterol and CoQ_{10}.

According to Dr. Bredesen, whose MEND program (metabolic enhancement for neurodegeneration) has led to reversals of MCI and AD:

> *People will come in and they're trying to drive their LDLs so low. We see this all the time, where you have some [brain] atrophy and it's associated with having a very low cholesterol. Why? Because you're on a statin. . . . You're preventing your cells from doing the thing that's actually appropriate, so you end up with a brain that has shrunken without the appropriate lipid content. To explain to people that this is actually not good for your brain is not easy.*[27]

I cannot and do not suggest that you discontinue taking any medication on your own, but I give you my strongest urging to speak with your doctor and begin exploring that option if you are taking a statin to reduce cholesterol and are experiencing memory loss, brain fog, or other disturbing changes to your cognition or behavior.

The low-carbohydrate diet advocated in this book will go a long way toward aiding healthy brain function, but progress and improvement will very likely be hindered if cholesterol synthesis is being reduced inside the body. If your doctor is unconvinced, you are well within your rights, as a proactive patient engaged in your own health or that of your loved one, to arrive at your appointment armed with information to share that will affirm your new viewpoint. (If your doctor is uncooperative and unwilling to even consider this different viewpoint to help you on your journey to better health, you are also well within your rights to find a new doctor! See the note at the end of this chapter for finding a physician who will be more open-minded and receptive to a conversation about cholesterol and statin drugs.)

Cholesterol Primer: What Is Cholesterol, Anyway?

Because the dietary strategy recommended in this book is one in which you will be intentionally consuming more cholesterol, I'll go out on a limb and assume you're concerned about the effects of this on your blood cholesterol or that of your loved one. Therefore, it will be helpful for you to have a very basic understanding of some of the terminology you've probably heard associated with blood tests for cholesterol levels.

There is no such thing as "good" or "bad" cholesterol. There is only cholesterol. Cholesterol is a fatty substance—it's not water-soluble, which means it can't travel through the watery bloodstream on its own. In order to travel through the bloodstream, cholesterol is placed inside transport vehicles. To return to an earlier analogy, think of it like shipping containers loaded onto cargo ships: We can't put shipping containers directly onto the ocean; they have to travel on ships. Cholesterol works the same way, and the "ships," or transport vehicles, it travels in are called lipoproteins.

There are several different types of lipoproteins, but the two you are likely most familiar with are high-density lipoproteins (HDL) and low-density lipoproteins (LDL). You might have heard HDL referred to as "good cholesterol," and LDL referred to as "bad cholesterol." But remember: There is no good or bad cholesterol; there is only cholesterol. The reason LDL is considered "bad" is that, in general, it transports cholesterol from the liver (where it is manufactured) and delivers it to the rest of the body. And the reason HDL is considered "good" is that, in general, HDL takes cholesterol away from other tissues and brings it back to the liver for recycling or removal. But when you think about all the wonderful life- and health-supporting things cholesterol does for us, it seems like we should be calling LDL the "good cholesterol," doesn't it? After all, the LDL particles are helping to deliver nourishing cholesterol to places that need it. So why, then, are total cholesterol and LDL cholesterol so often used as markers for risk for cardiovascular disease? Sometimes these are the *only* things doctors look at when evaluating a patient's heart health, as if there were nothing more to the picture.

Considering that part of what makes up your total cholesterol is HDL (something "good,"), then looking at total cholesterol as a marker for heart disease is foolish. After all, the higher your "good cholesterol," the higher your total cholesterol.

> If you're still looking at LDL as the "bad" cholesterol, then you're about thirty years out of date.   —*Ken Sikaris*[28]
>
> The least accurate way of estimating your atherogenic risk on a standard cholesterol panel would be to look at total cholesterol or LDL cholesterol.   —*Thomas Dayspring*[29]

Blood tests for cholesterol have come a long way during the last several years. If your doctor is only testing for total cholesterol, HDL, LDL, and triglycerides, she is way behind the times.

It's not that these numbers are meaningless, but they are such a small part of the total picture, and this very limited look at things could be giving you misleading information about your heart disease risk and overall health.

Beyond those very basic numbers, two things you can now have measured are your lipoprotein particle number and your particle size. (For the sake of providing you with just enough information to give you a basic understanding of this without overwhelming you with technical jargon and minutia, I am simplifying matters here. For more detailed information, consider accessing some of the recommended resources provided in the back of this book.)

There are two main types of LDL particles: what are known as "small, dense" LDL (sometimes called "pattern B") and what are known as "large, fluffy" or "buoyant" LDL (called "pattern A"). The small, dense particles tend to accumulate in the artery walls more than the large, fluffy ones. Atherosclerotic plaques form behind the lining of the artery, not actually in the lumen of the artery itself (see figure 9.2). Generally, cholesterol is sent there when there's a tear or some other damage to the arterial lining. (Remember, cholesterol is a repair substance.) The smaller particles slide more easily behind tears in the lining than do the large ones, so "pattern B" lipoproteins are hypothesized to be more atherogenic than pattern A.

Aside from particle size, measuring your particle *number* can also be helpful, because even though it is the small, dense particles that tend to influence heart disease risk more strongly than the large, buoyant ones, it can also be a "numbers game." That is, even if you have mostly the large, fluffy LDL particles that tend to be more benign, if you have too many of them, they can still cause trouble. (Typical cholesterol tests measure the amount of cholesterol inside the particles, not the number of particles themselves. To return to the cargo ship analogy, they measure the amount of cargo being carried in a ship, rather than the number of ships. And when it comes to heart disease risk, the number of ships [particles] can sometimes be a more accurate indicator than the amount of cargo [cholesterol] inside them.)

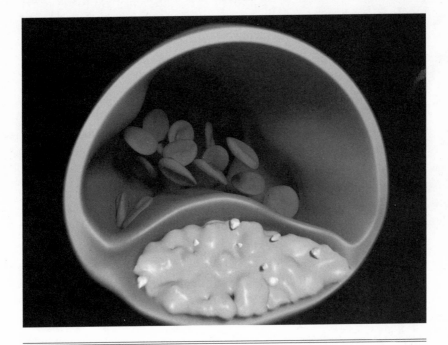

Figure 9.2 Atherosclerotic plaques form between the wall of the artery and the inside, or "lumen," of the artery, not in the middle of the artery itself, like grease in a kitchen pipe. Cholesterol, calcium, and other substances are drawn behind torn or damaged artery walls in order to strengthen and reinforce the tissue. They are there in response to damage, often from elevated blood glucose and insulin. Cholesterol in the artery wall is the result of arterial injury, not the cause. Image by iStock.com/selvanegra.

Beyond that, it's not usually just any lipoproteins that get stuck behind the artery wall, causing the narrowing that eventually leads to reduced blood flow and oxygen (and associated chest pain, shortness of breath, and, in the worst case, heart attack). It is usually oxidized lipoprotein particles that cause trouble. And as we'll explore when we cover dietary fats in chapter 12, high consumption of polyunsaturated fats can cause chain reactions of oxidation in the body. One thing that gets oxidized very easily (remember the free radical pinballs moving around, crashing into everything?) is lipoproteins. So a diet high in vegetable and seed oils can lead to atherosclerosis, regardless of total cholesterol levels.

Your total cholesterol level says nothing about the degree of atherosclerotic plaque in your blood vessels. And by the way, heart disease and heart attacks do not happen exclusively to people who have high cholesterol. Any cardiologist can tell you that plenty of patients with "normal" and even low cholesterol levels suffer from heart disease and cardiovascular disease.

Aside from the number, size, and degree of oxidation of the lipoprotein particles—the ships—something else that contributes to heart disease risk and cardiovascular complications is the condition of the blood vessels themselves—the ocean. Think of it like this: If you have an old, damaged, rickety, leaky boat, it's going to get into trouble even if the ocean is calm and the weather's clear, right? And on the other side: If you have a high-tech, modern boat in perfect condition with lots of safety features, it can still get into trouble if it's out on the ocean in the middle of a hurricane, with choppy seas, huge waves, and 100+-mile-per-hour winds.

I will paraphrase an excellent explanation of this from Mr. Ash Simmonds, a long-time low-carber who has put together a fabulous collection of published scientific literature related to ketogenic diets and health (including cholesterol).[30] As a takeoff on the previous example of a ship out on a stormy sea, this one involves cars on city roads. It will provide a helpful image for you to think about the issues of cholesterol particle number and the condition of the vasculature (arteries and other blood vessels).

If the roads in your city are narrow, torn up, poorly maintained, full of potholes, and badly signed, with bad traffic flow and unskilled or distracted drivers, then the number of cars on these roads is a huge issue. Nevertheless, even under such poor road conditions, things can flow somewhat smoothly if there's only a small number of cars. In this scenario, when the inevitable collisions occur, ambulances, police, and firemen can get through and attend to the damage without much issue. But on those same poorly maintained roads, if there are too many cars, there will be more crashes and subsequent pileups, and the emergency services either won't be able to get there in time to help, or they'll become part of the pileup themselves. (In other words, if the blood vessels are damaged and fragile, a small number of cholesterol particles might not be harmful, but a larger number might get you into trouble.)

Next, imagine a nice, wide, smoothly paved freeway that's well maintained and has good signage to direct traffic. Sure, the occasional accident will happen, but when it does, emergency services can get there quickly and easily, and they'll have plenty of room to deal with the situation. In this case, the total number of cars on the road doesn't matter much. (If the overall state of your vasculature is healthy, with very low levels of inflammation and oxidative stress, it is less likely that you will develop atherosclerosis, regardless of lipoprotein particle number.)

Please note: I am not saying there is no such thing as "too high" when it comes to either particle number or cholesterol content inside those particles. I am saying only that we cannot determine heart disease risk or risk for a coronary or ischemic event (for example, heart attack, stroke) by cholesterol numbers alone. They are simply one of a number of other factors that, taken together, present a more telling picture of the state of your cardiovascular health and total body health.

The science on this is continually evolving, but recent research now seriously questions the role of a "high" total cholesterol and a high LDL cholesterol in adverse health outcomes, especially in older people.[31] Thomas Dayspring, MD, one of the foremost lipidologists in the United States, has said that the majority of myocardial infarctions (heart attacks) are explained by insulin resistance, and that LDL cholesterol does not alarm him unless it's over 200 mg/dL—and that is *just* LDL, meaning *total* cholesterol could be well over that and still not be problematic.[32] Considering the sometimes debilitating side effects of statin drugs— including impaired cognition—I have to agree with Jimmy Moore and Eric Westman, who said of using statin drugs to lower cholesterol: "Calling this the single biggest blunder in the history of medicine is not overstating the case."[33]

Other Ways to Assess Cardiovascular Health and Heart Disease Risk

Cholesterol panels do offer useful information, provided they are comprehensive. Total cholesterol, HDL, and LDL are only a fraction of the full story. Consult your physician to inquire about advanced testing that measures many more parameters besides these very basic indicators. Other than lipoprotein number and particle size, there are other markers that can give useful insight into your overall cardiometabolic health.

I think it's reasonable to ask if we should be putting people through routine cholesterol screening at all. The preferred marker right now is LDL cholesterol. But levels of this are not a very reliable marker for heart disease, and most people who have heart attacks have normal or low levels of LDL cholesterol.

—*John Briffa*[34]

A helpful marker to keep an eye on is triglycerides. Triglycerides are often lumped in together with cholesterol on standard blood tests, but they are not the same thing as cholesterol. Triglycerides are fats—three fatty acids joined together to a molecule of glycerol. But even though they're fats, triglycerides measured in your blood provide more insight about your *carbohydrate* intake than your fat intake. High triglycerides are a marker for carbohydrate intolerance. If you have elevated triglycerides, you are better served by reducing your carbohydrate intake rather than your fat or cholesterol intake. Reducing all carbohydrates might be beneficial, but elevated triglycerides can sometimes be a marker for high fructose intake, specifically, from too much refined sugar, high-fructose corn syrup, or even from consuming very large amounts of fruit or fruit juice.

When we consume more carbohydrates than our bodies can immediately use or store in our liver and muscle glycogen reserves (which are limited and max out fairly quickly), the liver converts them into triglycerides (fats) for storage in our fat tissue. Yes, you read that correctly: Excess carbohydrates can be converted into fats. In fact, one of the quickest and most dramatic "side effects" of a low-carb diet is that elevated triglycerides decrease to healthier levels.

According to some of the top cardiologists in the United States, one of the best predictors for heart disease risk is your ratio of triglycerides to HDL. In general, the lower your triglycerides and the higher your HDL, then the lower your risk of heart disease. There's really no magic number, but if your HDL is higher than your triglycerides, this is a good thing. (Notice that this has nothing to do with your total cholesterol or LDL levels.) An ideal triglyceride-to-HDL ratio is 2 or below, though some researchers cite below 3.5 as satisfactory.

Other markers to pay attention to are C-reactive protein (CRP) or high-sensitivity C-reactive protein (hs-CRP), and homocysteine. These are markers for inflammation, and inflamed, damaged blood vessels are a greater harbinger for cardiovascular problems than elevated cholesterol. And of course, you'll want to have your hemoglobin A1c tested regularly, along with fasting blood glucose and insulin. Optimal ranges for these are provided in chapter 24.

Finally, two of the most useful tests for cardiovascular disease risk do not involve cholesterol at all, but rather, provide much more direct evidence of detrimental changes to blood vessels. The first is the carotid intima-media thickness test (CIMT). The CIMT is used to diagnose the extent of vascular disease in the carotid artery. It measures the thickness of the inner layers of the carotid artery and can show existing damage and disease well before symptoms arise. The second test is a coronary artery calcium scan (CAC). Even better than the CIMT, this is a direct visual image of vascular damage, this time in the coronary arteries. It allows physicians to measure the extent of calcification in the arteries surrounding the heart, and it's a far more reliable predictor of risk for heart attacks and other cardiovascular events than anything to do with cholesterol.

Cholesterol levels are only markers. They are surrogate indicators, and they do not, by themselves, predict cardiovascular disease risk. Markers are

> And how best to improve your triglyceride/HDL ratio? The striking reductions in plasma triglycerides and consistent increases in HDL-C in response to low carbohydrate diets are unparalleled by any other lifestyle intervention, or even drug treatment, and therefore represents the most powerful method to improve this ratio.
>
> —*Jeff Volek and Stephen Phinney*[35]

just that: markers. They are not diseases, in and of themselves. They are proxies that might or might not indicate a disease state. In contrast, the CIMT shows the amount of arterial thickening that has already occurred and might be a much better predictor for future cardiovascular events. (However, this is a measurement of the carotid artery, and the findings might not be indicative of the condition of the coronary arteries surrounding the heart.) The CAC is even more telling, as it shows the extent of atherosclerotic plaque that is actually currently present in the coronary arteries—and remember, the amount of cholesterol in your blood tells you nothing about the degree of this plaque deposition. Why rely on surrogate indicators that give you almost no actionable information when you can have the condition of your coronary arteries assessed directly?

If you're interested in learning more about cholesterol, heart disease, and unraveling some of the myths you have likely long believed, there are several excellent layperson-friendly books on the topic. You can find them in the recommended resources at the back of this book.

If you would like to find a physician who might be receptive to a conversation about protecting cardiovascular health through methods other than statin drugs, you can check the following websites, which list medical professionals who are familiar with low-carb and ketogenic diets. You might be able to find one in your local area

- http://paleophysiciansnetwork.com
- http://lowcarbdoctors.blogspot.com
- https://re-findhealth.com

CHAPTER 10

Carbohydrates: Starchy, Nonstarchy, and Not as "Complex" as You Think

When we think of carbohydrates, we tend to think exclusively of starchy foods, such as bread, pasta, rice, bagels, and potatoes. But, as I have mentioned, there is a world of other nutritious foods that are not starchy but are nonetheless classified as carbohydrates.

As explained earlier, there are three main macronutrients in the food supply: protein, fat, and carbohydrate. Think about foods like broccoli, spinach, blackberries, and eggplant. They're certainly not fats, and they don't seem like proteins, either. The only category left is carbohydrate, and that's exactly what these are. That's right: Lettuce is a carbohydrate! Cucumbers are carbohydrates! They just happen to not be starchy ones. These nonstarchy vegetables are high in water and fiber, and you can eat plenty of them while following this dietary strategy. Remember, this is a *low*-carb diet, not a *no*-carb diet. While limiting your carbohydrate intake from starchy foods, you may eat liberal amounts of the following, depending on your individual level of carbohydrate sensitivity:

- Alliums (includes onions, garlic, shallots, scallions, leeks, chives)
- Artichokes
- Asparagus
- Bell peppers— all colors (and all other peppers; for example, jalapeño, poblano, ancho)
- Bok choy*
- Broccoli* (also broccoli rabe, aka rapini)
- Brussels sprouts*
- Cabbage*—all varieties (napa,

savoy, green, red,   turnip greens,   to choose 100
radicchio, endive)   beet greens)   percent pumpkin,
- Carrots   - Jicama   not pie mix,
- Cauliflower*   - Kale—all varieties* which contains
- Celery   - Lettuce—all types   added sugar)
- Swiss chard   (romaine, arugula, - Radishes—
  (all colors)   iceberg, red leaf,   all varieties
- Cucumber   green leaf, Bibb,   - Snow peas
- Eggplant   spring mix)   - Spinach
  (all varieties)   - Mushrooms—   - Tomatoes—
- Fennel   all varieties   all colors and
- Green beans   - Okra   varieties
  (haricots verts)   - Pumpkin   - Turnips
- Greens (collards,   (if you use canned - Yellow squash
  dandelion, mustard,   pumpkin, be sure   - Zucchini

*Denotes a cruciferous vegetable. Raw cruciferous vegetables are hard to digest, and high intakes of raw cruciferous vegetables might interfere with healthy thyroid function. Do not consume large amounts of these raw. They are wonderful, highly nutritious foods. Just make sure to eat them cooked.

What about Fruit?

Fruit is delicious and nutritious. Remember, however, that it is "nature's candy." It is one of the sweetest naturally occurring foods we have easy access to, and because it's so tasty and sweet, fruit is very easy to overeat. You do not have to eliminate fruit from your diet entirely, provided that you are able to control your portions and stick to fruits that have a lower glycemic load. (Although you may safely avoid fruit altogether if you choose to do so. There are no nutrients present in fruit that you cannot obtain from other foods.)

Fruits to avoid

- Dried fruit (for example, raisins, prunes, dried cranberries, apricots)—these are very concentrated sources of sugar because the water has been removed
- Bananas and plantains (higher in sugar and starch, respectively)
- Grapes, apples, pears
- Tropical fruits (mango, papaya, pineapple, guava)

Carbohydrates to Limit or Eliminate Altogether

Starchy vegetables and legumes*

- Beans—all types (black beans, kidney beans, lentils, garbanzos [chickpeas], navy beans, pinto beans, lima beans, black-eyed peas)
- Beets
- Parsnips
- Peas
- Rutabaga
- Taro
- White potatoes, sweet potatoes, yams
- Winter squash (acorn, butternut, turban)
- Yucca

Grains and pseudograins*

- Amaranth
- Barley
- Buckwheat
- Corn
- Couscous
- Millet
- Oats
- Quinoa
- Rice—all varieties
- Rye
- Spelt
- Wheat— includes spelt, kamut, emmer, einkorn

*This also includes anything made from the beans and grains above: bread, bagels, cereal, oatmeal, granola, pasta, tabbouleh, rice cakes, crackers, rice pilaf, pita bread and pita chips, corn or wheat flour wraps and tortillas, pretzels, cakes, cookies, muffins, piecrusts, scones, pizza, refried beans, and so on. In time, there are some of you who might be able to add small amounts of these foods back into your diet as you gauge your carbohydrate sensitivity, but at the beginning, in order to allow the body to transition to being fueled by fat—and to generate ketones to fuel the brain—they are best avoided entirely.

Acceptable fruits

- Berries (raspberries, blueberries, blackberries, strawberries, unsweetened cranberries)—berries are the lowest glycemic fruits and have a relatively higher fiber and phytonutrient content compared to other fruits.

- Citrus fruits—consume these in their whole forms, not as juice: orange, tangerine, grapefruit, lemons, limes. (Small amounts of fresh-squeezed lemon or lime juice are permitted as condiments or added to beverages.)
- Small amounts of stone fruits (peaches, nectarines, plums, cherries), kiwi, and melon.

If you're asking yourself if you'll be missing out on important vitamins and minerals by cutting out starchy foods, fruit, and "healthy whole grains," the answer is an emphatic *no*. According to Dr. Keith Runyan, a physician who has type 1 diabetes and has followed a very low-carbohydrate diet in order to manage his diabetes:

> *The most common criticisms I have heard of the ketogenic diet, none of which have any basis in science, include the question, "Aren't you missing important nutrients by excluding or severely limiting 'healthy whole grains' and fruit?" My response is that all the nutrients found in grains and fruit can be obtained from meat, poultry, fish, eggs, non-starchy vegetables, nuts, and seeds, while avoiding the carbohydrates and gluten that accompany grain and fruit.[1]*

Avoiding Sugar: Be a Label Detective

Sugar goes by a multitude of names. Manufacturers use different names in order to disguise just how much of it is actually in their products. Now that you or your loved one will be avoiding sugar as much as possible, you will need to read labels carefully in order to identify sugar masquerading under its less incriminating nicknames. Be vigilant. Don't let clever marketing derail your progress.

Here is a list of sugars and other sweeteners that should be avoided. Note that this is just a sampling of the most common ones you'll see on food labels. Sugar goes by even more names than this. When in doubt about an ingredient, avoid it.

• Agave nectar	• Beet sugar	• Brown rice syrup
• Agave syrup	• Blackstrap molasses	• Brown sugar

- Cane sugar
- Coconut sugar
- Corn syrup
- Corn syrup solids
- Date sugar
- Dextrose
- Evaporated
  cane juice

- Fructose
- Glucose
- Glucose syrup
- Golden syrup
- High-fructose
  corn syrup
- High-maltose
  corn syrup

- Honey
- Invert sugar
- Maltose
- Maple syrup
- Molasses
- Palm sugar
- Sucrose
- Sugar

These sugars are best avoided as much as possible. However, some of the packaged foods that can help you or your loved one stick to a low-carb diet might contain small amounts of sugar, honey, and other sweetening agents. For example, bottled ranch and blue cheese salad dressings typically list sugar among the ingredients. However, the amount of sugar in a 2-tablespoon serving is typically just 1–2 grams. The same goes for deli meats. In cases like this, the presence of sugar (or corn syrup, or any other type of sugar) in the ingredient list on a packaged food is not necessarily a deal breaker. Very small amounts are acceptable if they fit within your total daily carbohydrate allowance; don't miss the forest for the trees and allow worry over the minutia to get in the way of implementing the most important tenets.

Counting Carbs and Net Carbs

Adopting this type of diet in a world where we're surrounded by inexpensive carb-laden junk food is difficult enough. I recommend beginning the diet without stressing out too much over the exact amount of carbohydrate you or your loved one are eating. For the most part, eating only those carbohydrate foods that are acceptable and completely avoiding the ones that are not will go a long way toward facilitating the shift in your body away from a glucose-centric metabolism and toward one fueled more by fats and ketones. However, if you find that you or your loved one are not consistently staying in ketosis or noticing improved cognition, it might be wise to track your intake for a while to see if you are inadvertently consuming more carbohydrate than you realize.

There are carb-counting books to help you get some idea of the carbohydrate content of the foods you eat, and there are also many good carb charts online, as well as resources for tracking food. If you find an online chart you like, consider printing out multiple copies—one to keep in the kitchen, perhaps, and others to keep in your purse, briefcase, or the glove box of your car, so you'll always have one handy when shopping for food, dining out, or preparing meals. The Ketogenic Diet Resource website, created by nutritionist Ellen Davis, provides charts that present this information for most of the foods that are allowable on this brain-boosting low-carb diet. (They are available at www.ketogenic-diet-resource.com/carb-counter.html.) These are very handy to refer to as needed if you are unfamiliar with a ballpark carbohydrate content for the foods you consume most frequently. You might also consider purchasing a food scale in order to keep track of portion sizes. These are inexpensive and can be found online or at most department stores and home goods stores.

The term "net carbs" is used to refer to the total carbohydrate content of a food minus its fiber content and sometimes also minus the sugar alcohol content. Because the fiber portion of food is not digested and absorbed, it is not likely to impact blood glucose and insulin. For this reason, many people who follow low-carb diets find that when computing their daily carbohydrate intake, they can subtract the fiber. That is, they can count the net carbs, rather than the total carbs. When you consume fibrous vegetables, nuts, and seeds, in effect this "buys you more carbs." You can consume a larger amount of foods that are high in fiber and still low in carbohydrate—for example, more spinach, kale, almonds, brussels sprouts, and sunflower seeds. Please note this does not mean that you can consume whole-grain products, bran cereals, granola bars, or the like, no matter how many claims the packages have about "high fiber." Counting net carbs means that you have a little more leeway with your food intake when you stick to foods that are high in fiber and also low in carbohydrate.

Sugar alcohols are a slightly different story. These are most commonly found in sugar-free or low-carb candies and chocolates. They can affect blood glucose and insulin responses, but the degree to which this happens varies from person to person. If you choose to consume foods that contain sugar alcohols, you will have to monitor your own results and see if they are suitable for you. (See chapter 14 for details on sugar alcohols and artificial sweeteners.)

It's up to you whether to count total carbs or net carbs. If you start out counting net carbs but find that you are not noticing any improvement in your or your loved one's cognitive function, consider switching to total carbs, as maybe you were simply consuming too many and you need to be stricter with your diet.

The biggest pitfall with counting net carbs is that it allows some people to feel justified in consuming what is essentially low-carb junk food. There are many bars, shakes, sugar-free chocolates, and other low-carb candies that have a low-carb designation only because they are loaded with sugar alcohols and fiber. Some people's bodies are more sensitive to these ingredients than others', and some people will experience spikes in blood sugar and insulin from consuming them.

Now that you've seen the wide variety of delicious, nonstarchy vegetables and low glycemic fruits you can enjoy on this plan, I hope the idea of avoiding grains, sugars, and starchy carbohydrates is less intimidating than you might have thought. In addition to carbohydrate, two other sources of calories fit into this nutritional strategy for supporting brain health and cognitive function. We'll focus on protein in the next chapter and then move on to fat.

CHAPTER 11

Protein: Primary Player in Our Bodies and on Our Plates

I n health and nutrition news for the lay public, fats and carbohydrates garner the lion's share of attention. The second half of the twentieth century saw a nearly across-the-board demonization of all fats, and then a shifting of the focus specifically to saturated fats. In the new millennium, the pendulum has begun to swing toward carbohydrates, with a menacing finger now pointing toward highly refined and processed sugars and grains. The macronutrient that seems to fly under the radar is protein. This is a shame, because adequate protein is critical for good health, and the general public is largely unaware of and greatly underappreciates the numerous beneficial roles of protein.

When you hear the word *protein*, you probably think first of muscle tissue. It's true that muscles are made predominantly of protein, but protein is also what makes up hair, skin, nails, blood vessels, tendons, ligaments, and even bones—they're not just calcium! The antibodies the immune system uses to fight off infectious disease and invading pathogens are also made from protein, as are many hormones, such as insulin, glucagon, human growth hormone, and others. As if all that weren't enough, amino acids (which come from protein foods) are also the building blocks for other hormones and some of the neurotransmitters we require for balanced moods, a positive mental outlook, and a healthy response to stress, such as thyroxine and triiodothyronine (T4 and T3 thyroid hormones, respectively), dopamine, serotonin, and epinephrine. And in case you're still not convinced of the crucial functions of protein-derived molecules in the body, the enzymes that control the myriad biochemical reactions happening inside us at all times are proteins. The digestive enzymes that break down the food we eat, the enzymes that facilitate the exchange of carbon dioxide and oxygen in the lungs, the enzymes that convert glucose to ATP—they're all proteins. In fact, the word protein is derived from the Greek *protos* ("first") or *prōteios* ("primary"), which underscores its fundamental importance for all living things, including humans.

The nutritional strategy presented in this book is not a high-protein diet. While it is possible that you will be consuming more protein than you're accustomed to, that doesn't make it a "high-protein" diet. It might be relatively higher in protein than the way you or your loved one were eating before, but you do not need to go out of your way to gorge on protein. (If anything, the macronutrient that is the main focus of this diet is fat.)

If you're interested in health news, it's possible you've come across headlines suggesting that a higher protein diet is harmful for the kidneys. It's true that individuals who already have compromised kidney function might need to limit their protein intake, but there is no evidence that increasing protein consumption would lead to kidney problems in otherwise healthy people, and it might even have benefits for cardiometabolic health.[1] Moreover, many researchers believe that current US government recommendations for protein intake might not be adequate to meet the needs of older individuals.[2]

Another concern regarding a relatively higher protein intake is the acid load it presents to the body. Upon digestion, all foods present the body with either an acid or an alkaline residue. Meats (including seafood and poultry), dairy products, cereal grains, and some refined sugars present an acid load; fats and oils are mostly neutral; vegetables and fruits present an alkaline residue.[3] It was long believed that a higher dietary acid load was harmful for bone health because calcium (an alkalizing mineral) would be leached from the bones in order to buffer the acidity. Many studies have proven this to be an incorrect interpretation of previous scientific literature. In fact, a higher protein intake might be *helpful* for bone strength, particularly in older individuals, who are the ones who might be most in need of this dietary shift in the first place.[4] Moreover, low protein intake is a risk factor for reduced bone density and increased rates of bone loss.[5]

Above all, bear in mind that, according to the Food and Nutrition Board of the US National Academy of Sciences Institute of Medicine, the acceptable range for protein intake as a percentage of total calories for adults is 10–35 percent.[6] You might remember from chapter 8 that none of the recommended macronutrient ratios call for protein to exceed 35 percent, so whichever proportions you choose to start this plan with, you will not have a "high" protein intake.

It is important, however, to consume adequate protein on a low-carb diet. You don't have to eat "a lot" of protein, but you do need enough. Remember: You need to eat enough protein to supply your muscles, organs, and other tissues with raw materials for repair, regeneration, and overall healthy function, not to mention for making hormones, enzymes, and immune system antibodies. It is especially important for older people not to skimp on protein. Our bodies naturally lose muscle mass as we age, but having active muscle tissue—and using it—is one of the most effective ways to maintain insulin sensitivity. So we want to hold on to as much muscle as we can. This would be true at any time, but it is especially true for an older person trying to regain insulin sensitivity and restore healthy cognitive function.

Fine-tuning with regard to protein consumption comes in when we consider the possibility of consuming excessive protein. Protein stimulates insulin secretion (which will decrease ketone levels), although not to the same degree as carbohydrate. For this reason, on very strict ketogenic diets, protein is typically restricted as well as carbs, which is why those diets might be upward of 75 percent to 80 percent fat.

So how much is "enough" protein, but not too much? It's virtually impossible to provide an exact answer. The recommended daily allowance (RDA) in the United States for protein is 0.36 gram of protein per pound of your body weight (or 0.8 gram of protein per kilogram of your body weight). This is the bare minimum; you should aim to consume at least this much, and many people will benefit from consuming more. Studies indicate that older people who consume less than approximately 0.5 gram of protein per pound of body weight [1 gram per kilogram] have an increased risk for physical frailty, and increasing protein intake in older people might help reduce frailty.[7]

Therefore, you do not want to drop below this amount unless you are significantly overweight. (In this case, aim for a protein intake closer to that which would be suitable for what would be considered a healthier body weight for your height.) Protein is extremely important for a multitude of functions in the body, and older people tend to consume too little of it.

The majority of calories on this low-carbohydrate diet should come from fat, but don't worry about overconsuming protein. Protein is very satiating and somewhat self-limiting. It is difficult to gorge on or overeat protein; your body will tell you when you've had enough. You'd almost have to force yourself to consume more than is suitable in one sitting. You will be fine going over 0.36 gram per pound (or 0.8 g/kg). Remember, this should be considered a minimum. If no noticeable improvement in cognition has occurred after a while of strictly implementing this low-carbohydrate strategy, consider testing for ketones. Some people's bodies will have a higher insulin response to protein than others', and protein might need to be reduced in those cases.

One thing to note is that 0.36 or 0.8 gram is grams of *protein*, not grams of food by weight. For example, a large egg that weighs approximately 40–50 grams on a food scale (a little over an ounce) contains just 6 or 7 grams of protein. A chicken breast that weighs 100 grams (approximately 3.5 ounces) contains 31 grams of protein. (You can find the protein content of commonly consumed protein sources at www.ketogenic-diet-resource .com/low-carb-food-list.html.)

Proteins That Are Good to Consume

Ideally, the animal proteins you consume will come exclusively from cattle, hogs, chickens, sheep, and other animals that are raised on pasture or are supplemented with feed rations that are biologically appropriate for them, as well as from seafood that is wild-caught. If these highest quality foods are not realistically within your budget, do the best you can. You are trying to restore healthy cognitive function and undo years of metabolic damage driven in large part by detrimental aspects of the modern diet. Isn't this worth spending a bit more on groceries? (See chapter 16 for a primer on food quality.)

The following sources of protein are suitable—all cuts and varieties, including steaks, chops, roasts, ground meat, and sausages. There is no need to purchase lean meat only. Animal fat is encouraged in this dietary strategy, and you should not at all shy away from fatty cuts of meat. The fat is especially encouraged if you purchase meat produced from grass-fed or pastured animals.

- Beef
- Bison/buffalo
- Cold cuts/
  lunch meat*
- Cottage cheese—full
  fat (usually labeled
  as 4 percent fat in
  the United States)
- Eggs—with the yolks
- Lamb/mutton
- Organ meat/offal—
  liver, heart, tripe,

tongue, kidneys,
plus liverwurst,
knockwurst, pâté
- Pork—including
  sausage and
  bacon—yes, you
  are allowed to eat
  bacon on this plan!
- Poultry—chicken,
  turkey, duck, and
  other fowl—no need
  to buy skinless!

- Seafood—all
  varieties of finfish
  and shellfish
  (canned tuna,
  salmon, sardines,
  and mackerel are
  excellent budget-
  friendly choices)
- Veal
- Venison, elk,
  rabbit, and other
  game meats

*Regarding cold cuts and processed meats: Bacon, sausage, and lunchmeat (cold cuts) are acceptable, but pay attention to the ingredients. These are often cured with sugar, brown sugar, or dextrose. This is fine as long as the carb count is 2–3 grams or less per serving. (Even though the meats are cured with sugar, the amount that ends up in the finished product is usually small.) Owing to potentially questionable additives and preservatives, cold cuts should not be staples of your diet, but small amounts are okay. They're convenient and familiar, but compared to other cuts of meat, they're not especially cost-effective or nutritious.

Read labels, especially on anything packaged or processed. Check for hidden carbohydrates among the ingredients, like wheat flour, sugar, corn-starch, corn syrup, and dextrose.

Regarding protein powders and shakes: For individuals who have trouble consuming an adequate amount of protein in the form of whole foods (such as older individuals who have trouble chewing or digesting meat), protein powders such as whey, pea, rice, or hemp, are acceptable as long as the carbohydrate content is low. A 30-gram serving should contain no more than 3 grams of carbohydrate, and there are some available that are as low as 1–2 grams per serving. Smoothies can be made with protein powder and coconut milk or unsweetened nut milk and MCT oil, for a ketone boost. (See chapter 21 for tips on supporting digestive function.)

Proteins to avoid

- **Prepared or packaged meat products that contain significant amounts of carbohydrate.** These include meatballs, meat loaves, stews, pot roasts, and protein-based entrées that use fillers, binders, or flavor and texture enhancers that contain wheat flour, breadcrumbs, cornstarch, corn syrup, sugar, and the like. (A carbohydrate count of 2–3 grams or less per serving is okay, but watch your portions so you don't inadvertently consume more carbohydrate than you realize.)
- **Breaded meats**, such as chicken nuggets, chicken tenders, or anything that comes in a starchy wrap, such as meat-based burritos, tortillas, and tacos, and anything deep-fried and coated in flour-based batter, such as tempura, deep-fried fish, or chicken wings. Meats that are grilled or roasted (no breading) are acceptable.
- **Beans** are a source of protein, but they contain far more carbo-hydrate than protein and therefore are best avoided. (Look at the labels on canned beans and bags of dried beans. You will see that they're relatively high in protein for plant foods, but they are even higher in carbs.) This doesn't mean beans are bad for health or that they are not nutritious. It simply means that they're not appropriate for a diet specifically designed to limit carbohydrates. This includes all beans and products made from them: black beans, kidney beans, lentils, chickpeas (garbanzos), soybeans, navy beans, hummus, falafel, refried beans, and baked beans. Depending on your individual level of carbohydrate tolerance, small amounts of beans might be acceptable. I recommend avoiding them for the first several weeks while your body adjusts to running primarily on fats and ketones, and then perhaps introducing small amounts of them later on. (A small amount of hummus, made with tahini and olive oil, is a nice treat that is high in healthy fats, and no pita chips are necessary; you can enjoy hummus with a crudité of raw vegetables, or use pork rinds to mimic the crunchy texture of chips.)
- **Soy.** Do not consume imitation meat products made from soy. Soy is one of the most common food allergens, and many people don't even realize they're sensitive to it. Soy is difficult to digest, and heavy consumption can lead to bloating, gas, diarrhea, upset stomach, and other unpleasant signs of digestive distress. Small amounts of traditionally prepared soy (fermented) are permissible,

but the highly refined and isolated soy protein products that are used to create things like "soy chicken" and "soy cheese" are not the same as the small amounts of traditionally prepared soy that are recognized as promoting health among Asian cultures. Do not consume soy protein shakes or soy milk, as high amounts of soy might interfere with healthy thyroid function.

Red and Processed Meats: Not the Dietary Devils They're Made Out to Be

As if it wasn't hard enough to wrap your head around the need to avoid what you're accustomed to hearing are "healthy whole grains," now a nutritionist is telling you that it's A-OK to eat red meat, and even processed meats like bacon, sausage, ham, and salami. What is the world coming to?!

I realize this might be quite a paradigm shift for you, so let's lay to rest your fears about consuming some of the foods you've been cautioned to avoid for most, if not all, of your life. If you eschew beef or pork for religious or cultural reasons, you may continue to do so. These foods are not required in order to follow a low-carb diet; I am simply setting the record straight for individuals who would like to partake of and enjoy these foods but have been avoiding them because they believe they're detrimental for health. They're not. Let's see why.

Many people have banished red meat and pork from their diet because of . . . wait for it . . . "artery-clogging saturated fat." The first thing to learn is that while beef and pork do contain saturated fat, the predominant fat in pork is monounsaturated (with a moderate amount of saturated and a small amount of polyunsaturated), and beef contains almost equal amounts of monounsaturated and saturated fat. In fact, the specific type of mono-unsaturated fatty acid that makes up the largest component of pork fat is oleic acid, the very same one believed to be responsible for the supposed health benefits of olive oil. (So the next time you hear the phrase "heart-healthy olive oil," think *heart-healthy lard!*) Dairy products are far higher in saturated fat than beef, pork, and lamb are, and the most highly saturated fats we typically consume don't come from animals at all but from tropical plants, such as coconut and palm oils.

Beef and pork are both highly nutritious. Not only are they wonderful sources of protein, but they're loaded with vitamins and minerals, too.

Table 11.1. Nutrient Content of Select Animal Protein Foods

Nutrient	Rib eye steak (beef)	Pork tenderloin	Beef liver	Lamb heart
Vitamin A	0%	0%	522%	0%
Thiamin (B₁)	4%	63%	12%	11%
Riboflavin (B₂)	7%	23%	201%	70%
Niacin (B₃)	36%	37%	87%	22%
Pantothenic Acid (B₅)	5%	10%	69%	14%
B₆	26%	37%	51%	15%
B₁₂	29%	9%	1,386%	187%
Folate	2%	0%	65%	0%
Iron	10%	6%	34%	31%
Zinc	32%	16%	35%	25%
Phosphorus	20%	27%	48%	25%
Copper	4%	6%	730%	30%
Potassium	9%	12%	10%	5%
Selenium	41%	54%	47%	67%

Source: Condé Nast, *SELF Nutrition Data*, accessed August 1, 2016, http://nutritiondata.self.com.
Note: Percentages are the daily values (% DV) for adults or children aged four or older, based on a 2,000-calorie-per-day reference diet.

When we hear that phrase—"vitamins and minerals"—we tend to automatically and exclusively think of vegetables and fruits. But the truth is, ounce for ounce, animal foods pack a nutritional punch that's difficult for plant foods to match. Table 11.1 shows the approximate percentages of select nutrients in approximately 3.5 ounces (100 grams) of various forms of red meat, pork, and organ meat. And keep in mind that 3.5 ounces is a relatively small portion of protein, so the amount you would typically consume in one sitting would provide higher amounts of nutrients than you see in the table (except maybe for liver. As you can see, liver is one of nature's most potent multivitamins, but unless you're a big fan of the flavor, it's not easy to consume a large amount of it at once).

It is time to put an end to the demonization of red meat and pork, which is based more in political expediency than in sound science. Pork, beef, lamb, and other red meats and game meats are extremely nutrient-dense foods that have nourished healthy and robust populations for centuries.[8] Also, the effects of consuming larger amounts of red meat—or any animal protein, for that matter—might be quite different in the context of a low-carbohydrate intake from the effects that are coupled with a high-carbohydrate intake and other aspects of the modern diet.[9] It's also possible that data indicating detrimental effects from consuming red meat are confounded by the fatty acid composition of the meat—that is, meat from animals that are fed high amounts of grains in the modern feedlot system has a different fatty acid profile than meat from animals that are fed the biologically appropriate diets for which they're adapted, such as cattle on grass pastures, and wild game meats in their natural habitat.[10] Meat from wild game animals (elk, moose, venison) and grass-finished ruminants have proportionally less saturated fat and more mono- and polyunsaturated fat (including the important omega-3 fats we'll talk about later). However, even this issue is unlikely to be responsible for the associations between red meat and poor health outcomes. It is far more likely that research using epidemiological data from large population groups is not able to completely separate intake of red meat from intake of sugar, refined grains, and isolated vegetable and seed oils. The impact of eating meat in the absence of these other factors could be a world apart from the impact of eating meat in their presence. All of this being said, if you are still wary of consuming meats that are higher in fat, lean meats are associated with beneficial effects on cardiovascular health, body weight, and other areas of concern.[11] And, of course, you are not required to eat these items. Should you prefer to continue avoiding them, you can construct a perfectly wonderful low-carbohydrate diet without red meat, pork, and processed meats, focusing instead on seafood, poultry, dairy products, and other meat sources, such as goat or wild game. But the bottom line is, protein is so important for overall health and wellness that you should not feel guilty or ashamed if the only meat you can afford is what's available at your local grocery store.

As for processed meats, much of the research regarding the possible negative influences on health from consuming processed meats is confounded by concurrent carbohydrate intake. That is, the majority of processed meats are consumed along with starch or sugar. Think about it: We eat bologna on sandwich bread, hot dogs on buns, bacon served alongside pancakes or toast and orange juice. As low-carb researcher Richard Feinman, PhD, wrote, "Basic biochemistry suggests that a roast beef sandwich may have a different effect than roast beef in a lettuce wrap," and "red meat on a sandwich may be different from red meat on a bed of cauliflower puree."[12] It is difficult to tease out the effects of consuming processed meats in the absence of starch and sugar. One thing's for sure: the healthy and long-lived Greeks, Italians, and Spaniards in the Mediterranean weren't consuming low-fat lamb sausages, or fat-free prosciutto and chorizo.

For readers who say, "But I'm a vegetarian! Is it essential to consume animal proteins on this plan?" we'll answer this question in detail in chapter 20, when we address implementing a low-carb diet for vegetarians and vegans.

CHAPTER 12

Fat Is Not a Four Letter Word! The Critical Importance of Fat in the Body

As you know by now, the low-carbohydrate nutritional strategy outlined in this book requires a much higher intake of dietary fat than you are likely used to consuming. More importantly, you also know by now that this is a higher fat intake than you are accustomed to hearing is "safe" or "healthy" according to many respected health organizations and perhaps even your own doctors. Therefore, it is crucial that you develop a new understanding of the role of fats in the human body. After establishing an appreciation for the critical importance of fats for good health, we will go into detail regarding which types of fats to emphasize in this brain-boosting diet, which ones to minimize consumption of, and which ones to avoid as much as possible.

The first thing we must do in order to gain an appreciation for the myriad benefits of fats is divorce ourselves from the automatic connotation we have of fats being "bad," "dangerous," or "unhealthy." In fact, even though dietary fat and stored body fat are the same things in terms of their chemical structure, in order to separate the knee-jerk association we have between fat in our foods and the excess accumulation of body fat on our hips, thighs, and bellies (called *adipose tissue*), let's use the term *fatty acids* when referring to the very helpful things fats do for us.

Functions of Fatty Acids in the Body

Just as we saw with cholesterol, fats have been demonized, vilified, and accused of all sorts of crimes against good health. But the truth is, fat is a vital structural component of the human body, not to mention the myriad other critical roles fats fulfill in physical, mental, and cognitive health. Here's a sampling of just a few of the important things fatty acids do for us:

- Serve as rich sources of energy—better than carbohydrates (carbohydrates provide only 4 calories of energy per gram; fats provide 9 calories of energy per gram)
- Facilitate the absorption of fat-soluble vitamins and nutrients (including vitamins A, D, E, K, and the carotenoids, such as lutein, lycopene, and beta-carotene)
- Serve as essential building blocks for the structure of cell membranes and plasma membranes
- Provide insulation and protective linings for the organs of the body (for example, lung surfactant is rich in saturated fat)
- Serve as structural components of myelin, the protective sheath that surrounds nerve cells and facilitates effective neuronal communication
- Serve as building blocks for molecules involved in a healthy inflammatory response—both inflammation and the resolution of inflammation (prostaglandins, leukotrienes, thromboxanes)
- Are required for healthy liver and gallbladder function, including production and appropriate secretion of bile, which emulsifies fats and aids in digestion
- Help slow the digestion and absorption of food, contributing to an appropriate postprandial (after-meal) hormonal response—particularly when taken in a mixed meal containing carbohydrates (the presence of fat in a meal tends to reduce the glycemic response in the body, which helps to moderate blood sugar and insulin levels)
- Contribute to soft, supple skin
- Last, but not least: Make food taste delicious! Who doesn't prefer their vegetables with a pat of butter melted on top? Think you don't like brussels sprouts? That's probably because you've never had them roasted with olive oil or bacon fat!

As you can see, fatty acids bring a lot to the table—no pun intended. We cannot be healthy without fat in our diets. Let me say that again: We cannot be healthy without fat in our diets. However, it's not enough just to consume any ol' fats. We have to pay attention to the *types* of fats we consume. Just as it's important to eat a variety of animal and vegetable foods because they provide different vitamins, minerals, and other nutrients, it's important to consume different types of fat, because they contribute to different processes in the body. In addition, there are specific fatty acids that have very important physiological functions, and if we don't get enough of them, those functions will be compromised.

Too much of certain fatty acids and not enough of others can lead to imbalances that contribute to chronic pain, fatigue, premenstrual syndrome, dry skin, acne, premature aging, and conditions involving chronic inflammation. We will explore additional special types of fat in the next chapter, but before we do that, we've got to set the record straight about dietary fat as a whole.

The Facts about Different Types of Fat

Fat is the most important ammunition in the nutritional arsenal against Alzheimer's disease and cognitive impairment. Fat is the key nutrient on this diet, and it will make up the largest source of calories. You read that correctly: Fat is a nutrient, and a very important one at that. The dietary strategy presented in this book is one that is powered by fat. Remember: Because the goal is to transition the body and brain to fuels other than glucose, we need to provide the body and brain with those other fuels, and they come in the forms of fat and the ketones that result from the metabolism of fat.

Conventional medicine and the mainstream media are both slowly—very slowly—coming around to the idea that dietary fat has been wrongfully vilified for several decades. Since the 1960s, we have been advised to follow diets low in fat—saturated fat, in particular—and to emphasize carbohydrates in our diet. The current epidemics of obesity, type 2 diabetes, heart disease, metabolic syndrome—and Alzheimer's disease—in the industrialized world can be laid directly at the feet of these misguided, scientifically unsound, and unproven recommendations.

According to Robb Wolf, an authority on Paleolithic nutrition and ancestral health:

> The assumption that fat makes people fat and causes heart disease makes sense, but that does not make it true. . . . High-carb pundits keep pedaling this failed approach. . . . We have over fifty years of failed governmental policy to keep track of and millions of lives lost in the process.[1]

Mainstream nutritionists, dietitians, and medical practitioners now recognize that fat is an essential part of a healthy diet. However, they remain behind the times when it comes to the types of fat they think are beneficial. Despite mounting scientific evidence to the contrary, they continue to insist that saturated fats—especially those that come from animal sources, such as butter and lard—are responsible for heart disease, obesity, and a host of other modern chronic illnesses. They recommend that we limit our intake of animal fats and instead use vegetable oils, such as soybean, corn, canola, and cottonseed oils. It is encouraging that the tide is turning and all fat across the board is no longer seen as dietary public enemy number one. However, it is disheartening that only the "politically correct" sources of fat—such as avocado, olive oil, salmon, and walnuts—have been vindicated, while animal fats and highly saturated plant fats—such as tallow and coconut oil—continue to be demonized.

In order to set the record straight about this extremely important topic and to give you the courage to implement a diet that is high in the very foods you have been cautioned against for much of your life, we are going to have to get slightly technical. If you are going to proceed with confidence in this dietary strategy, it is important that you understand just a little bit about the science of fats and oils, and the

> The vilification of saturated fat by the health and medical communities is one of the biggest scams that has ever been perpetrated on the American public.
>
> —*Jimmy Moore and Eric Westman*[2]

crucial role of fats in the human body. (The word *lipid* is a fancy way to say *fat*. The word *fat* usually refers to lipids that are solid at room temperature, such as butter and bacon fat, while *oil* usually refers to lipids that are liquid at room temperature, like canola and corn oil. I will use the word *fat* to encompass both fats and oils but will differentiate when necessary.)

Let's take a good look at the facts about fats. This will help you to make informed choices at the grocery store, in restaurants, and in your own kitchen. I promise, this will be much easier than your high school chemistry class!

Types of Fats

There are three types of fatty acids:

1. Saturated
2. Monounsaturated
3. Polyunsaturated

Fatty acids are long chains of carbon atoms strung together, with hydrogen atoms attached to them. (As a very simplified visual, picture a string of Christmas lights.) The differences between the three types of fatty acids have to do with their molecular structure: Saturated fats have no double bonds between their carbon atoms, monounsaturated fats have one double bond somewhere along the chain ("mono" meaning *one*), and polyunsaturated fats have two or more double bonds ("poly" meaning *many*). This is important because the number of double bonds a fatty acid has affects how that fatty acid responds to heat, light, and air and how it interacts with other substances inside our bodies.

The presence of double bonds is what makes a fatty acid susceptible to oxidation upon exposure to heat, light, or air. With regard to fats, when you hear "oxidation," think *rancidity*. If you've ever had a container of nuts sit around too long and it developed a horrible, offensive odor and flavor, that's rancidity, and it is a sign that the fragile polyunsaturated fats in the nuts have become oxidized and are no longer safe to eat. You can also think of oxidation as detailed in chapter 5—recall the free radical pinballs that crash into structures inside the mitochondria as well as outside the cells, stealing electrons and creating oxidative damage. Among the things free radicals oxidize are the fatty acids that make up our cell membranes—specifically, they oxidize the unsaturated fatty acids. (The more double bonds a fatty acid has, the more fragile it is, and the more susceptible to damage via oxidation.) Remember, fatty acids aren't just things that occur in our foods; they are structural components of our bodies, too.

Because they have no double bonds, saturated fats are the most stable. They undergo little to no oxidation.[3] Therefore,

There is simply no sound science behind the prevention message that reducing saturated fat in your diet will lower your risk of heart disease.   —*Cassie Bjork*[4]

they are the safest fats to use for cooking, where they are exposed to all three of the potentially oxidizing elements: heat, light, and air.

Monounsaturated fats have just one double bond, so they are okay to use for medium-heat cooking but should not be used with very high heat. (The most common monounsaturated fat you are familiar with is olive oil. Avocados, macadamia nuts, and other nuts and seeds are also high in monounsaturated fat, but remember, lard—rendered pork fat—is high in monounsaturated fat, too! That's right: Lard, the fat we are accustomed to hearing in lockstep with the phrase "artery-clogging saturated fat," is predominantly monounsaturated.)

Polyunsaturated fats have multiple double bonds—multiple points that are susceptible to damage by oxidation. For this reason, they are the most chemically unstable and the least suitable for high-heat cooking—or, really, for any cooking. The supposedly "heart-healthy" polyunsaturated vegetable oils we have been advised to cook with (such as corn and soybean oil, rather than the safe, stable saturated fats) are actually the worst things to use for cooking.

The Murky Manufacturing of Vegetable Oils

Now that we know it's predominantly the saturated and monounsaturated fats that we want to use for most cooking applications, let's go one step further and explore what is involved in the manufacturing of isolated and refined vegetable oils, to truly understand that not only do we want to avoid cooking with them but also that they're not safe for consumption in large amounts, even when they're not heated.

Let's start off with a thought experiment regarding fats and oils.

Here's the challenge: Name the five fattiest foods you can think of. Really, take the time to think of them. Very fatty foods—at least five of them.

Did corn make your list?

No?

How about soybeans?

Also no?

I'm not surprised. See, corn and soybeans are not especially fatty, are they? If someone were to ask me to name the fattiest foods I could think of, I would probably include lard, beef tallow, and ghee. But that's cheating. Those are pure fats. No protein and no carbohydrate. So let's say I had to name five whole foods that are very high in fat. I'd go with bacon, cheese, bone marrow, chitterlings, and macadamia nuts.

Of course corn and soy aren't high in fat. Corn is a grain and soy is a legume—two plant categories not generally regarded for their high fat content. And the one thing all the different nutritional camps seem to agree on—whether it's low carb, low fat, Paleo, vegan, vegetarian, or based on standard government nutrition advice—is that we should eat fewer processed foods. So if corn and soy are not high in fat, take a moment to consider how much processing is required in order to produce edible oils from them. How do they get seemingly endless gallons of clear, odorless oil from sources that don't contain all that much fat to begin with?

The answer is, it takes a lot of processing and refining. The oils are extracted from the grains, legumes, or seeds using mechanical and chemical means, such as pressing, crushing, grinding, and hexane solvents. They must then be filtered, bleached, and deodorized in order to neutralize or remove offensive flavors and odors. Much of the nutritional content that might have been present in the whole food source or even the initial cold-pressed oil is long gone by the time the eye-, nose-, and palate-pleasing oil is bottled and stocked on store shelves. And remember, these oils—corn, soybean, cottonseed, safflower, grapeseed—are highly polyunsaturated. They have already been subjected to temperatures and pressures that damage and oxidize them during the extraction and refining process, and then they are typically bottled in clear plastic containers and exposed to harsh light in grocery stores, twenty-four hours a day in some cases. And to put the final nail in the coffin of any nutritional value or health benefit that might have somehow still remained in these oils, we subject them to high temperatures yet again when we put them in our frying pans. Due to the long-standing demonization of animal fats, these vegetable oils are also the ones typically used in fast-food restaurant deep fryers, where they remain at high temperatures for many hours. Fried foods are not inherently bad for health; the problem is the type of oil they're fried in.

Another point to consider is the phrase "vegetable oil." If we classify all plant foods as vegetables, then, yes, soybeans and corn could be considered "vegetables." Nutritionally speaking, however, soybeans are legumes, and corn is a grain. Neither likely comes to mind when you hear the word "vegetable." You more likely think first of green things, like spinach, broccoli, asparagus, or brussels sprouts. A second after that, you might think of some of the brightly colored vegetables: eggplant, red bell peppers, carrots, beets, tomatoes, and so on. But soybeans? Probably not.

Now that you know that "vegetable oil" is industry-speak for the fat they somehow wrench out of corn, cottonseeds, and soybeans, start reading labels on foods at the store. You'll find these oils everywhere: salad dressings, margarines and other "vegetable oil spreads," nondairy creamers, bread, peanut butter (except for the "natural" varieties that contain only peanuts and salt), crackers, microwave entrées, cookies, cakes, biscuits, and just about everything else that comes in a box, bag, bottle, or tub. Mayonnaise is a good example—even the ones that say they're made with olive oil are still predominantly soybean oil. Manufacturers add a tiny bit of olive oil to the formula so they can give it a health halo and announce proudly in large letters on the label that it's "MADE WITH OLIVE OIL," while sweeping under the rug the fact that it's mostly soy. Another edible oil of questionable origin is cottonseed oil. Cotton is for wearing, not for eating!

More Fat Facts:
Animal, Vegetable, Saturated, Unsaturated

Now that we have learned about the incredible feats of mechanization and manufacturing required to produce the vegetable oils that are supposedly "heart healthy," we know that, based on their chemical structure, it is actually the saturated and monounsaturated fats that we want to use for most of our cooking and eating. So let's get an idea of how some common fats and oils break down in terms of their composition (see table 12.1). All fats and oils consist of combinations of saturated, monounsaturated, and polyunsaturated fatty acids. There are no fats—either from plants or animals—that are entirely saturated or entirely unsaturated.

Building upon what we learned in the previous section, we have a new understanding of "good fats" and "bad fats." This understanding is based on clear-cut biochemistry and human physiology. Facts about how these fatty acids respond to exposure to heat, light, and air during processing, bottling, and storage lead us to very different conclusions from what we're accustomed to hearing on the news or reading in health magazines.

As you can see, the nutritional therapy strategy suggested in this book recommends nearly the opposite of what we've been told to consume for several decades. The fats I emphasize for restoration of health and cognitive function are the saturated fats and monounsaturated fats, and I caution

Table 12.1. Fatty Acid Composition of Select Fats and Oils

Type of fat or oil*	% Saturated	% Monounsaturated	% Polyunsaturated
Coconut oil	91	6	3
Butter	66	30	4
Lamb tallow	58	38	2
Palm oil	49	40	10
Beef Tallow	49–54	42–48	3–4
Lard	44	45	11
Duck fat	35	50	14
Chicken fat (schmaltz)	31	49	20
Cottonseed oil	29	18	52
Peanut oil	16	56	26
Olive oil	15	73	10
Soybean oil	15	22	62
Sesame oil	15	41	43
Corn oil	14	27	59
Sunflower oil	13	18	69
Grapeseed oil	11	16	73
Safflower oil	9	11	80
Flaxseed oil	9	17	74
High oleic sunflower oil	9	81	8
Canola oil	7	65	28

Source: Mary Enig, *Know Your Fats*.
* The fatty acid composition of animal fats will differ slightly, based on the animals' feed (for example, grass versus grains).

against cooking with the supposedly "heart-healthy" vegetable oils that make up the bulk of the dietary fats most Americans consume today.

The preceding recommendations are specific to cooking. But what about oils you might use for cold applications, such as homemade dressings, marinades, and finishing garnishes? The following oils—cold pressed and unrefined—are safe to use for those purposes:

- Almond oil
- Avocado oil
- Extra-virgin olive oil
- Flaxseed oil
- Hazelnut oil
- Macadamia oil
- Pumpkin seed oil
- Sesame oil
- Walnut oil

Be sure to store these oils in airtight containers (preferably glass, metal, or dark/opaque plastic), in a cool, dark place, away from heat, light, and air. Do not store them on the counter, on top of the fridge, or near the stove.

We need to rid ourselves of any residual fear that fat intake is somehow bad, causes us to get fat, or causes heart disease. Enjoy the fat on your T-bone steak or coconut oil used to sauté your vegetables. . . . I find it astounding that many of my immediate physician and cardiologist colleagues cling to the outdated belief that total and/or saturated fat intake are somehow related to heart disease risk. Reassessment of the data used to justify such arguments, as well as more recent clinical studies, demonstrates that total and saturated fat intake have nothing to do with heart disease risk.

—*William Davis*[5]

What about Consuming Foods That Contain These Polyunsaturated Fats?

Polyunsaturated fats can be a healthful thing to include in a brain-boosting diet. We do not need to avoid them altogether, and there's no need to fear consuming them in their whole-food form—that is, as they occur naturally in foods, with their full complement of antioxidants and other synergistic nutrients. As explained earlier, the otherwise healthful fatty acids these foods contain can be rendered harmful by the high temperatures and pressures used when they are turned into isolated oils via extraction, refining, and processing. Consumed in their natural state, however, they are a nice addition to the diet and bring with them helpful vitamins, minerals, and fiber.

Here's a list of whole foods naturally high in mono- and polyunsaturated fats that are recommended on a low-carb diet:

- Almond butter (no added sugar)
- Almonds
- Avocados
- Brazil nuts
- Cashews (go easy; slightly higher in carbs)
- Flaxseeds (should be freshly ground before use)
- Hazelnuts (also called filberts)
- Macadamia nuts (mostly monounsaturated)
- Olives (mostly monounsaturated)
- Peanuts (go easy; higher in carbs)
- Pecans
- Pistachios (slightly higher in carbs)
- Poultry
- Pumpkin seeds (pepitas)
- Seafood (finfish and shellfish)
- Sesame seeds or tahini (sesame seed paste)
- Sunflower seeds
- Walnuts

The Old Way of Thinking about Fat

Good Fats

- Mono- and polyunsaturated fats
- "Heart healthy"
- From nuts, fish, avocado
- "Politically correct" vegetable oils

Avocado
Canola oil
Corn oil
Margarine
Olive oil
Safflower oil
Salmon
Soybean oil
Walnuts

Bad Fats

- Saturated fats
- "Artery clogging"
- From animals— especially red meat
- From some tropical plants

Bacon fat
Beef tallow
Butter and ghee
Cheese
Chicken skin
Coconut oil
Duck fat and chicken fat (schmaltz)
Heavy cream
Lard
Palm and palm kernel oils

It is not necessary (or, really, even possible) to completely avoid refined polyunsaturated vegetable oils. They are everywhere. Don't drive yourself crazy trying to eliminate them from your diet altogether. If you want to attempt that, that's fine, but a little bit of these oils will not hold back progress, and they will not interfere with the transition to a metabolism based on fats and ketones.

Your intake of these oils will naturally decrease by virtue of cooking more of your own foods from scratch, from whole, unprocessed ingredients. The majority of our intake of these oils comes in the form of manufactured foods, like crackers, cookies, cakes, premade sauces, condiments, microwave dinners, nondairy creamers, and the like. Because you will no longer

The New Way of Thinking about Fat

Best Choices for Cooking

- Mostly saturated or monoun-saturated fats and oils
- Animal fats from grass-fed or pastured animals
- Dark bottles, stored away from heat and light
- Organic when possible

Avocado oil
Bacon fat
Beef or lamb tallow
Butter (low-medium heat)
Coconut oil
Duck and chicken fat
Ghee
Lard
Olive oil
Palm oil
Peanut oil (occasionally)
Sesame oil (occasionally)

Worst Choices for Cooking

- Polyunsaturated oils
- Partially hydrogenated oils (trans fats)
- Margarine and shortening
- Transparent, clear plastic bottles

Corn oil
Cottonseed oil
Flaxseed oil (fine for cold uses)
Grapeseed oil
Safflower oil
Soybean oil
Sunflower oil (small amounts of high-oleic sunflower oil are okay)

be eating most of these items, your polyunsaturated oil consumption will be reduced by default. And of course, you will be eating real butter, instead of margarine and other "buttery spreads" that are typically made from corn, soy, and cottonseed oils. (You should avoid even the tub spreads that claim they have no trans fats or are labeled as "heart healthy." Do not consume these. Use real butter!)

The other main sources of these oils in the modern diet are salad dressings, mayonnaise, and bottled sauces (not to mention they're usually loaded with sugar and often gluten or other thickening agents). The simplest way to avoid consuming too many of these oils from these products is to make your own. (You can use olive oil or cold-pressed nut oils for vinaigrettes, or use cream, sour cream, or full-fat yogurt as the base for creamy dressings. See chapter 15 for details on condiments that are appropriate for this dietary strategy.) If you do not want to put forth the modest effort to make your own condiments, that's all right. If your main intake of isolated polyunsaturated oils comes from salad dressing and mayonnaise and not manufactured foods high in carbohydrates, that's okay, and it will not likely compromise your progress. However, I still must caution against using soybean or corn oil for any application involving heat. Do not purchase bottles of vegetable oil for cooking. Olive oil is fine, but when you see "vegetable oil" on the label, it is invariably from soy or corn.

Pick your battles: We are looking to limit total consumption of these polyunsaturated oils (except as they occur naturally in the whole foods listed earlier), so it is better to have a small amount from condiments than to use those oils for cooking in addition to getting them from dressings and sauces. Again, try not to let yourself become a victim of "paralysis by analysis" and allow overstressing about the details to stand in the way of taking the more important steps, such as greatly reducing carbohydrate intake.

Trans Fats—Steer Clear!

In addition to limiting intake of isolated and refined polyunsaturated oils, there are other types of fat that are best avoided entirely. These are trans fats, and avoiding them is one of the few issues the disparate nutritional philosophical camps agree on.

Trans fats are created when unsaturated fatty acids are chemically manipulated to make them act more like natural saturated fats. The process is called *hydrogenation*, and you can recognize the presence of trans fats in a food product by the words "partially hydrogenated" in association with a vegetable oil in the list of ingredients—for example, partially hydrogenated soybean oil in crackers, or partially hydrogenated rapeseed (canola) oil in peanut butter. (Partially hydrogenated oils are responsible for the "waxy" feel that coats your mouth when you eat peanut butter, margarine, cake frosting, crackers, cookie cream fillings, and other foods that contain them.) The rise of these man-made fats in the food supply paralleled the demonization of saturated fats, because one of the things hydrogenation does is make vegetable oils—which are normally liquid at room temperature—into solids or semisolids. The main purpose of this is to increase the shelf life of the products that contain these oils, as well as to improve their texture and mouthfeel. Because they provide similar tactile properties to saturated fats (which are naturally solid at room temperature), using trans fats allowed food manufacturers to replicate the taste and feel of saturated fats in their products while proudly advertising that they were made with vegetable oils. This was a boon for food manufacturers, particularly in the United States, where corn and soybeans are both heavily subsidized crops, making corn and soybean oils very inexpensive ingredients to include in manufactured foods. A boon for the food companies' bottom line, but a total bust for human health. Consumption of trans fats is associated with a host of poor health outcomes—particularly, adverse effects on the cardiovascular system.[6] There are multiple mechanisms by which trans fats exert their detrimental effects, but one of them is that they might be incorporated structurally into cell membranes.[7] Recall from our exploration of cell membranes that in order for cellular functions to be carried out properly, their membranes have to be constructed of the right materials. Moreover, animal studies indicate that high consumption of trans fats reduces levels of DHA (docosahexaenoic acid) in the brain.[8] DHA is an omega-3 fatty acid that plays an important structural role in the brain. (We'll go into detail on omega-3 fats in the next chapter.)

Industrially produced trans fats are relatively easy to avoid if the vast majority of your food comes from whole, unprocessed ingredients that you prepare and cook at home. Through eliminating packaged convenience foods and refined carbohydrates, your consumption of trans fats will decrease dramatically without any deliberate effort on your part. However, you must still be vigilant when grocery shopping. Labeling laws in the United States allow foods that contain less than 0.5 gram of trans fat per serving to claim zero grams on the nutrition facts label. The key phrase here is *per serving*. Some of these foods will have serving sizes that are unrealistically small for the sole reason of enabling the manufacturers to claim that their foods contain zero grams of trans fat. So don't automatically trust the numbers on the label; always read the ingredient list, and if you see the words *partially hydrogenated*, do not debate, do not think twice, do not hesitate. Put it back.

At the risk of complicating matters, however, I should add that not all trans fats are harmful. There are the industrial trans fats created through the hydrogenation process, but there are also trans fats that occur naturally in the meat and dairy products from ruminant animals, such as cows, sheep, goats, and deer. (In fact, the scientific name for one of these special fatty acids—*rumenic acid*—pays homage to its biological source, the rumen.) These natural trans fats have a slightly different chemical structure from the industrially produced trans fats, and this slight difference leads the natural fats to have profoundly different effects in the body. In stark contrast to the man-made trans fats, the ruminant trans fats have been shown to confer health benefits, rather than harm.[9] The research is mixed, however, with some of the more promising effects of the natural trans fats being more pronounced in animals than in humans.[10] This might be due to the fact that clinical experiments typically employ these fats in supplement form, rather than as they occur in their intact food source, such as beef tallow or butter from grass-fed and finished cattle and dairy cows. (The concentration of these potentially beneficial fats is higher in grass-finished animals than those who are fed grain. Grain-fed animals produce some natural trans fats, but the amounts are higher in animals whose rations are predominantly grass.[11]) There are likely synergies between the naturally occurring trans fats and other nutrients present in the whole food that are unable to be replicated in a laboratory or factory that manufactures supplements.

You do not need to go out of your way to seek out these naturally occurring trans fats. The takeaway here is that you don't need to go out of your way to avoid them, either. If you come across a health publication decrying the dangers of trans fats, it's important for you to understand the difference between the man-made and naturally occurring varieties so that you are not scared away from consuming some of the foods that can generously nourish the brain.

Saturated Fat—Delicious, Not Deadly!

As I mentioned earlier, mainstream nutrition and dietetics have made it so that the words *saturated fat* rarely appear without being preceded by the phrase "artery-clogging." Owing to over half a century of fearmongering regarding the consumption of this type of fat, these four words have practically merged into one: *arterycloggingsaturatedfat*. We could say the same thing about "whole grains" and "heart-healthy"—*hearthealthywholegrains*. Both are misguided.

Anyone who's lost a significant amount of body fat by following a low-carbohydrate, high-fat diet can confirm that fat in our foods doesn't automatically become fat on our bellies, hips, thighs, and backsides.

> There is no significant evidence for concluding that dietary saturated fat is associated with an increased risk of CHD [coronary heart disease] or CVD [cardiovascular disease].
>
> —*Patty Siri-Tarino and colleagues*[12]

Nor does fat in our foods automatically become lodged in our arteries and "clog" them. A great deal of research has been done in recent years that has largely exonerated saturated fat of the heinous health crimes it has been accused of. This doesn't mean you need to go out of your way to gorge on saturated fat while following this plan, but you no longer need to avoid it or fear it. Numerous studies and analyses have been published in recent years that not only redeem saturated fat's reputation but actually point a damning finger at the role of excessive carbohydrate consumption as a contributor to cardiovascular disease. According to a Harvard University meta-analysis of studies looking at the potential association between saturated fat and cardiovascular disease, "Despite the conventional wisdom that reduced dietary saturated fat intake is beneficial for cardiovascular health, the evidence for a positive, independent association is lacking."[13] The authors of this analysis also wrote, "Recent evidence indicates that limitations in carbohydrate intake can improve all features of atherogenic dyslipidemia."[14] "Atherogenic dyslipidemia" is the fancy way of describing a pattern in cholesterol and triglycerides (blood fats) that indicates an increased risk for heart disease. As for the detrimental role of carbohydrates, the authors said, "Replacement of [saturated fat] with a higher carbohydrate intake, particularly refined carbohydrate, can exacerbate the atherogenic dyslipidemia associated with insulin resistance and obesity that includes increased triglycerides, small LDL particles, and reduced HDL cholesterol."[15] In other words, when people cut down on the amount of saturated fat they eat and replace it with refined carbohydrates, their cardiovascular health gets worse.

What this all means is, in dutifully following conventional recommendations to reduce the amount of saturated fat in our diet and replace it with a greater amount of carbohydrate, we might have actually worsened the problems we were trying to solve. Replacing saturated fat with even those "heart-healthy whole grains" can be problematic for some individuals—particularly those who are insulin resistant or have other metabolic problems that affect their carbohydrate tolerance. Whole grains might be fine when consumed fresh and in their truly "whole" form, such as in a salad or pilaf of barley or hard red winter wheatberries, but even these "whole grains" can be considered to be refined carbohydrates when they're milled into microscopic flour particles and combined with sugar and preservatives and made into bread, chips, fiber bars, breakfast cereal, and other processed foods. It is telling that what used to be called a "beer belly" is now often referred to as a "wheat belly." (Some doctors even call it an "insulin pouch"!)

Contrary to what you've been hearing for many years, there is now a growing realization that refined carbohydrates are much more insidious culprits for heart disease risk than are saturated fats. According to a team led by Dr. James DiNicolantonio, a cardiovascular disease researcher with Saint Luke's Mid America Heart Institute, "When saturated fats are replaced with refined carbohydrates, and specifically with added sugars (like sucrose or high fructose corn syrup), the end result is not favorable for heart health. Such replacement leads to changes in LDL, high-density lipoprotein (HDL), and triglycerides that may increase the risk of CHD [coronary heart disease]."[16] One study even showed that among overweight older women, diets higher in cheese and meat were *less* atherogenic (harmful for heart health) than a low-fat, higher-carb diet.[17] According to Harvard University–based researchers, "dietary efforts to improve the increasing burden of CVD risk associated with atherogenic dyslipidemia should primarily emphasize the limitation of refined carbohydrate intakes and a reduction in excess adiposity."[18] ("Excess adiposity" is science-speak for obesity, and it's no coincidence that low-carbohydrate diets are quite effective for fat loss.)

Apart from switching out saturated fats for carbohydrates, conventional dietary advice also recommended that, instead of saturated fats, we substitute unsaturated fats—for example, cooking with soybean, canola, corn, or olive oils instead of butter, ghee, lard, and tallow. But the story we saw with the unintended and harmful results of increasing carbohydrates in lieu of saturated fats is echoed here: Consumption of large amounts of polyunsaturated fats, mostly in the form of isolated oils (as opposed to these fats in their whole food matrix, such as in seafood, poultry, nuts, and seeds) is associated with greater risk for compromised cardiovascular health.[19] It's like a police drama show on TV: Saturated fats have been framed for crimes committed by excess carbohydrates and polyunsaturated fats. Poor, innocent saturated fats have been in the jailhouse for a long time now, but they're finally being exonerated. As Glen Lawrence, PhD, said:

> *The lack of any clear evidence that saturated fats are promoting any of the conditions that can be attributed to PUFA [polyunsaturated fatty acids] makes one wonder how saturated fats got such a bad reputation in the health literature. The influence of dietary fats on serum cholesterol has been overstated, and a physiological mechanism for saturated fats causing heart disease is still missing.[20]*

Beyond all this, research on saturated fats is frequently confounded by these fats being lumped together with the industrial trans fats. Both are sometimes referred to as "solid fats," because they're solid at room temperature. But remember, while the saturated fats in dairy, beef, pork, and coconut are solid naturally, the polyunsaturated vegetable oils only become solid as a result of partial hydrogenation. And while the various warring nutritional factions don't all see eye to eye on saturated fats, general consensus among medical and nutrition professionals—whether they support low-carb diets, Paleo, low-fat, vegetarian, vegan, or some other type of diet—is that the trans fats have got to go. On the other hand, healthy, robust populations have been nourished by saturated fats from dairy products and meat for centuries, long before our modern epidemics of heart disease and obesity began. According to Donald Miller, MD, "It seems everything our grandparents and great-grandparents did was right! Having a lot of butter, meat, cheese, and eggs in your diet is the way they stayed healthy. The obesity rate a hundred years ago was just 1 in 150. Now that we've cut that stuff out of our diets and replaced it with carbohydrate, polyunsaturated fatty acids, and trans fats, two-thirds of the population is overweight or obese. It's really an incredible epidemic."[21]

One final note: For many years, we've been advised to reduce saturated fats in our diet and replace them with complex carbohydrates and unsaturated fats. The latter were specifically recommended because replacing saturated fats with polyunsaturated fats in the diet reduces total serum cholesterol, at least in some people. But as we now know, high cholesterol does not automatically correlate with heart disease or heart attacks, so what's the rationale for reducing cholesterol? There is none. It disappears. According to researchers who recently reexamined data from past studies exploring potential links between saturated fats and heart disease, "Available evidence from randomized controlled trials shows that replacement of saturated fat in the diet with linoleic acid [a polyunsaturated fat] effectively lowers serum cholesterol but does not support the hypothesis that this translates to a lower risk of death from coronary heart disease or all causes."[22] In plain English: Eating more polyunsaturated fats instead of saturated fats lowers cholesterol, but having a lower cholesterol level doesn't protect against death from cardiovascular events. So why bother?

Again, you need not intentionally gorge on saturated fats, but if you've been avoiding butter, cheese, bacon, cream, coconut oil, fatty rib eye steaks, and other foods rich in saturated fats due to concerns about heart health, you no longer need to be afraid to consume these delicious things. *Bon appétit!*

CHAPTER 13

Special Fats for the Brain

I n the previous chapter, we explored the differences between saturated, monounsaturated, and polyunsaturated fatty acids. Within these categories, there are specific types of fat that are especially beneficial for brain health and will be particularly important for you or your loved one to include in this high-fat diet intended to nourish those struggling neurons. The first is a class of saturated fats known as *medium-chain triglycerides*, and the second is the class of polyunsaturated fats known as *omega-3 fats*.

Medium-Chain Triglycerides: Cuckoo for Coconut!

By now, you have probably noticed an emphasis on coconut products in this book, especially coconut oil. Recall from chapter 2 that there's a good reason coconut products have a special place on a low-carbohydrate diet specifically intended to nourish the brain with ketones. Coconut oil, full-fat coconut milk, coconut butter, and other full-fat coconut products are rich in medium-chain triglycerides (MCTs), which bypass some of the normal digestive process and instead are more readily converted into ketones. As we covered earlier, MCTs can serve as a source of ketones even in the absence of carbohydrate restriction.

However, even though these oils can elevate ketone levels in the presence of a substantial amount of dietary carbohydrate (and high insulin levels), the real benefit—the one-two punch, if you will—comes from a combination of carbohydrate reduction and liberal use of MCT-rich products. Consume coconut products and MCT oils liberally, but do so while *also* restricting carbohydrates and engaging in other insulin-reducing practices for the maximum potential benefit. In the absence of dietary carbohydrate reduction, consuming MCTs will help a little bit, but by itself, this won't work miracles. Your health or that of your loved one is too important to go halfway. Foods rich in MCTs should be consumed in addition to, not instead of, carbohydrate reduction.

Look for organic, unrefined, extra-virgin coconut oil. (Sounds like a mouthful, but these are actually very easy to find at nationwide health food stores and well-stocked supermarkets, and even the best-quality ones are surprisingly affordable.) These oils will have a very pleasant coconut flavor and aroma. If you don't like the taste of coconut but still want to experience the "keto boost" coconut oil offers, look for refined coconut oil. It is nearly free of coconut flavor and odor, and you will still get the benefits of the MCTs. (As a highly saturated fat, coconut oil is safe for cooking, but it has a relatively low smoke point compared to other fats. Some people find that the refined version is better for high-heat cooking.)

Isolated MCT oils are now available at health food stores and online, and you may choose to experiment with them, particularly if you don't enjoy the taste of coconut. Moreover, MCTs make up only a small percentage of the total fatty acids in coconut. (The rest are short or long-chain fats, with short, medium, or long referring to the number of carbon atoms in the fatty acid chain.) Purified MCT oil is 100 percent MCTs and might be more effective at improving cognition—at least acutely. Coconut is simply a more budget-friendly choice with wider applications in the kitchen.

> MCTs are not dependent on the same regulatory factors that control LCT [long chain triglyceride] entry into cells and mitochondria; so MCT are promptly oxidized [burned] in muscle cells or used by the liver to make ketones. Thus, depending on the dose, ingestion of MCTs can result in rapid elevation of ketones.
>
> —*Jeff Volek and Stephen Phinney*[1]

Because of the ability of MCTs to generate ketones even in the presence of high insulin levels and a high-carbohydrate intake, if you are able to convince your loved one to implement no other strategies from this book, I encourage you to get coconut or MCT oils into them by hook or by crook, any way you can. The mere presence of ketones for fuel in the brain won't do much to arrest or reverse disease progression, but it might improve cognition in the short term, which can improve quality of life for the Alzheimer's sufferer and perhaps even more, for their caregivers. Using these special fats and exogenous ketones is really just a short-term fix—but it's better than nothing.

There are many ways to introduce coconut products and MCT oil into the diet:

- Add coconut or MCT oil to your coffee or tea. (This might sound odd at first, but it's quite delicious. Think of it as a "brain boost" first thing in the morning.)
- Use coconut oil as your go-to cooking oil for frying eggs, sautéing vegetables, searing meat, and stir-frying. If you prepare food for the individual afflicted with Alzheimer's, be generous with the oil!
- Use coconut milk in homemade curries or smoothies. (Always use full-fat, not "light" or reduced fat coconut milk. Remember—you want the fat.)
- Use coconut oil or coconut butter (sometimes sold as coconut "manna") in homemade chocolate treats using unsweetened cocoa or 85 percent dark chocolate.
- Use unsweetened, dried, shredded coconut flakes as a breading for chicken cutlets, seafood, or simply have a few spoonfuls as a snack. Use them raw or toast them for a few seconds in a dry pan. They'll get crunchy and will take on a delicious, nutty flavor.
- Take a spoonful, straight up!

A word of caution: Avoid consuming large amounts of coconut or MCT oil before bed. These special fats are such a good source of ketones and quick energy that some people find it difficult to fall asleep if they consume too much of them late at night. (On the other hand, some people don't experience this effect. You will have to experiment and see how these oils affect you or your loved one.) Additionally, if you are not accustomed to consuming coconut oil or MCT oil, I recommend starting slowly. Some people experience loose stools or digestive upset if they consume too much of these before their body has gotten used to that amount of easily absorbed fat. Start with small amounts, and increase gradually.

Understanding the Omegas: Omega-3, Omega-6, and Their All-Important Ratio

In the previous chapter, we addressed some of the reasons it's best to avoid consuming large amounts of refined polyunsaturated vegetable oils. We also clarified that it's okay—beneficial, even—to eat polyunsaturated fats as part of the whole-food matrix they naturally occur in, such as nuts and seeds, seafood, and poultry. Going a little deeper, the category of polyunsaturated fatty acids includes many subclasses of fats. Two of these are called essential fatty acids (EFAs). The reason they are "essential" is because we cannot make them from other substances in our bodies; we must get them from our diet. These two essential fatty acids are *linoleic acid* and *alpha-linolenic acid*. Linoleic acid is the "parent omega-6" fatty acid, and alpha-linolenic acid is the "parent omega-3" fatty acid, from which other forms of omega-6s and -3s, respectively, can be synthesized. We need both of these for good health, but we need them in very small amounts relative to our total food intake. (In scientific shorthand, omega-3s and -6s are abbreviated as n-3 and n-6, or ω-3 and ω-6, respectively.)

If you've ever read health- and nutrition-related articles, you've probably come across the terms *omega-3* and *omega-6* before. You might have also heard that omega-3s are "good," and omega-6s are "bad." This makes a good sound bite, but it oversimplifies things to the point of being inaccurate. The reason that we're told to decrease our intake of omega-6 fats and increase our intake of omega-3s is that excessive omega-6 intake tends to provoke inflammation, while omega-3s are generally anti-inflammatory. Remember, fats aren't just a source of energy; they have regulatory and signaling functions in the body, including inducing, moderating, and resolving inflammation.

The truth is, omega-3s and -6s are both inflammatory and anti-inflammatory, and both are necessary for good health and a proper inflammatory response. Not all inflammation is bad. Without inflammation, theoretically, we could bleed to death from a paper cut. Acute, short-term, controlled inflammation is a protective mechanism when we experience physical trauma, such as a cut, bruise, scrape, burn, or serious injury. Really, inflammation is only harmful when it is chronic, long-standing, and unresolved—and this can happen for a variety of reasons, including poor diet, unidentified food sensitivities, psychological stress, smoking, and more.

Omega-3 fats are critical for brain health because the brain is literally made out of them. DHA (docosahexaenoic acid—try saying that three times fast!), an omega-3 fat found in fatty cold-water fish, organ meats, and egg yolks, is a key structural component in the brain. (DHA might account for as much as 40 percent of the fatty acids in cell membranes in the brain.[2]) Picture trying to build a log cabin without a supply of wood, and you'll have some idea of how difficult it would be to support a properly functioning brain without adequate DHA. DHA is so important for brain health, in fact, that researchers studying the relationship between certain fats in the body and the development of Alzheimer's have written, "A change in diet emphasizing decreasing dietary carbohydrates and increased EFAs, such as DHA, may effectively prevent or delay AD."[3] They also said, "Diets deficient in ω-3 may be associated with decreased synaptic membrane DHA levels, membrane lipid peroxidation . . . synaptic loss . . . and inefficient function of membrane proteins such as glucose transporters."[4] Synaptic loss, oxidation of the fats in membranes, and inefficient functioning of glucose transporters: These are some of the very factors contributing to cognitive impairment and Alzheimer's disease.

Owing to their role in the physical structure of neurons and other brain cells, as well as their properties as precursors for signaling molecules in the inflammatory response, omega-3 fats truly are indispensable for healthy cognitive function. Data is mixed, but overall, higher concentrations of omega-3 fats in red blood cells (used as a marker for whole-body status) are correlated with higher total brain volume and higher hippocampal volume, with the hippocampus being one of the more severely affected and atrophied brain regions in Alzheimer's disease.[7] The normal aging process is known to result in brain atrophy (a shrinkage of brain volume), but a lower level of omega-3 fats in the body might result in brain volume loss greater than is expected in normal aging, specifically in the hippocampus.[8]

> Insufficient intake of DHA and low levels of DHA in the hippocampus may have a role in cognitive decline in the elderly and/or AD. —*Stephen Cunnane and colleagues*[5]
>
> Dietary intake of ω-3 long-chain PUFAs and consumption of fish, which is the primary source of DHA (the most abundant component of membrane phospholipid in metabolically active areas of the brain . . .), may also reduce the risk of incident AD. —*Roger Lane and Martin Farlow*[6]

It is a perfectly good idea to increase your intake of omega-3 fats, such as fatty fish, flaxseeds, chia seeds, and omega-3 enriched egg yolks, but the other side of this coin—and no less important—is reducing your intake of omega-6 fats (such as from corn, soy, safflower, and cottonseed oils). As stated above, omega-3s and 6s are both "essential," but that doesn't mean we need them in exactly the same amounts. Although the precise ratio we should consume is currently a matter of debate, experts agree that, overall, we are consuming far too much n-6 relative to n-3. This is an unavoidable outcome of the modern diet, which is high in vegetable oils that are concentrated sources of omega-6 fats. According to the University of Maryland Medical Center, the typical American diet contains between fourteen and twenty five times as much n-6 as n-3.[9]

> Mainstream medicine made a terrible mistake when it advised people to avoid saturated fat in favor of foods high in omega-6 fats. — *Dwight Lundell*[10]

Human physiology, experimental evidence, and the anthropological record indicate that we are biologically suited to consume no more than four or five times as much omega-6 as omega-3. (The ratio might even be closer to two or three times as much.[11]) However, thanks to the generous inclusion of soybean, corn, and cotton-seed oils in the modern diet, our intake of omega-6 fats has been skewed to as much as twenty or twenty-five times as much as our omega-3 intake.[12] According to the Food and Nutrition Board of the US National Academy of Sciences Institute of Medicine, the acceptable range of intake for omega-6 fats for adults is 5–10 percent of total calories.[13] On a diet of 2,000 calories per day, the middle of that range—7.5 percent—would account for 150 calories, or 16.7 grams of omega-6 fat. You could easily exceed this amount

It has been estimated that Paleolithic hunter-gatherers ate roughly equal amounts of n-6 and n-3 fatty acids. However, the modern Western food supply is much richer in n-6 fatty acids due to the use of grains both in the diet and as animal feed. This has greatly altered the ratio of dietary n-6 to n-3 fatty acids from roughly 1:1 for Paleolithic hunter-gatherers to ~20:1 for a modern diet. —*Samuel Henderson*[14] with nothing more than a generous serving of salad dressing, to say nothing of everything else you might eat that day. This heavy imbalance between omega-6 and omega-3 fats is associated with a host of poor health outcomes, including heart disease, chronic pain, debilitating PMS, and arthritis.

Now that we know we want to increase our intake of omega-3 fats and decrease our intake of omega-6 fats, let's see what the main sources of these are in the modern diet. Since both omega-6 and omega-3 are polyunsaturated fatty acids, the biggest sources of both are plant oils. (Remember, animal fats are predominantly saturated and monounsaturated. They do contain small amounts of polyunsaturated fats, but since we get far more polyunsaturated fatty acids from plant oils, let's stick with looking at those. See table 13.1.)

Animal foods do contain small amounts of both omega-6 and omega-3 fats. Wild-caught fish is the richest source of animal-based omega-3 fats, but you will also find small amounts of these essential fatty acids in beef, lamb, bison, poultry, and dairy products. However, the EFA content of animal foods is heavily influenced by the animals' diet. Meat, fat, and dairy

Table 13.1. Omega-6 and Omega-3 Composition of Select Oils

Type of oil	% Omega-6	% Omega-3	Ratio of n-6 to n-3
Safflower	75	0	75
Grapeseed	70	0	70
Sunflower	65	0	65
Corn	54	0	54
Cottonseed	51	0	51
Sesame*	42	0	42
Peanut*	32	0	32
Soybean	51	7	7.3
Walnut	52	10	5.2
Canola*	20	9	2.2
Flaxseed	14	53	0.26

Source: Mary Enig, Know Your Fats.

* The predominant fatty acids in peanut, sesame, and canola oils are monounsaturated, but they still contain a fair amount of polyunsaturates, hence their inclusion here. They are suitable for occasional use in cooking.

products from grass-fed and grass-finished cows, bison, and lamb will be higher in omega-3 fats and other nutrients than foods from animals that are grain finished.[15] The same goes for the yolks of eggs that come from pastured hens that consume greens and grubs as they peck around in a field, or from hens whose diet is supplemented with flaxseed, chia seeds, or fish meal.[16] (See chapter 16 for more information on these issues.)

As you can see in table 13.1, due to modern food-processing techniques and the subsidies that make corn, cottonseeds, and soybeans such incredibly cheap raw materials for food processors to use, some of the most prevalent oils in the modern diet are high in omega-6. You will see combinations of these oils in almost all mass-marketed condiments and nearly every packaged food with a long shelf life: salad dressings, mayonnaise, cookies, cakes, crackers, supermarket in-house-made baked goods, potato chips and other snack foods, canned frosting, roasted nuts, and more. And don't forget the large bottles of corn and soybean oil sold as "vegetable oil" that we discussed previously.

Even if you eat a substantial amount of fish every week, if you also consume large amounts of processed foods, your omega-6 intake is likely significantly higher than your omega-3 intake—much higher than the four-to-one or five-to-one ratio we want to stay below. And if you don't have a high omega-3 intake, the imbalance is even worse.

Some people choose to increase their omega-3 intake by taking fish oil supplements. If you do not regularly consume fatty fish or eggs that come from chickens whose feed is supplemented with a source of omega-3 fats, I suggest taking a high-quality fish oil or cod liver oil supplement. I must emphasize high-quality, however. I do not recommend large bottles from the corner drugstore. We are trying to heal from a long time of accumulated damage to the brain; this is not the time to compromise on quality. If it is within your means, I recommend seeking a medical or nutrition practitioner who knows of reputable companies that regularly test their batches for safety and purity, and whose inventory hasn't been sitting around for months in warm warehouses or exposed to bright lights in stores twenty-four hours a day, where the oils might become rancid.

Also, keep in mind that when I say "fatty fish," this means *eating the fat and skin of the fish*, especially salmon, sardines, or mackerel. If you are buying skinless fish, you are losing one of the best sources of this important fat. Think about it: The skinless salmon fillets you typically see at the store (or are served in a restaurant) are extremely lean. But the valuable omega-3s we are specifically consuming fish to get are in the fat. If you consume canned mackerel or sardines (which I recommend as a wonderful, budget-friendly source of omega-3s), I suggest favoring varieties with the bones and skin rather than the boneless, skinless versions. Remember, the important fats we're looking for are just that: fats. The skins of these fish are rich in fat, and the bones will provide calcium and other minerals. (The bones in canned fish are very soft and are as easy to chew as the flesh. They're not hard and will crumble easily in your mouth—not unpleasant at all. Eat the bones!) If you buy canned salmon and mackerel, I even recommend drinking the liquid you would normally drain out of the can. You'll notice this liquid appears shiny and oily—that's because some of the fat from the fish has leached out into the canning water. And since we want this fat, drink the water! Otherwise you will literally be pouring valuable nutrients down the drain.

Is Fatty Fish the Only Way to Get Omega-3 Fats?

No. The reason I emphasize fatty fish for omega-3 intake is because even though we can get some omega-3 fats from plant sources (such as flaxseeds, chia seeds, and walnuts), the type of omega-3 we get from plants is different from the type we get from animal foods. The plant form of omega-3 is called alpha-linolenic acid (ALA). This is the parent omega-3 mentioned earlier. It is the raw material from which we ultimately end up with EPA and DHA—the fats that are so critical for brain health. But converting ALA into EPA and DHA in the body requires a very complicated biochemical process with many steps along the way. Most people's bodies do not make this conversion very effectively, and this is made even worse if they eat a lot of omega-6 fats. Omega-3 and omega-6 fats both go through these conversion processes, and they "compete" for many of the same helper molecules required along the way. The greater the amount of omega-6 in the diet, the more it will crowd out omega-3 for these limited helper enzymes.

If you prefer to avoid seafood or are allergic to it, then I recommend increasing your intake of the plant sources of omega-3. Fortunately, flaxseeds, flax oil, chia seeds, and walnuts all fit just fine into a low-carbohydrate, high-fat diet, and although alpha-linolenic acid is not as potent as EPA and DHA, it's better than nothing—particularly for individuals who consume no seafood. (Walnuts are a source of omega-3, but they have about five times more omega-6, so they're fine to eat in small amounts, but don't rely on them as your primary source of omega-3s.) In cases of seafood allergy or aversion, I would also emphasize seeking out eggs from hens with omega-3 fortified feed (or better yet, hens raised outdoors on pasture, consuming grass, worms, and insects in addition to their grain feed), as well as meats from grass-fed and grass-finished animals. These might not be as important for individuals who do consume a substantial amount of fatty fish, but for those who don't, seeking these specific foods might ensure a higher volume of EPA and DHA than most people could expect to produce from the plant sources of omega-3.

Perhaps just as good a reason to consume fish and shellfish as their omega-3 content is their nutrient content overall. Shellfish, in particular, are an excellent source of several key nutrients for brain health and cognitive function (see table 13.2), and of course, you are no longer wary of their cholesterol content.

In looking at table 13.2, you can see shellfish and crustaceans are just loaded with micronutrients. Their B_{12} content is outstanding, and recall from the discussion of myelin in chapter 3 that B_{12} is absolutely critical for healthy neuron structure and function, and many older people have

Table 13.2. Percent Daily Value (%DV) of Nutrients per 3-Ounce Serving

Nutrient	Oysters	Clams	Mussels	Lobster
Vitamin C	18%	31%	19%	—
B_{12}	408%	1401%	340%	44%
Riboflavin	22%	21%	21%	3%
Niacin	15%	14%	13%	5%
Iron	43%	132%	32%	2%
Phosphorus	21%	29%	24%	16%
Zinc	188%	15%	15%	17%
Manganese	52%	43%	289%	3%
Copper	114%	29%	6%	82%
Selenium	187%	78%	109%	52%

Source: Condé Nast, *SELF Nutrition Data*, accessed April 28, 2015, http://nutritiondata.self.com.

Note: Percentages are the daily values (% DV) for adults or children age four or older, based on a 2,000 calorie per day reference diet.

low levels of this vitamin, leading some researchers to speculate that inadequate B_{12} might actually be a contributing factor to dementia. Selenium is a mineral required for proper recycling of glutathione—often called the body's "master antioxidant," as well as for production of thyroid hormones. Oysters, in particular, are an excellent source of highly bioavailable zinc, and many older people with compromised cognitive function are deficient in zinc. Zinc is present in plant foods—pumpkin and sesame seeds, peanuts, and some types of beans are good sources—but the body absorbs zinc more readily from animal and seafood sources than from plants.

Additional Dietary Considerations: Dos and Don'ts on Dairy, Gluten, Sweeteners, and Sugar Alcohols

Staying within the basic framework of a diet low in carbohydrate and high in fat is simple. However, there are some additional issues you might be wondering about, such as dairy products, gluten, and the use of artificial sweeteners and sugar alcohols. In this chapter we will explore the place these items have in this nutritional strategy for fueling the brain.

Dairy—Say *So Long* to Skim Milk!

The issue of whether to include dairy in your diet should be guided by your sensitivity to the small amounts of lactose—"milk sugar"—in the products. Some dairy foods are higher in lactose than others, but many dairy foods are wonderful sources of mostly fat and protein, and including dairy can make sticking to this plan for the long term much easier and more enjoyable. If you choose to include dairy products, emphasize full-fat options, rather than low-fat, nonfat, or skim. Remember, fat is the most important macronutrient on this diet. This is not a low-fat diet, so there is no need to consume reduced-fat dairy products. In fact, the fat is encouraged.

As with all foods, different dairy foods stimulate insulin to different degrees. In general, the higher in fat and the lower in carbohydrate and protein a food is, the less it will stimulate insulin, and since the goal of this dietary strategy is to keep insulin levels low in order to facilitate the synthesis of brain-boosting ketones, you should always favor dairy foods that are higher in fat.

If you are lactose intolerant or sensitive to the casein protein in dairy products, you may avoid dairy and still reap the benefits of this nutritional strategy. Including delicious high-fat dairy foods such as butter and cream can make it easier to follow this plan, but you can certainly get plenty of nourishing fat and protein from other foods.

Permissible dairy foods

- Butter
- Ghee (clarified butter—butter that has had the milk solids removed)
- Heavy cream or heavy whipping cream
- Light cream (sometimes labeled "table cream")
- Half-and-half—in small amounts; it's better to use light cream or heavy cream, but half-and-half is permissible for people who prefer its texture.
- Cream cheese—plain or flavored with scallions, chives, or other herbs—avoid fruit flavors or honey nut varieties, which typically have added sugar or corn syrup.
- Sour cream
- Cottage cheese—read the labels for additives; many contain starch-based thickeners and stabilizers that can increase the carbohydrate content. Favor the full-fat variety, usually sold as 4 percent in the United States.
- Cheese—all types: hard, soft, aged, blue—from cows, goats, or sheep. Long-aged and hard cheeses tend to have the lowest lactose content, as the sugar is consumed by the bacterial cultures during the aging process. Fresh cheeses will have a slightly higher carbohydrate content.
- Full-fat, plain yogurt or Greek yogurt—in small amounts. (You may add cinnamon, berries, or artificial sweetener if desired.) Due to the presence of live bacteria, the carbohydrate content of yogurt is less than what appears on the label. The live and active cultures in yogurt convert some of the lactose to lactic acid, which is responsible for the sour, tangy flavor, and for turning liquid milk into semisolid yogurt. According to experienced low-carb researchers, a ½ cup of plain yogurt contains only about 5 grams of carbohydrate.[1]

Dairy foods to limit or avoid entirely

- Liquid milk—in all forms and flavors (whole, 2 percent, 1 percent, skim, chocolate)
- Ice cream
- Milk shakes (including bottled chocolate and strawberry milk smoothies available in supermarket dairy sections)
- Fat-free, low-fat, and fruit-flavored yogurts—yogurt is commonly thought of as a "health food," but these concoctions contain far too much sugar for this dietary strategy. One 6-ounce cup might contain almost 30 grams of carbohydrate! (If you choose to consume yogurt, stick to the aforementioned plain, full-fat version. Even the sugar-free varieties might still be high in total carbohydrate.)
- Any reduced-fat, low-fat, or fat-free dairy products. Eat the fat!

A note about dairy substitutes

- **Nondairy creamer:** If you enjoy cream in your coffee or tea, use real cream! Avoid flavored nondairy creamers. These look like cream, but they are usually oil-based, made from soybean or cottonseed oils, and are loaded with sugar. (Many of these have 5 grams of sugar in just a 1-tablespoon serving, and it's easy to consume far more than that. Moreover, even though there are nondairy creamers that are labeled "sugar-free," these still often contain corn syrup or other sweeteners, and you'd be surprised at the carbohydrate content.)
- **Margarine:** Do not consume margarine or any other "vegetable oil spreads" designed to mimic the taste and texture of butter. Now that any lingering fears regarding saturated fat and cholesterol have been put to rest, please, use real butter. The problems with vegetable oil spreads are numerous, and these products are best avoided completely, whether you are following a low-carbohydrate diet or not.
- **Almond milk and other nut milks (rice milk, cashew milk, and so on):** These are suitable, provided you take care to purchase the unsweetened varieties. Be vigilant in looking at the labels; the sweetened and unsweetened versions often come in packages that are nearly identical. Almond, cashew, hemp, and rice milks are acceptable, provided the carbohydrate content is 3 grams or less per 8-ounce serving. Avoid soy milk, whether sweetened or not.

Do You Need to Go Gluten-Free?

Gluten is a protein found in wheat and related grains, such as barley, rye, and the "ancient" forms of wheat—spelt, emmer, einkorn, kamut, and triticale. In addition to the whole foods it is naturally present in, extra gluten is often used to enhance the texture and structure of other foods. Aside from the obvious—bread, pasta, bagels, crackers, cookies, and anything else wheat-based—isolated gluten might be found in bottled sauces, dressings, and other condiments, packaged foods, processed meat items (chicken nuggets, prepared meatballs, and so on), and more. Some individuals experience unpleasant effects when they consume gluten, which can be anything from acute intestinal distress and discomfort to more mild but still uncomfortable effects, such as abdominal bloating, gas, headaches, skin manifestations (dermatitis herpetiformis, psoriasis, atopic dermatitis), and even neurological and psychological effects such as anxiety and ataxia.[2] In fact, studies suggest sensitivity to gluten might be a primary driver of schizophrenia, and some researchers even use the term "gluten psychosis."[3]

The most well-known condition related to gluten sensitivity is celiac disease, in which an overt allergy to gluten causes an attack on the lining of the small intestine. (Due to the resultant compromise in digestive function, individuals with celiac disease often experience gas, bloating, diarrhea, and undesired weight loss due to impaired absorption of nutrients from food.) However, there is increasing recognition in the medical community that celiac disease is simply one manifestation of sensitivity to gluten, and that there is a spectrum of what is called *non-celiac gluten sensitivity* (NCGS), which gives rise to "gluten-related disorders" that lack the gastrointestinal effects of celiac disease but affect other parts of the body.[4] Many individuals with conditions resulting from NCGS are unaware that an everyday foodstuff might be causing their symptoms because they've never attempted to go any significant period of time without consuming it. The modern Western diet and the convenience foods many of us have come to rely on emphasize wheat and other gluten-containing foods: breakfast cereal or toast in the morning, a sandwich at lunch, pretzels or pita chips for a snack, pasta for dinner. Some of us are absolutely inundated with gluten—and the refined carbohydrates it typically comes wrapped up in.

The dietary strategy outlined in this book can be a gluten-free diet, but it is not gluten-free by definition. You may choose to adopt a completely gluten-free diet if you desire, but this is not absolutely necessary. There are a number of gluten-containing products that can be quite helpful on a low-carb diet, such as very low-carb, high-fiber bran crackers. The long-term goal is to phase these things out entirely, but if you are not ready to jump in headfirst, these things can help ease the transition as you gradually reduce your carbohydrate consumption. They can also provide a "safer" (that is, lower-carb and much less insulin-stimulating) alternative to regular bread or crackers when you absolutely must have something to satisfy a craving for that taste or texture.

Because of the low-carbohydrate nature of this diet, you will automatically be consuming far less wheat and gluten than you are accustomed to. By eliminating (or cutting dramatically back on) bread, pasta, bagels, pizza, cookies, crackers, muffins, cereal, fiber bars, pretzels, and the like, you will be drastically reducing the amount of wheat and gluten you consume.

If you are interested in following a completely gluten-free diet, you will need to be even more vigilant when reading labels, as gluten and other wheat derivatives are found in almost every processed, packaged food available in supermarkets. It even hides in places you would never suspect, such as shampoo, lipstick, lotion, and other cosmetics. However, if you choose to make your low-carb diet completely free of gluten, the trace amounts of gluten in these nonfood items should have no impact on your metabolism and fueling your brain. These incidental exposures to gluten are a grave concern for people with severe gluten sensitivities, but if you are avoiding wheat simply as part of an overall low-carb diet, you do not have to avoid these "environmental" glutens and need not be concerned about low-level exposure to gluten via cross-contamination in restaurants or packaged foods that are produced on shared equipment with gluten-containing items.

A Note on Artificial Sweeteners

There are two main categories of sweetening agents outside of what we think of as sugars (for example, white or brown sugar, honey, maple syrup, molasses): artificial sweeteners and sugar alcohols. Artificial sweeteners are noncaloric substances that contribute a sweet taste to foods. There are several kinds, sold under different brand names. The most common in the United States are:

- Sucralose: most commonly marketed as Splenda (yellow packets)
- Saccharine: most commonly marketed as Sweet'N Low (pink packets)

- Aspartame: most commonly marketed as Equal or NutraSweet (blue packets)
- Acesulfame potassium (sometimes called Ace-K on labels)

Almost all artificial sweeteners are packaged along with dextrose, a sweetener usually made from corn. It is used as a filler—because the artificial sweeteners themselves are so extremely concentrated, they are needed in just tiny amounts, so dextrose is added to the packets to give them some bulk. As with any carbohydrate, some people will be more sensitive to even these small amounts of dextrose than others. For this reason, if you choose to use artificial sweeteners, I recommend using the lowest amount you feel you need to in order to still comply with (and enjoy!) your diet. You can also find liquid versions of these artificial sweeteners, and the liquids typically don't contain fillers or bulking agents.

The use of artificial sweeteners is a controversial subject. They are not prohibited on the low-carbohydrate diet outlined in this book, nor is liberal use of them encouraged. You must decide for yourself whether these substances have a place in your diet or that of the person you care for. Ideally, you will break yourself completely of the need to consume anything sweet tasting. However, this is a tall order. Maybe even impossible. (We're only human!) I believe that small amounts of sweetening agents can make a low-carbohydrate plan much easier to stick to, and if employing artificial sweeteners or sugar alcohols means the difference between you or your loved one giving this strategy a try, versus throwing your hands up in defeat before you even start, use them! Don't let food perfectionism and puritanism prevent you from embarking on a nutritional strategy that could be life-changing for you or the Alzheimer's sufferer you care for. You can start with an amount that will make this diet manageable for you and cut back over time.

The main drawback to artificial sweeteners and sugar alcohols is that for some people, the sweet taste—even an artificial one—will lead to cravings for more and more, until eventually they "fall off the wagon" and end up eating large amounts of genuinely sugary or starchy foods. If you find that you can have a small amount of an artificially sweetened food or beverage and not give in to cravings for more—specifically, cravings for foods that will wildly throw off your blood glucose and insulin levels—then I believe these things can be a helpful adjunct in keeping you on your diet.

On the other hand, studies suggest that artificial sweeteners do affect insulin levels. This occurs mainly because simply having a sweet sensation in the mouth—whether from sugar or an artificial sweetener—might stimulate the pancreas to secrete insulin with the expectation that a carbohydrate-containing food is being consumed.[5] However, the findings are inconsistent, and moreover, the metabolic and physiologic effects of these substances might be different in individuals consuming a low-carb diet than those following a more typical high-carb diet. Much of the data is inconclusive and a lot remains to be determined regarding the precise mechanisms by which artificial sweeteners might affect physical processes in the body as well as the psychological aspects of dependence on sweet foods.[6] Other research indicates artificial sweeteners do not affect blood glucose, insulin, or appetite-related hormones the way caloric sugars do.[7]

However, some of the most experienced researchers and physicians who have used low-carb and ketogenic diets to help thousands of people reclaim their health do not prohibit artificial sweeteners on their programs. And in terms of supporting cognitive function, I believe that any of the artificial sweetening agents will have fewer detrimental effects than consumption of large amounts of real sugar and natural sweeteners, all of which will absolutely stand in the way of moving over to a fat-based, ketone-producing metabolism.

Sugar Alcohols and Stevia—Better Choices

Unlike artificial sweeteners, sugar alcohols do provide calories, but fewer than regular sugar. Sugar alcohols are not completely metabolized by the human digestive system, so they don't have the same impacts on blood glucose and insulin as regular sugar. They do still have an effect; it's just milder than for more traditional sweetening agents. Large consumption of sugar alcohols might also interfere with ketone production. Additionally, because they are not fully absorbed, remnants of them pass undigested into the large intestine, where intestinal bacteria feed off them, producing gas and other unpleasant side effects. (Products that contain sugar alcohols typically have a note on the label warning consumers that excessive consumption can lead to loose stools or diarrhea. Sometimes it is referred to as a "laxative effect." This is not uncommon, but it should not be a problem if you stick with small amounts. Just be aware of this potential outcome if you or the person you care for overindulge.) Finally, individuals vary in their sensitivity to sugar alcohols: Some will experience a larger fluctuation in blood glucose and insulin than others. If you choose to make these a part of your diet in significant quantities, you might wish to monitor yourself and see how they affect you.

There are many different sugar alcohols in use in products commonly available at the grocery store. You can recognize them in ingredient lists by words ending in "-ol":

- Xylitol
- Sorbitol
- Mannitol
- Erythritol
- Lactitol

Note: Erythritol typically does not cause the unpleasant gastrointestinal side effects of other sugar alcohols.

Because the degree to which these sugar alcohols are metabolized differs, they have different glycemic indices and, therefore, different effects on blood glucose and insulin levels. According to data gathered by Jeff Volek and Stephen Phinney, prominent low-carb researchers and authors, in table 14.1 is an overview of the most common sugar alcohols as they compare to sucrose (table sugar).

As mentioned earlier, the most insidious thing about these sweetening agents is that they might induce cravings for additional sweet foods. If you can have a small amount and be satisfied, and you don't find yourself

Table 14.1. Sugar Alcohols

Sugar alcohol	Calories/gram	Sweetness	Glycemic index	Absorption (g/100g)
Sucrose (sugar)	4.0	100%	60	100
Erythritol	0.2	70%	0	90
Xylitol	2.5	100%	13	50
Maltitol	2.7	75%	36	40
Isomalt	2.1	55%	9	10
Sorbitol	2.5	60%	9	25
Lactitol	2.0	35%	6	2
Mannitol	1.5	60%	0	25

Source: Jeff Volek and Stephen Phinney, *The Art and Science of Low Carbohydrate Performance* (Lexington, KY: Beyond Obesity, 2012), 61.

craving more and more, then these can really help you stick to this plan. Additionally, sugar alcohols are not plagued by the controversy and mixed findings that surround artificial sweeteners, so apart from the potential for gastrointestinal effects, you might feel more comfortable using the former instead of the latter. There are many other sweeteners available online and at well-stocked supermarkets if you are interested in trying alternatives to the more common varieties:

- Swerve (brand name for erythritol available in packets, granulated, and powdered [confectioner's style] forms)

- Truvia (brand name for a mixture of erythritol and stevia)
- Zsweet (brand name for a mixture of erythritol and stevia)
- Xylitol

- Sweet One (made from Ace-K)
- Stevia—several different brands, flavors, and versions available (as powder, liquid, or tablets)

Depending on your point of view, stevia is either a "natural" sweetener or it's as refined and processed as any of the others. Stevia comes from a plant whose green leaves are very sweet. You can find stevia powder that is just these green leaves, dried and pulverized into a powder, with nothing added and no bleaching or refining. However, much more often you will find stevia extract—a white powder made from stevia. Stevia is also available as a liquid and in various flavors that are nice for adding to coffee, unflavored seltzer, or plain yogurt. The important thing to note about stevia is that it is extremely concentrated. You only need a tiny bit—a tiny bit—to equal the sweetness of sugar. Many people complain that stevia has a bitter aftertaste; however, it is likely that they are simply using too much because they're unaware of how powerful it is.

Stevia is excellent for use in coffee, tea, and other simple applications, such as homemade whipped cream or chocolate pudding, or adding to plain yogurt for a sweet, low-carb dessert. There are many different brands and forms of stevia available. Experiment to see which you like best if you choose to use stevia. Nowadays, you can find it in powdered or liquid form at most well-stocked supermarkets, health food stores, and online. Stevia is not recommended for low-carb baked goods that require the bulk sugar normally provides. For this purpose, erythritol is best, or consider using regular sugar, honey, blackstrap molasses, or maple syrup, if you must, in the smallest quantity possible to give you the desired texture and flavor. Remember, it's not that any of these are prohibited outright; it's just that the total amount of carbohydrate in them can add up very quickly, and it's simply not worth it. (One tablespoon of maple syrup provides 13 grams of carbohydrate all by itself, and a tablespoon of honey brings 17 grams!) However, if you're making grain-free muffins or quickbreads, for example, the total amount of sugar in one small portion might be fairly low. So if you prefer to use natural sugars rather than sugar alcohols or other sweetening agents, be mindful of your portions and the total carbohydrate load.

Low Carb Libations—You Know What to Eat, but What Should You Drink?

Water is the best beverage—no contest! But if and when you need something else, choose from the following:

- **Herbal tea:** Hot or iced (be sure it contains no sugar).
- **Flavored seltzers:** As always, read labels and make sure the carb content is zero.
- **Coffee, tea (black or green):** Caffeinated beverages are permitted. Do not use sugar or honey in your coffee or tea. (A very small amount is acceptable if you prefer to avoid artificial sweeteners.)
- **Chai tea:** This becomes a delicious treat as a latte when you add heavy cream or coconut milk and (if desired) your choice of zero-carb sweetener. Drink it hot in cold weather and iced during the summer.
- **Sugar-free and artificially sweetened powdered drink mixes:** Heavy consumption of artificial sweeteners is not encouraged, but these drinks can satisfy your sweet tooth while staying on plan if you are not ready to give up sweet drinks cold turkey. Most of the brands available in major supermarkets contain aspartame or sucralose. You can find others that are sweetened with stevia and erythritol in health food stores or online.
- **Diet soda:** Again, if you are comfortable consuming artificial sweeteners, small amounts of diet soda are permitted. Aspartame is the most common artificial sweetener used in diet sodas and iced teas, but there are brands available online and in health food stores that use sucralose, stevia, erythritol, or combinations of these.

Beverages to avoid entirely

- **Fruit juice:** Juice is prohibited on this diet. Juice is liquid sugar. Even organic juice with no added sugar—it's still liquid sugar. There's no quicker way to wreck your blood glucose and insulin levels than to have concentrated sugar enter your body in a form that doesn't even need to be chewed.
- **Liquid milk:** As discussed earlier, liquid milk contains a high amount of lactose, the "milk sugar." If you desire a creamy, milklike beverage, choose unsweetened almond, rice, hemp, or coconut milk, and be sure to watch the carb count per serving. Also consider making milk by adding water to heavy cream, although the carbs can add up quickly depending on how much cream you use. I recommend using full-fat coconut milk and watering it down a little. (Not only will you have a good substitute for milk, but you'll also get those brain-boosting medium-chain triglycerides.)

A Special Note about Alcohol

Alcohol is not permitted at first. In time, you might be able to add small amounts of wine or light beer back into your life, but at the beginning, while you are helping your body transition to using fats and ketones, alcohol is best avoided completely. If you choose to consume alcohol anyway, please be aware that the change in your nutrition will make you much more sensitive to alcohol. Alcohol will affect you more quickly and more strongly than you are used to. Go slowly! You will feel the effects more severely, and you might not realize it until you've already had too much. Additionally, if you choose to imbibe, make the best choices you can for your metabolism and brain health:

- Avoid juices, sugary mixers, and schnapps.
- Stick with small amounts of wine or light beer.
- Regarding hard liquor (for example, rum, vodka, whiskey, gin)— these are actually fairly low in carbohydrates; it's the juice and sweet mixers the liquor is added to that are most problematic, so be careful about what you mix distilled spirits with if you choose to consume them.

What about Condiments?

Just because you're following a special diet doesn't mean your food has to be bland and tasteless. As long as you are careful to avoid high amounts of sugar, corn syrup, high-fructose corn syrup, and starchy thickeners (most commonly cornstarch), you can take advantage of a wide variety of sauces, marinades, and other condiments. Be sure to read labels when purchasing these items: Many contain high amounts of sugar, high-fructose corn syrup, honey, and other sweetening agents.

Here is your guide to permissible condiments and flavorings:

- **Mayonnaise:** Use full-fat, not light, reduced-fat, or imitation products. Light versions almost always contain added sugar or corn starch to make up for the flavor and texture lost with the removal of fat. There is simply no need to avoid high-fat foods with this nutritional approach.
- **Mustard:** All kinds are okay—yellow, spicy brown, Dijon, coarse grain—but avoid honey mustard and other sweetened varieties. They contain honey, sugar, or high-fructose corn syrup. The carb count should be 0 grams or 1 gram per teaspoon.
- **Vinegar:** All types are okay—balsamic, red wine, champagne, apple cider. Large amounts of balsamic vinegar might negatively impact blood glucose, however. It's higher in sugar than the other vinegars, but consumed in reasonable amounts, it's fine.
- **Hot sauce:** Choose plain or original flavors. Some flavored varieties are sweetened; if you choose something off the beaten path, be sure to read the label and look for added sugars.
- **Salad dressing:** Choose full-fat, low-carbohydrate dressings—ranch, blue cheese, creamy Caesar, or nonsweet vinaigrettes. Avoid French, Thousand Island, Catalina, and vinaigrettes that contain sugar, high-fructose corn syrup, fruit purees, and other sweeteners. No fat-free or light varieties. Go for the full-fat—you're allowed now! The salad dressings you choose should have no more than 2 grams of carbs per 2-tablespoon serving. (Better yet, simply make your own using olive or avocado oil and your choice of vinegar and herbs, season with salt and pepper, and use mustard to thicken and emulsify. For creamy dressings, use sour cream, plain yogurt, or mayonnaise as the base.)

- **Fresh-squeezed lemon and lime juice:** A splash of these adds wonderful zing to a finished dish.
- **Extra-virgin olive oil and toasted sesame oil:** A drizzle of these oils makes a delicious finishing for many dishes.
- **Soy sauce or tamari** (wheat-free soy sauce)
- **Thai-style fish sauce**
- **Reduced-sugar ketchup:** Most common brands of ketchup are made with high-fructose corn syrup or sugar and contain about 4 grams of carbohydrate per tablespoon. This might not be problematic if you can limit yourself to just 1 tablespoon, but that's an unrealistically small serving size for most people, and it's easy to consume two or three times as much. Some supermarkets stock a reduced-sugar ketchup from the Heinz brand, which is made with sucralose. If you prefer to avoid artificial sweeteners, you can find unsweetened ketchup (such as Westbrae brand) at health food stores and online. Or you can simply make your own, using no sweetener at all. Homemade ketchup requires nothing more than tomato paste, distilled white or apple cider vinegar, onion powder, and water. Add minced raw garlic and a little cayenne pepper for a "grown-up" ketchup with a kick!
- **Pickles and pickle relish:** These are often made with high-fructose corn syrup. (What isn't, these days?!) Some popular brands have sugar-free varieties (usually made with sucralose), or simply read the labels and find pickles that are unsweetened altogether. (Even better, make your own fermented pickles, sauerkraut, or kimchi to bring some more beneficial bacteria into your gut.)
- **Salsa:** Pay close attention to labels, and note carbs per serving. Avoid salsas that contain corn, black beans, or mango and peaches—these are higher in carbohydrates. Stick to salsas with the basic ingredients: tomatoes, onions, bell peppers, chilies, vinegar, herbs. Salsa should have no more than 3–4 grams of carbs per 2-tablespoon serving, and you will be able to find many that are just 2 grams.
- **Pesto:** Make sure it's just olive oil, basil, herbs, cheese, and nuts, with no sweeteners or thickeners added. You'd be amazed at what they add sugar and potato starch to!
- **Barbecue sauce:** Unfortunately, you will need to avoid all mass-produced barbecue sauces. Read labels next time you're at

the store: They all contain high-fructose corn syrup or some sort of sugar—usually as the very first ingredient. If you absolutely must have the flavor of barbecue sauce, the best way to get it will be to make your own. Try using a lower-carbohydrate tomato sauce and doctoring it up to match the barbecue flavor you enjoy, by adding ground cloves, cumin, onion powder, Worcestershire sauce, liquid smoke, and other savory seasonings. Sugar-free barbecue sauces are difficult to find in the supermarket, but well-stocked stores might carry it, and of course, you can purchase it online.

- **Any and all herbs and spices without added sugar:** Garlic powder, cumin, oregano, basil, sage, ginger, thyme, rosemary, salt, black pepper, chili powder, turmeric, paprika, curry powder, unsweetened spice blends, and so on. They're all fine! Fresh and dried herbs are both acceptable. If you purchase seasoning blends, read the label to look for added sugars. Tiny amounts are okay, as long as the total carb count per serving is still very low, and be mindful of how much you use.

—CHAPTER 15—

Low Carb in the Real World

By this point, you've realized that the low-carb, higher-fat way of eating I advocate for supporting healthy cognition is quite different from how you or your loved one might be accustomed to eating, and it's quite different from how others around you likely eat. But the truth is, there's nothing strange about this type of diet at all. There are no special shakes, bars, or meal replacement items; it's just real food, minus most of the starch and sugar. This means you will not need to go out of your way to purchase special ingredients or abandon enjoyable visits to your favorite restaurants. Because this way of eating requires nothing out of the ordinary, you or your loved one will have no problem dining out, eating on the go, and making delicious food at home. This chapter will give you some tips on how to do just that.

Prepping Your Kitchen for Low-Carb Cooking

Sticking to a low-carb diet will be easy if you have suitable foods on hand at all times. This doesn't mean that you need to create weekly meal plans in advance; it just means that creating appropriate low-carb meals "on the fly" is a breeze, as long as you keep your fridge, freezer, and pantry stocked with certain staples and go-to foods. Doing this will allow you to put together perfectly suitable meals without a specific plan.

Think of it like a wardrobe: Ladies, whatever your size or shape, you likely have a go-to dress for special occasions that is flattering and always makes you feel good. You have a wide variety of shirts, pants, skirts, and accessories to choose from, depending on the occasion, so that no matter what your day holds, you can put together an appropriate outfit in minutes. Gentlemen, you probably have at least one or two good black, dark blue, or gray suits hanging in the closet that are ready to go at a moment's notice (or maybe with one or two days' notice for a quick run to the dry cleaner!). You also have athletic shoes, dress shoes, sandals, and maybe a sports watch, a dress watch, and a nice pair of cufflinks. You've got some dress shirts, jackets, ties, casual weekend wear, and an old, ratty T-shirt you wear to fix the car or clean the gutters. Because you have articles of clothing that cover all the bases, creating a look suitable for any occasion is a snap.

Preparing delicious and satisfying meals that are appropriate for your low-carbohydrate lifestyle is no different. When you have a good variety of basics on hand, plus a few accessories to jazz things up, cooking is an absolute pleasure—and you won't miss the starches one bit. Food shopping, cooking, and eating on a ketogenic or low-carbohydrate diet isn't difficult; it's just different.

Here are some suggestions to get you started on building your low-carb kitchen. Additional ideas can be found on the Ketogenic Diet Resource website (www.ketogenic-diet-resource.com/low-carb-grocery-list.html).

Stock your freezer

- Bacon
- Beef
- Chicken
- Lamb
- Pork
- Seafood
- Turkey
- Vegetables (plain, no sauce or breading)

Fill your fridge

- Leftovers! Cook once, eat two or three times. When you take the time to cook, prepare more than you will eat in one sitting. This will ensure that in a pinch, you have something ready to go when you're pressed for time or simply don't feel like cooking.
- Bacon fat (reserved from cooking bacon; use for sautéing greens, frying eggs, and other applications)
- Butter (preferably organic, from pastured/grass-fed cows—spending a little extra on the best-quality fats is worth it)
- Cheese (preferably real cheese, full fat, from grass-fed cows; avoid imitation cheeses and "pasteurized process cheese foods")
- Eggs—consider keeping two or three dozen on hand; you will go through them quickly, so save yourself the trouble of having to run to the store so often. It's also a good idea to keep a few hard-boiled eggs on hand at all times, ready to go for a quick and easy snack.
- Heavy cream, light cream, or half-and-half

- Low-glycemic vegetables: Keep some raw and cut up for simple snacks (bell peppers, celery, radishes, jicama, cucumber, fennel, mushrooms); leftover steamed, roasted, or grilled vegetables also make great snacks.
- Low-sugar lunchmeat (cold cuts)—roast beef, turkey, pastrami, but also fatty ones (for example, salami, prosciutto, sopressata)
- Mustard
- Olives
- Salad dressings (full fat, 2 grams of carbs or less per 2-tablespoon serving)
- Sour cream
- Unsweetened ketchup

Pantry essentials
- Assortment of vinegars (apple cider, red wine, balsamic)
- Canned fish—tuna, salmon, sardines, mackerel, oysters. Stock up when they're on sale; they won't go bad, and they're an excellent snack or part of a meal.
- Canned tomatoes (crushed, whole, diced, stewed, plain, fire-roasted—keep a variety on hand for quick and easy meals)
- Chicken, beef, or vegetable broth or stock (for soups)
- Coconut milk (always full fat, organic if possible)
- Coconut oil
- Dark chocolate (85 percent or higher)
- Desiccated (dried) coconut flakes (unsweetened)
- Nuts and seeds—all nuts and seeds are fine, but go easy on peanuts and cashews, as these are slightly higher in carbs. (Nuts and seeds can also be stored in the fridge or freezer to prolong their freshness if you don't expect to consume them in a timely fashion.)
- Olive oil (preferably organic, in a dark bottle or metal tin; store it in a cool, dark place, away from direct light)
- Pork rinds (a great snack on their own or with homemade dip from sour cream, cream cheese, or guacamole)
- Sesame oil or peanut oil (for occasional stir-frying)
- Spices and herbs (no sugar added); salt and pepper
- Canned pumpkin (Be sure to buy 100 percent pure pumpkin, not pumpkin pie mix. The pie mix has added sugar. Plain pumpkin

is pleasantly sweet on its own, and although it is slightly high in carbohydrate, its high-fiber content helps to mitigate the impact on blood sugar and insulin. Canned pumpkin makes a great low-carb dessert, sprinkled with cinnamon and topped with homemade whipped cream.)

Cooking Tips for Convenience

One of the keys to sticking to a low-carbohydrate diet is having delicious foods prepared ahead of time and ready to go. It's much easier to make appropriate choices and reach for beneficial foods when these things are on hand and already cooked, just waiting for you. You will be less likely to reach for "convenience foods"—which are almost always sugary and starchy—when real foods are equally convenient, thanks to prep work and cooking you did in advance. (This is true of any diet, not just one that restricts carbohydrates.)

Cook in Big Batches

It takes almost no extra effort to cook a large amount of food than a small one. If you're grilling a steak, grill two or three at a time. This way, the next day (and the day after that!), you'll have steak that's already cooked. All you'll need to do for another meal is slice it up and serve it on top of a big green salad loaded with low-carb vegetables and maybe some blue cheese crumbles, or simply eat it cold as a snack. (You could even dice it up and use it in an omelet. The possibilities are endless.)

Grill or Bake Extra Chicken

Cold chicken breasts make excellent snacks. Just cut them into strips and dip them in ranch dressing, onion dip, or guacamole. Better yet, consider switching to bone-in, skin-on chicken thighs or leg quarters. They are far more economical . . . and flavorful! Plus, they're a little higher in fat than skinless breasts, and it's important to have a high ratio of fat in your meals. (Bone-in chicken is a snap to bake. Just sprinkle with your choice of seasoning blend and bake at 350°F [180°C] for thirty to forty-five minutes, depending on the size of the pieces. It's mostly hands-off time, freeing you to attend to other things.) If you happen to have a large oven, consider roasting two whole chickens at once. You can have one the day you make it, and use the second one for a high-fat chicken salad or hash in the following days.

Steam, Grill, or Roast a Huge Pile of Vegetables

Store them in the fridge. They can be eaten cold as a snack, or reheated as a side dish with a meal. An added bonus to steaming or roasting large amounts of low-carb vegetables at one time is that you can use some of the leftovers during the next few days in omelets or frittatas, added to meat loaves, or even just tossed in a bowl with cooked ground beef, turkey, or pork, and your choice of sauce or seasoning, for a quick and super-simple meal. I promise, low-carb cooking is much easier than you might think it is! Like I said: not difficult, just different.

Cook a Few Dozen Eggs at a Time

Don't waste your time soft- or hard-boiling one, two, or three eggs at a time. Think more like one, two, or three dozen. When kept refrigerated and still in their shells, they last quite a while, and eggs are one of the brain's very best snacks!

Make Meals Designed for Large Quantities

Cook once, feed yourself and your family for days. Think stews, chili, pot roast, and soups. Buy a large cut of meat, and put it in a slow cooker with some vegetables. Make two or three large meat loaves at once; they can be sliced and eaten cold for lunch or a snack.

Remember what they say: *Go big, or go home!*

Regarding Recipes and Cookbooks

I've included a list of cookbooks and recipe websites dedicated to low-carbohydrate and ketogenic cooking in the recommended resources at the back of this book. But you might be surprised at how much low-carb cooking you already do without even realizing it. So much of your routine cooking might be perfectly suitable for this nutritional strategy and you just don't know it. Omelets, beef stews, roast chicken, roasted or stir-fried vegetables, tuna and egg salads, baked salmon—these are all low-carb! The truth is, low-carb cooking isn't anything special, scary, or out of the ordinary. It's the same wholesome, real food that you're already perfectly comfortable preparing, minus the starchy items.

The best place to find fantastic low-carb recipes is the cookbooks you already own. Additionally, if you have a public library in your area, you might be surprised at the extent of the cookbook section; many public

libraries have excellent cookbook offerings, and you'll have no trouble finding cookbooks that are specifically for low-carb diets. That being said, many
recipes for home-cooked dishes are already low-carb. You don't need to go
out of your way to find specialized low-carb or ketogenic recipes and cookbooks. In fact, many cookbooks authored by popular celebrity chefs—none
of whom would remotely be considered "low-carb chefs"—have plenty of
recipes that are perfectly suitable for your brain-reviving, low-carbohydrate
diet. As you specifically look for dishes that contain meat, poultry, seafood,
lots of low-starch vegetables, and cheese and other high-fat dairy, you will
find endless interesting and delicious possibilities—no pasta, rice, corn,
potatoes, beans, or flour required! Vegetarian cookbooks are good sources
for recipes on how to prepare vegetables in new ways to keep you excited
about your diet. (Simply skip the recipes that contain beans and grains, or
use cauliflower as a substitute. Long-time low-carbers have perfected the
art of making "cauliflower rice," cauliflower hummus, and even mashed
cauliflower as a substitute for mashed potatoes. Some well-stocked supermarkets now even sell bags of "riced" cauliflower for easy use in recipes.)

A Note about "Treats"

Low carb is sometimes defined loosely. That means that when you flip
through low-carb cookbooks or look at recipes online, some recipes will
be higher in carbs than others. Use common sense and your best judgment
when determining whether a particular recipe is suitable for you or the
person you care for. Many of the books and websites you'll come across
will contain recipes for sugar-free desserts and treats, usually using ingredients like almond flour and coconut flour (instead of wheat flour). You
will be amazed at the amount of recipes out there for low-carb cookies,
cakes, quickbreads, muffins, cupcakes, and so on. There is room for these
things on a healthy low-carb diet to support brain function, but please
don't fall into the trap of making these items a regular part of your diet.
Low-carb treats should be approached the same way as regular treats: as
treats, meaning they are not for everyday consumption, and not in large
amounts. Remember: We are trying to stop, slow, and possibly reverse years
of compromised cognitive function due, in part, to insulin and glucose
dysregulation. Consuming too many of these imitation sugary foods will
stand in the way of progress. That being said, some of these items genuinely
are low in carbohydrate and high in fat, and for people who truly miss the

taste and texture of their old favorites, these things can make staying on plan much easier and more enjoyable.

Outfitting a Low-Carb Kitchen

In order to set yourself up for success in implementing this low-carbohydrate diet, there are a few tools I recommend having in your kitchen. These will help you prepare delicious meals that are appropriate for this diet, as well as make things in advance and store them so they'll be ready to go in a pinch.

Electric Egg Cooker

This is the best $30 you'll ever spend as a low-carber. This appliance will allow you to make up to seven hard- or soft-boiled eggs at a time, and they will come out perfectly every time, whether you prefer them soft (with gently cooked whites and runny yolks), medium, or hard (rubbery whites; dry, powdery yolks). Of course, you can boil a dozen or more eggs at a time in a large pot, but this device takes all the guesswork out of it. (I recommend a simple one from the Krups brand. I have used it nearly every day for several years, and it is still going strong. You can find it at most department stores, discount chains, and kitchen and bath stores and online from several retailers.) If you're an old hand at making hard-boiled eggs and have mastered the elusive craft, keep doing what you're doing. But if you're one of the many who are mystified by the process and whose hard-boiled eggs are nearly impossible to peel and are of unpredictable consistency, then this inexpensive device really is a gem, particularly considering the large role that eggs play in a low-carb diet to support brain health.

Slow Cooker

A slow cooker (also commonly referred to by one of the brand names, Crock-Pot) is indispensable for creating nutrient-dense, nourishing, low-carb meals with almost no effort whatsoever. Tough cuts of meat that are difficult to eat are ones that are especially delightful when made in a slow cooker—for example, oxtails, beef or veal shanks, beef tongue, brisket, and short ribs. Some of these cuts are very rich in collagen, gelatin, and connective tissue, all of which are especially beneficial for anyone with joint pain and digestive complaints, which are common in Alzheimer's sufferers because of advanced age. But almost any kind of meat can be cooked perfectly in a slow cooker: chicken breasts, pork tenderloin, chuck roasts, ribs, pork shoulder, and more. All that's required is a little bit of liquid (water, stock, broth, or even coffee) and some vegetables (carrots, onions, and celery work especially well, as do canned tomatoes).

Beyond being able to create delicious meals with very little effort, a huge benefit slow cookers offer is making large amounts of food at one time. Because most of the foods that are suitable for this nutritional strategy are whole, unprocessed foods that need to be prepared or cooked (rather than purchased in a bag or box, ready to go), you will find that it is helpful to make large amounts of food that will provide you with leftovers for a few more meals or snacks. You might even consider purchasing two slow cookers. Even the most impressive, high-tech models are relatively inexpensive and are available at nationwide discount stores. For those on an even tighter budget, the simpler, nondigital standard models are a low-carber's best bargain.

Storage Containers

Purchase glass, ceramic, and BPA-free-plastic food storage containers in a variety of shapes and sizes. These will be your go-to vessels for storing the leftovers your cooking endeavors will create, and also for storing foods that can be prepared ahead of time for easy snacking, such as celery sticks, sliced raw bell peppers, cucumbers, radishes, cheese cubes, sliced steak, and so on. Also be sure that you have a variety of smaller ones for convenient transport—this will allow you to take food with you on long car trips, or carry breakfast, lunch, or dinner with you if you'll be away from home for mealtime.

A note about plastic: Please avoid heating anything in plastic, even if it says "heat safe," or "microwave safe." Do not purchase vegetables that are advertised as "steam in the bag." Remember, this nutritional strategy is designed to heal the brain and body. When plastics are heated, potentially harmful compounds might leak into the food. For the same reason, I also caution against storing hot food in plastic containers. (For example, pouring piping hot soup or stew into a plastic container.) For this purpose, I recommend glass, or simply waiting until the food has cooled down a bit before putting it into plastic for storage. Plastic containers are lightweight and wonderful for keeping things in the fridge and freezer. It is not necessary to completely rid your life of plastic; just wait until foods are no longer hot before storing them in plastic, and place them in a different vessel for reheating. I recommend avoiding use of plastic containers when heat is involved; for microwaving, consider using glass, ceramic, or porcelain. All of this is, of course, up to you, and you should do what you are comfortable with.

Large Soup or Stock Pot

Soups and stews make great go-to meals for low-carbing. A large pot is an essential in any kitchen!

Blender or Immersion (Stick) Blender

Many recipes that pack a low-carb nutritional wallop call for a blender or immersion blender. This is a fantastic way to make creamy soups using steamed broccoli, cauliflower, asparagus, summer squash, and other vegetables that can be puréed and then thickened with cream, coconut milk, or sour cream.

Metal Steamer Insert

This is invaluable for making steamed vegetables (broccoli, brussels sprouts, zucchini, yellow squash, carrots, asparagus, etc.). You can find them online or at most department stores and discount stores. Microwave-safe plastic steamers are available if you're comfortable using them for this purpose.

Metal Roasting Pan or Cookie Sheet

Use this for roasting vegetables (onions, summer squash, brussels sprouts, broccoli, asparagus, peppers, eggplant, cauliflower, fennel, radishes). For people who claim they don't like vegetables, my guess is they've never had them roasted with bacon, or with good olive oil, salt, and pepper. Roasting vegetables at a high temperature brings out their natural sweetness, and the right seasoning helps to make them irresistible. If people are accustomed to being served vegetables that are soggy, mushy, bland, and boiled beyond recognition, it's no wonder they're not big fans. A change in cooking technique is all it takes to convert a veggie hater into a veggie enthusiast.

10-Inch or 12-Inch Glass Pie Plate

Crustless quiches are one of the most delicious low-carb meals out there. Eggs, cheese, onions, mushrooms, herbs, greens, roasted peppers—whatever you have on hand works. Quiches are a great way to use up leftover vegetables. Just throw 'em in! They're highly nutritious and can be eaten hot or cold any time of day.

Salad Spinner

You can wash salad greens in your sink, but I've found this tool to be quite handy, both for ease of washing and adequately draining lettuce and other greens, and also for storing them in the fridge. Salad greens seem to last a little longer when kept in this vessel after washing and spinning. Salads are a good vehicle for liberal amounts of dressing made from olive oil, avocado or macadamia oil, and nutritious add-ins, such as walnuts and blue cheese crumbles.

A Word about Dining Out

As the nutritional strategy outlined in this book is so different from the way you're likely accustomed to eating—and from the way most people are accustomed to eating—you might be asking yourself whether you can eat at restaurants while following this plan. The answer is YES! Provided you are careful about what you order, you can absolutely enjoy dining out while restricting carbohydrates. Fighting Alzheimer's with this dietary strategy will not prevent you from experiencing a nice meal with friends and family. Don't be shy about customizing your order and asking for substitutions when necessary. As people become more health-conscious and food allergies are becoming more common—not to mention the increased popularity of low-carb and Paleo diets—waitstaff are not put off or surprised by special requests. They are quite familiar with the modifications you will ask for, and servers will not look at you funny if you ask them not to bring the bread basket.

General Tips

Here is a guide to selecting appropriate foods that will allow you to continue getting the brain-nourishing benefits of your unique diet.

- Choose simply prepared dishes—grilled, baked, steamed, or roasted meat, poultry, seafood, and nonstarchy vegetables, or salads.
- Avoid all obvious starches and sugars, such as pasta, rice, bread, potatoes, corn, beans, soda, and desserts.
- At restaurants where free bread or rolls are provided before the food is served, request that the waitstaff not bring those to the table. Ask for something else if it is the type of restaurant that is likely to have something available; sometimes olives or pickles can be served instead of starches and grains.

- For full entrées, many restaurants offer your choice of a vegetable plus a starch as side dishes. Simply ask for a double portion of vegetables instead of the starch (for example, double steamed vegetables instead of a potato or pasta).
- For dessert, if you absolutely must have something sweet (or if you don't want your loved one to feel left out), see if fresh fruit is available. Berries are the best choice, and they can be served plain or with heavy cream, sour cream, or unsweetened whipped cream.

Tips for Specific Cuisines

Mexican: Fajitas are a great choice—just ask the server not to bring the tortillas, and ask for extra vegetables (peppers and onions) instead of rice and beans. Fajitas are just grilled meat and vegetables, and you can enjoy sour cream, cheese, guacamole, and pico de gallo as condiments. (Just be sure there's no corn in the pico de gallo). At the Chipotle restaurant chain, you can get meat, lettuce, cheese, and vegetables in a bowl rather than in a flour wrap.

Middle Eastern/Greek: Choose kebabs or other grilled meat dishes. Ask for extra vegetables or meat instead of rice or pita bread. Avoid stuffed grape leaves (which usually contain rice) and anything else with beans or high starch. These cuisines are famous for grilled meat specialties; take advantage of that, as well as marinated feta cheese, olives, and seared halloumi cheese. Small amounts of hummus are okay, but avoid the pita. Use raw cucumber slices or cherry tomatoes for dipping.

Indian/Afghan/Pakistani: These are somewhat similar to the Middle Eastern cuisines discussed above. Avoid rice and naan bread. Favor curries and dishes of grilled or roasted meat and vegetables; avoid chickpeas and potatoes.

Chinese/Japanese/Thai: Ask for your dishes to be prepared steamed or with no sauce. (Sauces typically contain sugar and cornstarch. Use soy sauce, hot mustard, or wasabi as condiments.) Great choices for Chinese takeout are steamed chicken or shrimp with mixed vegetables. Some restaurants also offer grilled chicken or beef on skewers. Avoid rice, noodles, wontons, dumplings, deep-fried foods, and tempura (due to the breading). Sashimi is wonderful; eat the fish but avoid the rice. For Thai restaurants, avoid noodle and rice dishes. Choose curries that contain meat or seafood and vegetables, spices, and coconut milk. Ask your server if the curries are thickened with flour or cornstarch; they might be able to leave those out.

Italian: You might get lucky and find a forward-thinking restaurant that serves spiralized zucchini "noodles" as a pasta substitute, but otherwise, pasta is not permitted. (Not even gluten-free pasta, as this will still be made from grains). Fortunately, most Italian restaurants have many other options that are suitable for a very low-carbohydrate diet. Choose salads, steaks, chicken, pork chops, or seafood with vegetables. Avoid bread and breadsticks, and ask for no croutons on your salad. Ask for extra nonstarchy vegetables instead of pasta or potatoes as side dishes.

Diner/American bistro: These restaurants usually have very diverse menus, and finding suitable options is easy. Just use the same logic as for anywhere else: no grains or other starchy carbohydrates, and no sweets for dessert. Fantastic choices are Cobb, chef, or Caesar salads (no croutons). Perfectly fine choices are bunless hamburgers or sandwiches. Always ask for nonstarchy vegetables instead of fries or other potato or pasta sides. You can often substitute a house salad for a starchy side dish. Other good selections include any type of roasted meat/chicken/fish, or a platter of egg or tuna salad on a bed of lettuce.

Breakfast: Stick with eggs, bacon, ham, and sausage. Avoid pancakes, waffles, potatoes, toast, bagels, muffins, fruit, juice, and jam/jelly. Western omelets are a great option (eggs, ham, onion, bell peppers), as are any type of omelets that contain eggs, meat, cheese, and low-starch veggies (peppers, spinach, mushrooms, onions, zucchini, and so on). Any other eggs are great, too: poached, scrambled, over easy, hard-boiled—however you prefer them. Avoid bottled ketchup, which contains high-fructose corn syrup. Use mustard, mayonnaise, or hot sauce as condiments.

Entrée salads: Customize your salad as necessary: no dried cranberries, fruit, or crunchy noodles. Stick with lettuce, spinach, and other greens. Suitable additions are chopped hard-boiled egg, bacon, cheese, avocado, ham, turkey, chicken, steak, salmon, olives, cucumbers, sliced peppers, radishes, and other nonstarchy vegetables. Use oil and vinegar or a high-fat dressing like ranch or blue cheese. Avoid Thousand Island, French, honey mustard, raspberry vinaigrette, and other sweetened dressings.

Chain restaurants: Chain restaurants like Applebee's, Chili's, Olive Garden, Outback Steakhouse, and others all have several suitable options. I have never encountered a restaurant that was not willing to substitute a double portion of nonstarchy vegetables for a starchy side dish.

Beware of Hidden Pitfalls

Don't be shy about asking your server for details on how foods are prepared. For example:

- Some restaurants add flour or pancake batter to their eggs to make omelets fluffier. Ask if this is the case, and if so, request that they prepare your eggs without that. (One way around this is to stick with your eggs hard-boiled, poached, or over easy/sunny-side up.)
- If there's a sauce with ingredients you're not sure of, ask the server to tell you what's in it. Many sauces contain sugar, corn syrup, cornstarch, or flour. It's best to stay with simply prepared dishes to avoid this.
- Be careful with condiments. Commercial ketchup is loaded with high-fructose corn syrup, and many salad dressings are high in sugar and corn syrup. Your best bets for condiments (if you need them at all) are mustard (any kind except honey mustard), mayonnaise, hot sauce, melted butter, olive oil, and vinegar (red wine, apple cider, balsamic). Full-fat, low-carbohydrate salad dressings are permitted—look at labels in supermarkets to get an idea of which types are best. The carb count per 2-tablespoon serving should be 2 grams or less.
- Prepare ahead of time! Most restaurants have their menus posted online. Look in advance to see what will be suitable for you so you'll have an easier time ordering. (Or so you can suggest a change of location if necessary.)

Eating on the Go

Just as with dining out, you should have no trouble finding suitable options to eat if you're on the road frequently or have a hectic schedule where you're running from one task to the next and don't always have time to prepare food or sit down to a full meal. Being pressed for time or being away from your usual cooking environment does not need to be an obstacle to sticking with a low-carb diet. Thanks to the expanding availability of appropriate foods just about everywhere, you'll be able to find something great no matter where you are.

Foods to grab on a quick run into a grocery store

- Salad bar (lettuce, peppers, mushrooms, olives, chicken, ham, bacon, turkey, tuna, cheese, radishes, hard-boiled eggs, cucumbers, carrots, sunflower seeds, and so on)
- Tuna or salmon in pouches or pop-top cans
- Nuts (plain, salted, or unsalted; avoid honey roasted)
- Pepperoni, salami
- Cold cuts and cheese
- Rotisserie chicken
- Deli department prepared egg salad or tuna salad

Foods to grab at a gas station or convenience store

- Hard-boiled eggs
- String cheese, cheese sticks
- Packets of cream cheese
- Beef jerky (choose plain or original flavor— BBQ, teriyaki, and others will have more sugar)
- Nuts
- Pork rinds
- Pepperoni
- Worst case scenario: hot dogs or burgers—no buns

In order to make sticking to a brain-nourishing low-carb, high-fat diet as easy and convenient as possible, you might want to consider keeping a supply of nonperishable foods handy in your car or desk drawer at work. Doing so will mean you're never caught in a circumstance in which you feel there is "nothing you can eat," and you opt for a high-carbohydrate item because you have no other options.

"Low-carb survival pack" to keep in your car, purse, briefcase, or desk drawer

- Pouched or canned tuna, salmon, sardines, mackerel, oysters, chicken
- Nuts, almond butter
- Beef jerky or meat-based snack bars
- Leak-proof container of coconut oil

And don't forget the supplies! It does no good to have great food available if you have no way of eating it, so keep a small stash of plastic silverware, napkins, paper plates, a can opener, and plastic storage containers where you have your "emergency foods" located.

Sweet Cravings

What can a dedicated low-carber trying to support brain health turn to when those sweet-demanding demons start rearing their ugly heads? Don't despair. Although it's best if you or your loved one can white-knuckle your way through cravings and just wait until they subside, sometimes they're just a little too strong. In those situations, there are options you can choose that will satisfy your sweet tooth while allowing you to continue getting the benefits of your low-carb diet without derailing your progress. For the times when you absolutely, positively must have something sweet, consider the following choices:

- ¼ cup of berries with whipped cream, sour cream, or full-fat plain yogurt
- Two or three dates stuffed with cinnamon goat cheese, cream cheese, or ricotta cheese
- Coffee or tea with cream, sweetener, and coconut milk or oil
- Canned pumpkin with cinnamon. Be sure to purchase 100 percent pure pumpkin and not pumpkin pie mix, which has sugar added.
- Red, orange, and yellow bell peppers, or cherry tomatoes, raw. In summer, when these are in season, you will be amazed at how sweet they are. Once you have been away from cookies, cake, cereal, and soda for a while, your taste buds will reacclimate to foods that are naturally sweet, and you will find ripe summer cherry and grape tomatoes to be as sweet as raspberries.
- Full-fat plain regular or Greek yogurt or cottage cheese with cinnamon
- Sugar-free candies—many brands, including Hershey's and Russell Stover, make sugar-free chocolates and hard candies that are readily available at your supermarket or corner drugstore. Remember that sugar-free chocolate typically contains large amounts of sugar alcohols, which might cause a laxative effect in some people.
- Sugar-free gelatin desserts. (Whole foods are preferred, but sugar-free gelatin can sometimes make the difference between having something low-carb friendly or straying from the plan. Try your

hand at homemade gelatin desserts using powdered gelatin, berries, and fresh-squeezed lemon or lime juice. They're easy to make, and you might find they require little to no sweetening at all.)

- Dark chocolate—85 percent or higher. You can now find 86 percent, 88 percent, and 90 percent from popular nationwide brands, such as Ghirardelli, Endangered Species, and Lindt. These are available at your local supermarket or corner drugstore. Even though these are sweetened with regular sugar, if you can stick to just one or two squares to satisfy a craving, the total amount of sugar in that small serving will be minimal.

CHAPTER 16

A Primer on Food Quality

This is a nutritional strategy intended to promote healing. Therefore, it is important that you buy the best-quality food you can afford. The Alzheimer's brain has been ravaged by the long-term effects of the poor-quality convenience foods that constitute so much of the modern diet, and in order to provide the most powerful elements for stopping and potentially reversing these effects, we need to go to the opposite end of the food quality spectrum.

If your current financial reality is such that you absolutely cannot afford anything other than what is on sale at the local supermarket, don't despair. Regardless of your budget, please keep reading in order to gain knowledge about the importance of choosing higher quality foods whenever possible.

Produce

Your produce should be local and organic whenever possible. Your very best source for these vegetables and fruits will be a local farmers' market. Many small-scale farmers grow their crops without the use of harmful pesticides, herbicides, and fungicides, but they are unable to claim that their produce is "certified organic," because the paperwork and monitoring required for certification by the USDA is too expensive and administratively burdensome. (These are small-scale growers; they need to spend their time and money on what's important—growing nutrient-dense foods—not on completing reams upon reams of forms to satisfy government bureaucracy.)

If you shop at a farmers' market and you are unsure about whether foods are organic, simply ask the vendors how they grow their produce. Even if organic is unavailable, you will still get a great nutritional bang for your buck by purchasing locally grown foods. In some produce, vitamins degrade over time, so the longer an item takes to get from the ground to your plate, the fewer nutrients it will deliver. This means that organic produce that was grown thousands of miles away (possibly in another country, or even on another continent) and took days, or possibly weeks, to get to the store, might provide you with fewer vitamins than a nonorganic food that was grown just a short distance away and picked only a couple of days before you see it at the farmers' market. Remember: We are trying to provide the struggling brain with as many concentrated nutrients as we can. Shop with that in mind.

Animal Foods

Even more important than the quality of your produce is the quality of your animal foods: the meat, poultry, dairy, seafood, and animal fats. Since these will make up your biggest source of calories, you should strive to make them as nutrient rich as possible. Again, the best source of these foods will be local livestock farms and fisheries that sell fish that are truly "wild-caught." Think of it this way: In just the same way that people get sick when they eat the wrong foods, animals get sick from improper diets. You can't get healthful foods from sick animals. Animals' anatomy, physiology, and digestive systems give us insights as to the types of diets they are biologically designed to thrive on. Here are some examples, based on the foods you are most likely to consume:

Poultry

Poultry (chickens, turkeys, ducks, other fowl) are omnivores. This means they can eat grains and grasses, but they are also well-equipped to consume worms, grubs, and other bugs they would naturally encounter when they are pastured—that is, allowed to roam freely on a grassy pasture, rather than being in indoor cages—or even "cage-free" but restricted to indoor barns with no access to sunlight, fresh grass, and insect larvae. (Don't confuse *pastured* with *pasteurization*, which is the process of heating milk and other foods in order to destroy pathogens.)

Despite clever marketing claims about "vegetarian diets" on egg cartons at the store, chickens—the ones raised for meat as well as the hens raised to lay eggs—are omnivores. They should be consuming insects and grasses in addition to their grain-based feed. Eggs from pastured hens will contain more nutrients in their yolks (including vitamins A and K₂, and the yellow-pigmented carotenoid lutein)—even more than ones that are labeled "cage-free" or "free-range." These terms are mostly unregulated and are largely meaningless. Should you choose to purchase eggs from a local farmer, you might notice the yolks are a much darker, deeper orange color than the insipid yellow you're accustomed to seeing in conventional eggs. Don't be alarmed. This is a good thing! This is a sure sign that the hens the eggs came from were truly pastured. You might also notice the shells are harder to crack—again, a higher mineral content in the shell is a sign that the hens consumed a better diet.

Be sure to eat the yolks! Egg whites are a good source of protein, but all the other nutrients—the vitamins and minerals, especially brain-boosting DHA and choline—are in the yolks. And by now, your worries about consuming cholesterol-rich foods are a thing of the past.

If you prefer to buy eggs from the local store, take heart. The manufacturers of brands of eggs sold at supermarkets are getting wise to these issues, and poultry feed is now often supplemented with flaxseed, chia, or fish meal, which increases the amount of omega-3 fats in the yolks.[1]

Beef

Forget açaí and gogi berries. Forget pomegranate juice and the latest "miracle fruit" discovered deep in the tropical rain forest. When it comes to delivering a nutritional knockout, grass-fed beef and the fat that comes with it are the true superfoods. When we hear the phrase "vitamins and minerals," we tend to think exclusively of fruits and vegetables, but the truth is, animal foods pack a huge nutrient wallop. Beef is loaded with B vitamins and minerals, but where grass-fed meats really shine is in their fat content. (And remember, fat will make up the majority of your calories, so it makes sense to get your fats from the best sources you can.)

Cows that eat grass concentrate the nutrients in that grass in ways humans can't. We can eat as many greens as we want, and we won't harness energy from them the way cows do. Meat that comes from cattle that consumed grass for their entire lives (grass-fed and grass-finished) has a different nutrient profile than meat from grain-finished cattle.[2] All cows start their lives on grass, but most spend their last weeks or months in large, industrial-scale feedlots, where they are fed soy, corn, and other grains, in order to fatten them up quickly for slaughter. You will find that grass-fed beef is leaner than grain-fed, but this doesn't mean it is lean. Depending on the cut, it will still have quite a bit of fat, and this fat is low-carb and nutritional ketosis gold.

The fat in grass-fed meat will be higher in omega-3 fats and lower in omega-6 fats than grain-fed.[3] Additionally, the meat and dairy products from grass-fed steers and dairy cows contain a unique type of fat called conjugated linoleic acid (CLA). (CLA is one of the naturally occurring beneficial trans fats discussed in chapter 12.) This special fat has shown promising potential for a variety of health concerns. Obviously, our concern here is cognitive decline, but perhaps this natural fat—which is virtually absent from the modern diet—has properties we haven't uncovered yet. This special type of fat is available almost exclusively in the fat of ruminant animals consuming their species-appropriate diets. (Beef from grain-fed cattle contains some CLA, but the amount is lower than in grass-fed beef. The same goes for omega-3s. Since beef fat is predominantly monounsaturated and saturated, and CLA, omega-3, and omega-6 are all polyunsaturated fats, the total amount of any of these polyunsaturated fats is still relatively low. Nevertheless, since the ratios of some of these fats might be important, it's not a bad idea to seek out meats from animals that have consumed a diet that results in better ratios.)

In cooking ground beef from grass-finished cows, there is no need to drain the fat. In fact, I encourage you to eat the fat. It is highly nutritious—not to mention delicious! Alternatively, if you do drain the fat, save it! Store it in a glass container in the fridge, and use it for sautéing greens or frying eggs, just like you would do with bacon fat. The same goes for cooking grass-finished steaks: no need to cut the fat off. Savor it! On a low-carb or ketogenic diet, fat is your friend!

Note: All of the above also applies to meat and fat from lamb, bison, and goat. It is less important to specify grass-fed for these animals, as almost all lamb, bison, and goats are grass-fed and grass-finished, but if you are unsure, ask the vendors when you buy these foods.

Dairy

Most of what applies to beef applies to dairy fats as well. Dairy products (butter, cream, cheese, and so on) should come from cows that are grass-fed. The fat will contain more CLA, more vitamin K_2, and more nutrients overall. Butter from grass-fed cows is low-carb gold just like grass-fed beef.

Consume it liberally. It's brain food! The healthy fats and cholesterol are exactly what the brain needs for repair. There are many suitable brands at health food stores in North America, but an even better option is to find a dairy farmer in your local area who produces butter or ghee from grass-fed cows. You will notice the butter will be much more yellow than the mass-produced brands of butter you're likely accustomed to. This is because when cows consume grasses, the chlorophyll, carotenoids, and other pigments that give grasses their eye-catching green colors become concentrated in the animals' fat. You can see this reflected in the color of butter as well as in the fat surrounding the meat of grass-finished animals. Tallow and suet from grass-finished animals will have a yellow hue to it, while that from grain-finished animals will appear more white. (*Note*: The yellow color does not apply to imitation butters, in the form of margarines and vegetable oil spreads. These typically have vibrant color added to make them more pleasing to the eye, but the nutrients are not there.)

Pork

If you've been eschewing pork because you're worried about its fat content, worry no more! Pork is an excellent source of protein, and just like beef, it's loaded with vitamins and minerals. And the fat from pastured hogs is yet another low-carb gold mine. It's delicious and is mostly monounsaturated and saturated. Moreover, as mentioned in chapter 11, the specific type of monounsaturated fat that predominates in pork is oleic acid, the very same one that predominates in olive oil and is the darling of the much celebrated, yet ill-defined Mediterranean diet. (Sauté your greens in reserved bacon fat—if you think you don't like kale or spinach, you will!) Seek out rendered lard from local farmers. Do not be afraid to consume bacon or sausages, as long as you trust the ingredients. We have been warned against consuming these kinds of "processed meats" because of links to various health conditions, but those associations are much more likely due to the wacky chemical preservatives and additives used in the mass-marketed national brands. Moreover, those studies are confounded by the concurrent consumption of carbohydrates. (For example: bologna or salami on sandwich bread, and sausages served alongside pancakes or toast at breakfast.)

When you buy bacon and sausages from small-scale local farmers, there will be little to none of those questionable ingredients. All you'll be getting is the meat, the top-quality fat, some salt, herbs, and spices. If you purchase bacon from pastured hogs and throw the fat away, you are doing yourself a grave disservice. Save the fat! Pour it into a glass ramekin and store it in the fridge. It will last a very long time without going "off"—not that it'll be around that long. You'll find all kinds of delicious ways to use it.

If you avoid pork for religious or cultural reasons, obviously, you may continue to do so. I am simply setting the record straight for those who enjoy pork products but have been avoiding them for health reasons, as this is not necessary.

Organ Meats (Offal)

If you're feeling adventurous, organ meats (also called "offal") are packed with nutrients. In fact, they're typically richer in nutrients than muscle meat. Beef liver is the superfood of yesteryear. Its vitamin and mineral content leaves most other foods in the dust. Liver from humanely raised animals that consumed biologically appropriate diets are nature's vitamins. Chicken or duck liver pâté or a liver mousse is a fantastic way to eat liver if you find pork, beef, or calf liver too strong. Pâté is a high-fat, ultra-nutrient-rich snack that you can enjoy as a dip for raw vegetable crudité or spread on grain-free or low-carb crackers or crispbreads. Heart is another nutrient-dense organ meat; if you find the texture of liver or kidneys off-putting, the texture of heart is more like that of other muscle meats because heart is actually a muscle. As an added bonus, because it's such a hardworking muscle, heart is loaded with CoQ_{10}. Ethnic markets (Asian, Hispanic, kosher) are good places to find liver, heart, tongue, kidneys, tripe, and marrow bones, and these cuts are usually more affordable than fancier steaks, chops, and roasts.

Seafood

Seafood is a wonderful choice for a low-carb diet designed to improve brain health. Choose fatty cold-water fish for some of the richest sources of omega-3 fats: salmon, sardines, mackerel. Do your best to purchase seafood that is truly "wild-caught." Just as beef cattle, hogs, and chickens are being concentrated into massive industrial-sized feedlots, fish are now being "farmed" in coastal pens, where they are fed rations that include pellets made from corn, soy, and wheat—foods that fish would never encounter in their natural marine habitats.[4]

It is important to seek out wild-caught fish for the same reason it's important to buy foods made from grass-fed and pastured land animals: They only produce the nutrients we expect them to produce when they consume biologically appropriate diets. For fish, this means eating seaweed and other marine plant life, smaller prey fish, krill, and plankton. One thing to take note of is that most fresh or frozen salmon you will find at the supermarket will say "color added" on the package. Truly wild salmon is naturally a very vibrant pink or red due to the tiny shrimp, krill, and other small marine organisms they eat. That pink or red color is the result of antioxidant nutrients that concentrate in the salmon flesh (for example, astaxanthin). Farmed salmon has a dull, lifeless, unappetizing color, which is why they add coloring to it—but just because they add color doesn't mean they add the missing nutrients.

Shellfish and crustaceans are another fantastic choice from the marine world. Shrimp is a rich source of cholesterol, the brain's best friend. Oysters, mussels, and clams are loaded with vitamin B_{12} and minerals, particularly zinc. They're also high in selenium and iodine, which are crucial for thyroid health, and selenium is required for recycling of glutathione, the body's most important internally produced antioxidant.

If you cannot afford the highest quality seafood, I still encourage liberal consumption of fatty seafood, as even the farmed varieties do still contain appreciable amounts of the crucial omega-3 fats. Canned salmon, sardines, and mackerel are very economical ways to include seafood in your diet.

Where Do I Find These Higher Quality Foods?

Your best bets for finding these foods are local farmers' markets or by driving directly to a farm with a store on the premises. If you do an online search for farmers' markets in your area, you will likely be surprised at how many you find. You can also search for local farms at Eat Wild (www. eatwild.com/products/index.html) and Local Harvest (www.localharvest. org/organic-farms/). Additionally, your local chapter of the nonprofit organization the Weston A. Price Foundation can connect you to farmers in your area who are producing these kinds of foods (www.westonaprice.org/ get-involved/find-local-chapter/). If there is no chapter in your immediate area, I recommend contacting the nearest one you can find. They will be able to recommend good food sources for you, and some of the farms they will be familiar with can ship their products nationwide.

What If I Can't Afford It?

If you cannot afford to purchase grass-finished meats and pastured eggs and poultry, THAT IS OKAY. Don't let that discourage you from following this nutritional plan. You will still experience the beneficial effects of the diet while eating the meat and dairy available at the regular supermarket. The major effects we are hoping to achieve with this nutritional strategy will come from a dramatic reduction in carbohydrate intake, coupled with increased dietary fat. The main metabolic change—making the switch to fueling the body primarily on fat and ketones, instead of glucose, in order to nourish the struggling brain—will occur as long as your macronutrients (fat, carbs, protein) are at the proper levels. As it relates to correcting the metabolic imbalances at the heart of Alzheimer's disease, it is far better that you eat whole, unprocessed, low-carb animal and plant foods from *any* source than that you revert to cereal for breakfast and pasta for dinner. Going the extra mile is simply a way to ensure you're getting the biggest nutritional bang for your buck. Don't let the struggle for food purity stand in the way.

If you'd like to prioritize how you spend your food budget, the highest priority should be getting the best-quality fats you can. This might mean buying butter, lard, or beef tallow from farmers with grass-finished steers, grass-fed dairy cows, and pastured hogs. Pastured hen eggs from a local farm might cost $5–$6 per dozen. This seems quite high compared to supermarket eggs that you can purchase for $2.99 or less per dozen, but do the math: At $6 per dozen, each egg costs just 50 cents. This is probably the single best food bargain ever. Egg yolks are loaded with cholesterol and choline, and are a good source of B_{12}—three nutrients absolutely critical for healthy brain function.

Another way to save on higher quality meats is to purchase them ground. Ground beef, pork, and lamb (and sausages made from them) are typically priced lower than steaks, chops, and roasts. For example, some grass-based farms sell ground beef for $5–$8 per pound, which might sound high compared to finding it on sale for $2.99 or $3.99 at the supermarket, but compared to cold cuts, these best-quality ground meats are a steal. (Turkey breast, roast beef, and ham embalmed with dextrose and corn syrup regularly go for as much as $7–$10 per pound at the supermarket deli counter!)

If you have a second freezer—or simply a lot of space in a single one—the most economical way to purchase the best-quality meats is to buy in bulk. If you have space to store a quarter beef or half a hog, you will be able to purchase several different cuts at lower prices than if you bought only a couple of individual steaks or chops. (You can also freeze butter. If you catch a good sale, stock up. Butter freezes wonderfully. Just make sure it's well-wrapped, as it can take on off-flavors if stored for too long and not tightly wrapped.) If you cannot imagine purchasing and storing that much food at once, consider pooling resources with neighbors, friends, and family who might be interested in joining you in acquiring the best-quality foods at a lower price. Speak to your local farmers about these buying options. They will be happy to help you!

PART THREE

Lifestyle Factors to Support Healthy Neurological Function

Alzheimer's disease is a multifactorial condition that requires a multifactorial intervention. While a diet low in carbohydrate and high in fat is the starting point and the cornerstone, it is not the only tool in the arsenal. In this section we'll explore issues beyond diet that will help support healthy neurological function. Lifestyle factors, such as sufficient sleep, physical exercise, and stress reduction, are equally important parts of this strategy to nourish the brain.

CHAPTER 17

The Importance of Exercise

H elping us to improve cardiovascular health and maintain mobility, strength, and flexibility aren't the only good things exercise does. One of the most important things exercise does for us is help us maintain insulin sensitivity, in part by "giving glucose somewhere to go." Consider physical activity—movement—an essential nutrient: *vitamin M*! It is well established in the scientific literature that exercise stimulates the insulin-sensitive glucose transporters in our muscle cells (called GLUT-4s). This means that when we exercise regularly, we can tolerate a higher carbohydrate intake than if we were sedentary. This does not mean, however, that regular exercise can take the place of a low-carbohydrate diet or that you can "buy yourself more carbs" by exercising. (This might hold true for a young, healthy, very athletic and insulin-sensitive person, but it is not true for an older individual whose cognitive function is declining.) It means that the combination of a low-carb diet with exercise is a double way to resensitize the body and brain to insulin. The insulin-sensitive GLUT-4s are also present inside the brain, and they are especially abundant in regions responsible for memory and cognition, such as the hippocampus.[1] Therefore, interventions intended to improve insulin sensitivity could potentially result in these brain regions taking up glucose more effectively.

After resistance training (weightlifting), muscle cells become more sensitive to insulin, but they also are able to absorb more glucose even in the absence of an insulin stimulus. In other words, the uptake of glucose by muscle cells is enhanced after intense exercise even without an insulin spike. Hard-charging athletes interested in increasing their muscle mass typically consume protein powders along with a dose of carbohydrate immediately after a workout, because insulin doesn't just facilitate glucose getting into the muscles; it helps amino acids get in, too. With this in mind, bodybuilders use a combination of protein and carbohydrate with the goal of building larger muscles. However, after an intense workout, muscles become more receptive to glucose and amino acids even without a carbohydrate-induced rise in insulin. We can think of this as exercise stimulating the muscles to become "sponges" that soak up glucose, regardless of the actions of insulin. Brain fuel metabolism researcher Stephen Cunnane and colleagues said it well: "Skeletal muscle is the main site of insulin-mediated glucose utilization in the body and so declining muscle mass (sarcopenia) in the elderly may be a factor contributing to the increased risk of insulin resistance associated with aging."[2]

Insulin resistance is extremely common in older people, as is a loss of muscle mass. So it makes sense that a condition related to insulin resistance—such as Alzheimer's—would be more common in older people. Some degree of muscle loss during the aging process is normal and to be expected, but we can slow and delay this deterioration by performing regular exercise and giving our bodies a reason to hang onto as much muscle as possible. Muscle tissue means more than just strong biceps or quadriceps. While strong, lean muscles might be aesthetically pleasing at any age, they are far more than just a way to show off in a tank top or bathing suit. Muscle tissue is extremely metabolically active, and building and keeping muscle mass for as long as we can is critical for healthy aging, both physically and cognitively. And the two things required for building and preserving muscle tissue are adequate protein intake and a physical stimulus.

With regard to utilizing glucose more effectively and lowering insulin levels, any type of physical movement is beneficial. Whatever you or the person you care for can manage, do it, and keep doing it regularly, whether that means walking, jogging, gardening, weightlifting, cycling, golf, shuffleboard, swimming, senior aerobics, senior stretching—anything. Just move.

As we age, we tend to be less physically active, so remain active if you already are, and if you're not, start getting active to whatever degree you can. Recall that mitochondria are the energy-generating factories in our bodies. And recall that optimal mitochondrial function is absolutely critical for a healthy brain. Muscle cells are loaded with mitochondria. (Of course they are; muscles perform hard work, and they need a lot of energy to power that work.) As one study's authors put it, "The chronic muscle disuse that accompanies aging or muscle wasting diseases provokes a decline in mitochondrial content and function, which elicits excessive

ROS formation and apoptotic signaling."[3] (Recall that ROS, or reactive oxygen species, are free radicals that damage mitochondria and other structures inside our cells. Apoptotic signaling refers to apoptosis, which is the death of a cell. So when we have significant loss of muscle mass, we might have more oxidative stress in the body, ultimately resulting in the death of cells. And we know that oxidative stress is certainly not limited to muscle tissue; it interferes with mitochondrial function and neuronal health in the brain as well.)

By staying active, you will give your body a reason to generate healthy new mitochondria. Exercise is one of the most powerful stimulators for "mitochondrial biogenesis"—that is, the body creating new mitochondria.[4] Aerobic endurance-type exercise (such as walking, jogging, cycling, or swimming) and resistance training both lead to mitochondrial biogenesis, so again, it is helpful to engage in whatever activity you are able to, although evidence suggests resistance training (or something else of a high intensity) might be slightly more beneficial for this purpose, particularly if combined with lower-level activity.[5] Hardworking muscle cells need lots of mitochondria in order to keep working hard. Mitochondria literally provide muscle cells with the energy they demand in order to do whatever they're doing: lifting a barbell, doing a push-up, or just carrying a heavy grocery bag from the car into the house. Physical movement gives the body the stimulus it needs to create more mitochondria and keep the ones it has in good working order.

Exercise has other beneficial effects for the brain apart from its role in stimulating mitochondrial biogenesis. Exercise has been shown to increase expression of signaling molecules that support memory and learning. One, in particular, called *brain-derived neurotrophic factor* (BDNF), is a key player in brain health and cognitive function, and Alzheimer's patients have reduced BDNF levels compared to healthy people.[6] Inducing an increase in BDNF is one of the primary ways by which exercise stimulates synaptic plasticity and improved cognition.[7] In a paper in the journal *Neuroscience*, a group of researchers wrote, "Brain-derived neurotrophic factor is a central player for the effects of exercise on synaptic and cognitive plasticity."[8] The effects of exercise on synaptic and cognitive plasticity—clearly, adequate exercise is as important for the brain as it is for the rest of the body. Regarding the connection between disturbed blood glucose and insulin handling, type 2 diabetes, and Alzheimer's disease, research published in

the journal *Experimental Physiology* concludes, "Brain-derived neurotrophic factor is likely to mediate some of the beneficial effects of exercise
with regard to protection against dementia and type 2 diabetes."[9] *Beneficial
effects of exercise with regard to protection against dementia*—it's hard to
state it any more clearly than that.

A major contributor to the processes of learning and
memory formation involves brain derived neurotrophic
factor (BDNF) signaling pathways. It has been known for
over two decades that physical activity or neuronal activity
markedly enhances BDNF gene expression in the brain
and that this increase in BDNF protein leads to activation
of signaling pathways that result in exercise-dependent
enhanced learning and memory formation.

—*S. F. Sleiman and colleagues*[10]

Moreover, elevated ketones—which you know by now are like rocket fuel
for the brain—might directly impact BDNF levels. Elevated ketones might
increase production of BDNF and be involved in exercise's positive effects
on memory, cognition, and synaptic transmission.[11] Memory, cognition,
and synaptic transmission: exactly the things that are compromised in the
Alzheimer's brain.

Physical activity—whether it's simply a walk around the neighborhood
or an all-out weightlifting session—induces myriad changes in the body
and brain. It shouldn't surprise us that exercise is one of nature's most effective and inexpensive antidepressants. It is beyond the scope of this book
to go into detail on the physiological adaptations exercise stimulates, but
it's no coincidence that exercise is a natural mood booster and seems to
also enhance memory and executive function.[12] Physical activity has been
shown to improve cognition in healthy older adults as well as those with
cognitive impairment.[13] One of the effects of exercise overlaps nicely with
those of a healthy low-carb diet—namely, improving the body's response to
insulin. The combined effects of proper nutrition and physical activity are
so powerful that scientists have said, "Exercise and dietary management

appear as a noninvasive and effective strategy to counteract neurological and cognitive disorders."[14]

Researchers have noted an inversely proportional relationship between the amount of physical activity an individual does and their risk for cognitive decline and dementia. That is, the more physical activity someone engages in, the lower their risk for dementia.[15] Exercise also seems to stimulate the growth of new neurons and the formation of new synapses in various regions of the brain, as well as increase the synthesis of neurotransmitters in parts of the brain involved in cognition, largely driven by an increase in BDNF and related compounds.[16]

However, lest you get the impression that you need to train for an Ironman triathlon in order to support healthy cognitive function, keep in mind that "too much" exercise might be just as damaging as too little. Intense exercise is a strong physiological stressor—that is, it is stressful to the body. That's the whole point of it, actually: It is in adapting to and recovering from this stress that our muscles become stronger and our cardiovascular systems become more efficient. People who work out intensely and frequently need to rest and recover just as intensely, with nutrient repletion and adequate calorie intake being a big part of helping the body recover. It is unlikely that the Alzheimer's sufferer you care for falls into the category of exercising too much (more likely they are too inactive), but I wanted to clarify this point in case younger people reading this were fearing that they need to quit their jobs in order to spend all day working out. As with antioxidants, as with water intake, so with exercise: Just because a certain amount is good doesn't mean more is always better, and there's usually a point of diminishing returns where more can even become harmful.

Walking is a fantastic way to keep yourself healthy. No special equipment or training required! Just lace up your tennis shoes, grab a friend, and go! Beyond that, if you are physically capable of doing so, you will get even better benefits from exercise that is more intense—something like lifting weights or moving your body more quickly. (Remember the notion of giving the mitochondria a challenge to adapt to and get stronger.) Exercise has also been shown to directly influence the health of mitochondria in the brain. Bottom line: Physical activity is crucial for maintaining metabolic and cognitive health and for helping to restore them if they've already been compromised. There might also be a role for regular physical activity in *preventing* cognitive decline and dementia.[17]

A Note for Those Unable to Exercise

If you or the person you care for is physically unable to exercise, you can still reap the benefits of this nutritional strategy. By far, the biggest "bang for your buck" comes from reducing insulin levels and generating ketones. Adding in exercise is just a way to up the ante and potentially make this nutrition and lifestyle strategy even more effective. However, if you are capable of performing any physical movements—even something simple, such as walking—please incorporate it as much as you can. If you or your loved one is able to exercise, then it should be a nonnegotiable part of this multipronged intervention to protect and preserve brain health. But an inability to engage in regular, vigorous activity is absolutely not a deal breaker with regard to healing the brain. So if the individual you care for is of very advanced age or has mobility issues that make even low-level activity an impossibility, don't despair. Exercise is only one arrow in the quiver; there are many more that you and your loved one can implement.

As always, before undertaking a program of physical movement, please check with your qualified health care providers to assess whether you are healthy enough to do so.

CHAPTER 18

Too Much Stress and Too Little Sleep Can Break the Brain

A low-carbohydrate diet and appropriate levels of physical activity are the cornerstones of a strategy to combat Alzheimer's disease and other forms of cognitive decline. But beyond those two pillars of this approach, there are other lifestyle factors that can affect cognitive function—for better or for worse. Two of the most powerful at work in Alzheimer's patients are stress and sleep.

Stress

Emotional and psychological stresses are lifestyle factors that can be managed to help reduce the damage in an Alzheimer's brain. Stress physiology is known to affect the entire body in myriad ways. Long-term high levels of psychological stress are associated with heart disease, diabetes, obesity, anxiety, depression, and more. One of the reasons psychological stress is associated with obesity and diabetes is that stress elevates levels of cortisol—one of the hormones responsible for the body's "fight-or-flight" response.

Cortisol is a *glucocorticoid* hormone. If you think that word sounds like glucose, you are correct! Cortisol's job is to provide our bodies with glucose in order to help us survive in a life-or-death situation. This glucose is supposed to give us a quick burst of energy—to allow us to literally stay and fight, or run (flee) for our lives, hence the aforementioned famous fight-or-flight phrase. In the ancient past, this was a great survival mechanism. If you were being chased by a wild animal, you would have needed lots of quick energy. But in modern times, we almost never face acutely life-threatening situations. More likely, we deal with common, everyday stressors that our minds and bodies are hard-wired to *interpret* as immediately dangerous, even though they are far from it.

It's important to note that when we say "stress," we are referring to anything that we *perceive* as stressful to us—so it doesn't have to be an actual life-or-death emergency. It could be something as simple as being stuck in an aggravating traffic jam, facing a tight deadline at work, or dealing with worrisome financial troubles or a difficult personal relationship. If these types of issues are a constant presence in your life or that of the person you care for, blood glucose will be somewhat difficult to manage unless and until you or your loved one learn some relaxation techniques to help you stay calm and cool.

Because of the role of cortisol in raising blood glucose, chronically high levels of stress can be the undoing of the best actions and intentions regarding a low-carb diet. Even if you are eating all the right foods and managing your carbohydrate intake, your progress might be stymied by high blood sugar due to stress. Stress will not affect blood glucose and insulin to the same degree that eating, say, a bagel would, but it will affect it somewhat. Your blood sugar might not be sky-high because of stress, but it might be slightly higher than it would otherwise be, even on a low-carb diet.

There are many ways to reduce and relieve stress. Common practices for this purpose include yoga, meditation, and deep breathing. If you are not interested in these pursuits, that's fine. (As they say, one person's pleasure is another's poison.) Just make an effort to regularly participate in activities that you do find relaxing. Perhaps it's reading, gardening, golf, taking walks in nature, watching comedy movies, knitting, cooking, or something of the like. Whatever it is that you enjoy doing that provides you with relaxation and joy, make it a frequent part of your life. Stress reduction is a key lifestyle factor in reversing the disturbed insulin signaling and other metabolic dysfunctions that underlie Alzheimer's disease.

Studies in animals indicate that stress has the opposite effect of exercise on brain-derived neurotrophic factor: While exercise increases BDNF, stress decreases it.[1] And we've just covered how important BDNF is for maintaining synaptic plasticity and supporting healthy cognition. The last thing we want is to be our own roadblock to healthy BDNF levels, so it's nice to know the way we respond to stressful situations is entirely under our control. It might not feel that way when we're right in the middle of something angering, but with deliberate intent, we can alter our emotional reactions and mitigate the effects of stress.

It's not surprising that a number of individuals with Alzheimer's disease were focused, driven, "type A" personalities in their younger, healthier years. The stereotype of the overworked, overstressed executive who falls ill "all of a sudden" is no coincidence. It's based in a significant body of truth. Individuals who pride themselves on always being "on," always being reachable, never taking a vacation, eating lunch (and breakfast and dinner!) at their desk, and getting a million and one things done at once do so at great risk to their long-term physical, emotional, and cognitive health. Family members of individuals with Alzheimer's, MCI, and other problems with cognition often confirm that their loved one was very productive at work or dedicated to raising the family at home, was always working for and taking care of others, but never took time for themselves. Their loved one was selfless, always putting themselves last. By not making rest, relaxation, and pursuit of some of their own interests a priority, these individuals might have unknowingly sacrificed their own long-term health. Contrary to what we tend to believe in modern American society, disconnecting from work, turning off the phone, hiring a babysitter, taking a vacation, having a "date night," and other ways to stop and catch your breath are not signs of weakness. They are, in fact, fundamental for good health, and we dismiss them at our peril.

Sleep

Following a healthy diet and making time for physical activity are important for maintaining insulin sensitivity and lean muscle tissue and for supporting healthy cognitive function. But it's not all about diet and exercise. Considering the powerful influence of circadian rhythms on multiple aspects of human physiology, getting to bed at a reasonable hour and getting a good night's sleep could be just as important. Insufficient sleep—particularly if it has been a long-term situation—might contribute to oxidative stress and neuronal loss in the brain.

Scientists are still elucidating the myriad crucial roles sleep plays in promoting health, but an absolute and unalterable requirement for sleep has been identified in every animal that has been studied. There are no exceptions. We all sleep, and we all *need* sleep. New reasons to get adequate sleep are identified all the time. A detailed discussion of the physiological details of sleep is beyond the scope of this book, but there are several important connections between sleep, healthy cognitive function, and loss of healthy cognitive function.

Modern industrialized society sometimes feels like a constant competition in which the winner is always doing more: Who can lift the most weight? Who makes the most money? Who drives the most expensive car or owns the biggest house? There's only one area where people like to brag about how *little* they do, and that's sleep. It's almost a badge of honor for people to brag about how late they stay up or how little sleep they need to function. (Never mind the coffee they inhale immediately upon waking or the energy drink they mainline when they start crashing in the late afternoon.) But racking up sleep debt isn't a contest. There's no blue ribbon for winning, and the consequences are no laughing matter. In fact, chronic sleep insufficiency can trigger serious metabolic effects, one potential long-term result of which is cognitive impairment.

Chronic sleep debt is associated with developing obesity, metabolic syndrome, and other health complications, including Alzheimer's. Moreover, disruptions in sleep patterns might also lead to decreased insulin sensitivity and elevated afternoon and evening cortisol levels, feeding into a vicious cycle of yet more sleep debt and hormonal dysregulation.[2] It is telling that the type-A, workaholic individuals described above are probably also likely to have chronic sleep debt. Whether they were staying up late to get more work done or because they did want to have time for themselves and long into the wee hours was the only time they could find, the result is that they might have spent years—decades, possibly—not getting adequate sleep.

Chronic sleep debt has very serious consequences for metabolic and cognitive health. Shortened sleep and fragmented sleep (waking up several times during the night) reduce insulin sensitivity and impair glucose tolerance, even among healthy young people, so imagine how much more dramatic the effects are in older people, whose bodies are naturally less resilient.[3] Combine this with the natural tendency for people to seek high-carbohydrate foods to provide a quick energy boost when they're tired, and the implications are obvious. A large body of evidence connects chronic short sleep with weight gain and obesity. Weight gain is the result of complex biochemical processes that can't be boiled down to something as straightforward as eating too much and moving too little. However, the conventional advice to "eat less and move more" isn't completely off base, and insufficient sleep might influence behavior in both of these areas: Too little sleep makes people hungry and tired—that is, more likely to eat *more* and move *less*.[4] If someone is tired and hungry, odds are against them being in the mood to hit the gym.

Obesity, however, is only one potential consequence of insufficient sleep. Far more nefarious issues can result. For example, due to the role of sleep in regulating insulin signaling and glucose handling, sleep dysregulation is closely associated with type 2 diabetes.[5] Many people with type 2 diabetes might have undiagnosed obstructive sleep apnea, which would impair their blood glucose control even in the presence of glucose-lowering medications and dietary modifications.[6] Some researchers even speculate that sleep apnea directly causes insulin resistance and type 2 diabetes because of the role of adequate quantity and quality of sleep in helping to properly regulate blood glucose control and the endocrine system as a whole.[7]

For the purposes of trying to reverse the metabolic damage that is preventing healthy cognitive function in an Alzheimer's sufferer, it's helpful to think of sleep as "fasting for the brain." Although the brain is quite active during the different phases of sleep, sleep is also when the brain clears out debris, old, worn-out cellular parts, and goes through a kind of "mini cleanse" each night. Sleep allows the brain to rest and reset, and don't forget, not getting enough sleep is stressful!

Beyond the easily recognizable feelings of anxiousness and irritability we experience when we don't get enough sleep, insufficient sleep is also associated with elevated cortisol levels and insulin resistance. Perhaps this is another sign of our prehistoric wiring at work: If we are not sleeping enough, our brains will assume there must be a reason. Maybe there's a threatening situation going on—a predator nearby or a conflict with a neighboring tribe—so it's in our best interest to stay awake and remain hypervigilant, with cortisol and glucose coursing through our bloodstream. Bottom line: Don't neglect sufficient sleep. Think of it as *vitamin S*—as important and necessary as any other vitamin or mineral.

The detrimental effects of chronic insufficient and poor-quality sleep on insulin sensitivity, blood glucose management, and stress physiology alone should make it clear that getting adequate sleep is near the top of the list of things that can help improve cognitive function. We all know we tend to think more clearly after a good night's sleep, and when we've been up tossing and turning all night, the next day is usually a struggle, both cognitively and emotionally. But for the specific purpose of improving cognition in someone with Alzheimer's or MCI, there's even more to the sleep story.

There are many ways by which waste products are transported out of the brain and central nervous system and delivered to the bloodstream for removal and excretion. One of these is called the glymphatic system.[8] The glymphatic system is most active during sleep and is largely disengaged during waking hours.[9] In fact, researchers speculate that the absolute biological requirement for sleep across all animal species might be due to the brain's need for this "down time" in order to eliminate potentially neurotoxic wastes.

Disturbed sleep patterns and disrupted circadian rhythms play a role in the pathology and progression of Alzheimer's disease, just as they do in obesity, insulin resistance, and metabolic syndrome.[10] Alzheimer's patients often have trouble sleeping and might wake many times during the night or find themselves awake or asleep at inappropriate times. It has yet to be determined for certain whether this altered circadian rhythm is a *cause* or an *effect* of the condition. It seems to be a little of both: Long-term poor sleep quantity and quality contribute to the development of Alzheimer's, and once the condition has taken hold and healthy neuronal communication is impaired, proper sleep becomes increasingly elusive.[11] So disrupted sleep patterns are both chicken and egg, but the preponderance of the scientific literature suggests that poor sleep is an initial contributing factor, which then spirals into a vicious cycle.

The role of poor sleep in affecting insulin sensitivity, stress hormones, and blood glucose management alone might be enough to explain at least some of the influence of disrupted sleep on Alzheimer's pathology. However, the detrimental effects are even stronger than these. Chronic sleep deprivation increases the deposition of amyloid plaques, and the accumulation of amyloid plaques seems to bring about disrupted sleep. Studies in mice indicate that more effective clearance of amyloid proteins results in normalization of the sleep-wake cycle.[12] Certainly, increased sleep duration might help the brain clear more plaques. The concentration of amyloid protein rises during wakefulness and falls during sleep.[13] That is, it shows a "diurnal" pattern. This is due in part to the heightened activity of the glymphatic system: Clearance of beta-amyloid proteins (which, if left to accumulate, form into the infamous plaques) occurs twice as quickly during sleep than during waking hours.[14]

Insulin-degrading enzyme (IDE) is another factor potentially affecting clearance of beta-amyloid proteins during sleep. Recall that two of the substrates for IDE (that is, the molecules this enzyme targets)—insulin and beta-amyloid—compete for the enzyme. However, the affinity of IDE for insulin is much greater than for beta-amyloid, such that whenever there are appreciable amounts of insulin in the body, the ability of IDE to break down the amyloid is reduced. One of the many things that occurs during sleep is a normalization—or, at the very least, a reduction—in insulin levels. In healthy people, during a long period of sleep, insulin levels will come back to a relatively low baseline. Even in someone who is insulin resistant, whose insulin levels are abnormally elevated nearly all the time, insulin levels might not completely normalize by the time they wake up, but they will be lower than typically found throughout the rest of the day. (The fasting insulin level first thing in the morning will still be high compared to that of a healthy individual, but relative to this person's usual high level, it will be at or near its lowest point.) At this point, because insulin levels are low, insulin is no longer a big source of competition for IDE, thus allowing the enzyme to focus on degrading the amyloid proteins. And remember, it is believed that Alzheimer's patients don't produce excess amyloid proteins; rather, the problem is that they accumulate and aggregate because they are not cleared away effectively.

With all this in mind, our affinity for catching a little shut-eye whenever we can might be an evolutionarily conditioned mechanism for ensuring that our brains have time to "take out the trash" on a regular basis. Overall, wastes are cleared more effectively from the brain during any kind of sleep than during wakefulness, so good sleep quantity and quality are key. There's also evidence that sleeping on one's side (as opposed to on one's back or stomach) makes waste clearance even more effective—at least in rodents.[15] We might not be able to say what the optimal sleeping position is for humans just yet, but one thing is for sure: Whatever posture someone assumes while they sleep, *being asleep* is the important thing.

Beyond the amount of sleep you or the person you care for gets, something to be mindful of is your sleep environment. Our hard-wired circadian rhythms expect us to be awake during daylight hours and asleep while it's dark. Lots of artificial light near bedtime and while we sleep can trick our bodies into thinking it's still daytime, and we will produce less melatonin—a key hormone that regulates circadian rhythms and helps us fall asleep and stay asleep. Try to remove as much artificial light as possible from your sleeping area. This means no bright digital clocks right near the bed, no streetlight flooding in from outside, and no electronic devices with bright screens just before you go to sleep. If a lot of light from outside comes in through your bedroom windows, consider purchasing "blackout curtains." These can be found at most home furnishing stores.

You might also consider establishing a routine for "sleep hygiene." In addition to turning off brightly lit electronic devices, this might involve turning the lights down an hour or so before you go to sleep, to wind down and ease your body into nighttime. If you are surrounded by bright lights—particularly overhead lights—right up until it's time to get in bed (or possibly even while in bed), it will be difficult for your body to get the signal that it's nighttime and time to go to sleep. (Use table lamps with softer lighting rather than harsh overhead lights if possible. If you have dimmer switches, use them!) If you have trouble falling asleep, I recommend sublingual melatonin lozenges or herbal teas intended to promote restful sleep. Getting sufficient exposure to sunlight during the earlier hours of the day can also help regulate your circadian rhythm and promote better sleep later that evening.

CHAPTER 19

Intermittent Fasting: Boost Ketones and Let the Brain "Clean House"

Another lifestyle strategy to consider implementing in order to help heal a struggling brain is occasional or intermittent fasting. After all the emphasis on food and nutrients earlier, it probably seems strange to read about *not* eating. But there's a method to the not-so-madness. People who engage in fasting for religious or spiritual purposes often report feelings of extreme clearheadedness and physical and emotional well-being. Some even feel a sense of "euphoria." They usually attribute this to achieving some kind of spiritual enlightenment or nirvana, but the truth is much more down to earth and scientific than that: *It's the ketones!*

During fasting, as blood glucose and insulin levels remain low, the body shifts to using fat as its primary fuel source, and upon metabolizing higher amounts of fat, the body produces higher levels of ketones. As we have established, ketones are a superfuel for the brain. When the body and brain are fueled primarily by fatty acids and ketones, respectively, the brain fog, mood swings, and emotional instability that are caused by wild fluctuations in blood sugar will be a thing of the past, and sharp, clear thinking becomes the new normal.

Fasting can be extremely therapeutic for an Alzheimer's sufferer, as well as for those with milder forms of cognitive decline and impairment. Digestion is a very energy-intensive process. We don't typically think of digestion as "exercise," and while it's certainly not the same as running a marathon, at the cellular level, digestion is quite a workout. (There's a reason we feel so sleepy after Thanksgiving dinner—or any large meal, for that matter—and it has nothing to do with the tryptophan in the turkey. Digestion requires a lot of energy, and with increased blood flow and nutrients being diverted to the digestive organs, there's less for the rest of the body.) During a fast, with no food coming into the body, the body is spared the task of channeling resources toward digestion. Instead, it can concentrate its energy on clearing out old cellular debris and repairing damaged tissue—crucial factors for restoring healthy cognition.

Fasting has been practiced throughout the ages for a host of reasons, and it might be particularly helpful for Alzheimer's victims due to the role of insulin-degrading enzyme (IDE) in clearing away the beta-amyloid proteins that muck up neurons, form advanced glycation end products, and alter the shape of neuronal synapses. Recall that insulin and beta-amyloid compete for the attention of IDE, but insulin is IDE's "favorite child." This means that as long as insulin levels are elevated (which they frequently are in the context of the high-carbohydrate modern American diet, especially among the millions with insulin resistance), IDE will prioritize clearing the insulin, thus allowing the beta-amyloid to accumulate. Only when insulin levels are low—such as on a very low-carbohydrate diet, and even more so, upon fasting—will IDE be able to focus on going after the amyloid proteins.

If you have tried fasting in the past for religious observance or other reasons and found it difficult, you might be pleasantly surprised at how easy it is once your body is adapted to running on fat. When you are fat-adapted, you are no longer subject to wild fluctuations in blood sugar, and it is these highs and lows that make fasting a daunting prospect to people who are dependent on constant carbohydrate feedings to keep their energy levels up.

A well-formulated low-carbohydrate diet should prevent hypoglycemia, so your biggest obstacles to fasting will likely be psychological, rather than physiological. In the modern industrialized world, we are accustomed to eating 'round the clock. We eat when we're happy, sad, bored, excited, stressed out, lonely, watching TV, celebrating, mourning, and just about anything and everything else. In order to fast successfully, try to divorce yourself from the notion that you are "supposed to" eat several times a day. It is okay—beneficial, in fact—to become reacquainted with feelings of hunger. For most of human history, large amounts of food were not readily accessible all throughout the day. Intermittent fasting was likely a regular part of human evolution, and it's possible our bodies—and brains—have come to expect periods of food scarcity. Because we are blessed with abundant food all year long in the twenty-first century, we now have to make a special effort to impose food scarcity upon ourselves for therapeutic purposes. We are wired for feast and famine, but thanks to the bounty of inexpensive food available everywhere we turn, we are living with feast, feast, feast.

One of the most prominent researchers into the biochemical mechanisms and effects of intermittent fasting (IF) has written that, in part, IF mimics the effects of exercise, such as increased levels of BDNF in the brain,[1] and "BDNF increases the resistance of neurons in the brain to dysfunction and degeneration in animal models of neurodegenerative disorders."[2] Fasting also reduces oxidative damage in cells, and fascinatingly, caloric restriction (of which fasting is simply the most extreme form) increases "numbers of newly-generated neural cells in the adult brain suggesting that these behavioral modifications can increase the brain's capacity for plasticity and self-repair."[3]

Caloric restriction and IF induce a plethora of beneficial biochemical changes almost too numerous to detail here.[4] For the specific goal of healing the Alzheimer's brain, one of the most important things fasting does is improve insulin sensitivity and facilitate the use of fats and ketones for fuel. Beyond that, fasting induces a kind of "stress" upon cells, but a good kind of stress. Exercise does the same thing. Many people engage in exercise for stress-relief purposes, and indeed, it can be very effective for this—at least, for psychological stress. At a cellular level, however, exercise is physically stressful. As mentioned previously, it is in *adapting* to this stress that the body gets stronger and more resilient. The brain is the same way. The beneficial adaptations to the biochemical "stress" of fasting help to protect neurons from degeneration and death.[5] Studies in animals show that many of these positive changes occur even without fasting, simply by going longer between meals. According to experts in these mechanisms, "Interestingly, increasing the time interval between meals can have beneficial effects on the brain and overall health of mice that are independent of cumulative calorie intake."[6] This means that even when total food intake is not reduced at all—the amount of calories consumed is the same—simply going longer between meals can induce some of these helpful effects. (Yes, it was a mouse study, but it is still informative.) So rather than the conventional advice you

might be accustomed to hearing about eating several small meals throughout the day, it might be beneficial to consume larger meals less frequently.

Another benefit of fasting is a process called *autophagy*. This is a fancy
science word that translates to "self-eating." In simplified terms, it is the body's
way of reusing, recycling, and just generally tidying up. The "self-eating"
part describes what happens inside tissues: When the body no longer has to
prioritize the monumental task of digestion—a process we typically engage
in three times a day, and some of us more than that—it can turn its attention to cleaning house. That is, it moves old, worn-out, and malfunctioning
cellular debris and either allows the body to get rid of it altogether or else
repurposes the various amino acids, sugars, and fatty acids for other tasks
or structural destinations. To be clear, autophagy happens inside us all the
time; it's a normal, beneficial process. It is simply upregulated during fasting
or dramatic calorie reduction.

Something to tack on to fasting that might enhance its impact is exercising during a fast. It is not recommended for older people to perform intense
exercise while fasting, but slower, low-intensity activity is a way to boost fat
metabolism and ramp up ketone production even further. Consider taking
a long, slow walk first thing in the morning, prior to consuming any food.
(You can have coffee or tea beforehand if you need that in order to "become
human." Add coconut or MCT oil to it, and you'll be a ketone-fueled beast!)

Just as with exercise, fasting is not required on this plan. It is simply
one more tool in the toolbox in the fight to regain brain health if you or
your loved one are well enough to do so. I will say again, however, that
once you are fat-adapted, fasting can be thought of as a time for the brain
to "clean house."

There are many ways to incorporate fasting into your lifestyle. You can
experiment with a full twenty-four-hour fast once a week, or once or twice
per month, or consider "intermittent fasting," which can be implemented a
few different ways:

1. Schedule dinner and breakfast such that at least twelve hours pass
   in between. For example, finish eating dinner at 7 p.m., and do not
   eat again until breakfast the following morning, no earlier than 7
   a.m. This is one of the strategies Dr. Bredesen, whom I introduced
   you to earlier, employs in the program he has used to reverse
   Alzheimer's disease. (This is why going for a walk or doing some

other physical activity in the morning prior to eating might be helpful; a nice walk outdoors in pretty scenery can help take your mind off the fast and enable you to delay breakfast a little longer.)

2. Eat your meals within a "compressed feeding window." That is, only consume food during a preset number of hours per day. For example, eat only between 10 a.m. and 6 p.m., for an eight-hour feeding window, or between 10 a.m. and 8 p.m. for a ten-hour feeding window.

During a fast, there are a limited number of foods and beverages you can consume and still consider yourself to be in a fasted state. The key thing to keep in mind is keeping blood glucose and insulin levels low. This means avoiding carbohydrate entirely and consuming little to no protein, but perhaps allowing yourself to have small amounts of pure fat, which perturb insulin very little to not at all, as long as they're consumed in the near absence of carbohydrate and protein.

Things you may consume during a fast

- Water—obviously!
- Coffee
- Tea—herbal, green, or black, whatever you like
- Small amounts of heavy cream (aka heavy whipping cream) for use in your coffee or tea
- Coconut oil and MCT oil—by themselves or added to a hot beverage
- 1–2 ounces of macadamia nuts, walnuts, or pecans
- Pure fat—occasional pats of butter, a spoonful of olive oil, coconut butter
- Broth (homemade bone broth or made with bouillon cubes)— good for important electrolytes, especially sodium

You might find some of what you see in the list above to be quite strange. But being able to have "just a little something" might be what enables you or your loved one to sustain a therapeutic minifast, which might otherwise be difficult. And remember, the key is to avoid anything that would affect insulin and blood glucose levels, so items that are pure fat or close to it are perfectly logical choices. When you are new to a very low-carbohydrate diet, taking a bit of pure oil on a spoon might be an extremely foreign concept to you, but as you progress with this diet and lifestyle, you might find—as many seasoned low-carbers have—that it's actually quite pleasant. If anything, you can consider a spoonful of coconut or MCT oil during a fast to be the ultimate "brain medicine"!

A Word of Caution

Fasting is not appropriate for everyone. As always, consult with your licensed health care provider before experimenting with a fasting strategy to determine whether it is appropriate for you or your loved one. Everyone should check with their doctor, but this is especially true for people with diabetes, as medication schedules might need to be tailored to avoid dangerous hypoglycemic events. Additionally, fasting is not recommended for elderly individuals who might already be underweight.

PART FOUR

Setting Yourself Up for Success:
Beyond Diet and Lifestyle

In this section, we'll go beyond diet and lifestyle and address other factors that will help you be successful in implementing this brain-nourishing plan. We'll cover what to expect as you adjust to the change in diet, ways to optimize digestive function to ensure you absorb the wonderful nutrients you'll be eating, and the importance of moral support for staying on the path. We'll also cover the critical issues of medication and contraindications for this type of diet.

CHAPTER 20

Your Roadmap for Making the Transition

The basics of adopting a brain-nourishing low-carb, higher fat diet are simple, but before you get started, there are a few important things you need to know about in order to modify the diet and lifestyle strategies to best suit your or your loved one's needs. In this chapter, we'll cover issues like medication, what to expect when you make such a dramatic change to your diet, how vegetarians and vegans can follow a low-carb plan, and whether there's anyone who should *not* follow this kind of diet.

Dive Right in or Make the Change Gradually?

Whether to jump in immediately and change the way you or your loved one eats overnight or to ease into this strategy gradually is a choice only you can make. You must do whatever you are comfortable with, but my recommendation is to get started immediately. We are in a race against nutritional and environmental damage that has been inflicted upon the brain for a very long time. In my opinion, there is no longer any time to wait.

However, if you are more comfortable making a gradual transition to lower carbohydrate consumption, then proceed accordingly. You would do well to record your typical carbohydrate intake for a few days so you get a baseline, or starting point, for how much carbohydrate you normally consume. You will need to determine for yourself how you will approach the incremental reduction if this is the method you choose. Perhaps you will start with 25 percent less for a week or two, then move to 50 percent less, then 75 percent. Or perhaps you'd prefer to consume low-carbohydrate meals for breakfast and lunch, and "save" your carbohydrates for dinner.

(This might be a better strategy than using your carb allotment for break-fast, as that runs the risk of inducing cravings for more as the day goes on. Also, remember that insulin levels are typically at their lowest first thing in the morning. This would be the *worst* time to spike them up via breakfast cereal, an English muffin, or a glass of juice.) Whatever strategy you choose, just make sure you are reducing the amount of carbohydrate you consume as time goes on. In order to reap the neurological and cognitive benefits of a low-carbohydrate diet, you will need to reach a level of carbohydrate intake that is low enough to keep insulin levels relatively low and generate at least some amount of ketones.

Another way to approach a gradual transition is to remove individual foods from your diet over time, so that after a while, the most detrimental foods are no longer part of your routine. For example, for the first week, change nothing but cutting out pasta (or rice, or bread, or whichever item you choose to start with). The following week, remove something else—beans, perhaps, or potatoes. Eventually, you will reach a point where your diet no longer includes any of these, but your switch to a low-carb protocol will have been more manageable and less intimidating for you.

Regardless of whether you dive right in or make a gradual transition, there are several issues you should be aware of before adopting your brain-supporting low-carbohydrate diet. We'll start with the two most important: (1) How the diet might interact with medications that are common among older individuals and diabetics (the two groups most likely to experience cognitive impairment or Alzheimer's), and (2) Who should not follow a ketogenic diet.

A Word about Medication

Upon implementing this nutritional strategy, the dramatic change to your diet will have powerful and quick effects on your physiology. This means that the pharmacology and metabolism of any drugs you are taking might be altered. It is critically important that you be aware of this and that you and your doctor or other licensed health care providers plan accordingly. *Note*: Do not alter your medication on your own. Work with your qualified health care practitioner in monitoring the changes to your body and to determine the appropriate course of action. But be proactive about this, because some important changes will happen very quickly—sometimes within just days of starting the diet.

Blood Pressure Medication
(Beta Blockers, Calcium Channel Blockers, and Others)

One of the most rapid changes upon adopting a low-carbohydrate diet is a reduction in blood pressure. If you have elevated blood pressure, this is, of course, a good thing. However, if you are currently taking medication to control your blood pressure, you must keep in mind that combining the medication with a low-carbohydrate diet could lead to a situation of dangerously low blood pressure.

If you or the person you care for are under a physician's orders to follow a low-sodium diet for hypertension, please note that insulin levels have a far greater influence on blood pressure than does dietary sodium. Insulin is one of the primary influencers of how the kidneys retain minerals and electrolytes—sodium, in particular—and a significant reduction in insulin levels, as would be expected on a very low-carb diet, leads to the body excreting more sodium than when insulin levels are high.[1] Moreover, increasing evidence points to *sugar*, rather than sodium, as the primary driver of hypertension, leading some researchers to write that we've been demonizing "the wrong white crystals."[2] It's no coincidence that many people who adopt a low-carb diet are able to stop taking their blood pressure medication, because the diet is such a powerful natural way to lower blood pressure.

Insulin and Oral Diabetic Agents

It should be clear by now that one of the hallmarks of a low-carbohydrate diet is a reduction in fasting as well as postprandial (after meals) blood glucose and insulin levels. You will very likely require much less insulin than you are accustomed to taking. The same might also be true for any oral medications you are taking to control blood glucose or insulin levels. You must keep this in mind when bolusing your insulin or you could potentially induce a dangerous situation of low blood glucose. (*Note*: Your understanding of what constitutes low blood glucose will change as a result of this diet. In the past, you might have begun to feel symptoms of a low while your glucose was in the 70s, 80s, or even 90s [mg/dL]. This is because your body might have been accustomed to running at 150–200 mg/dL or even higher. The truth is, blood glucose in the range of 70–80 mg/dL is perfectly normal and healthy, and as long as you have enough fatty acids and ketones fueling your body and brain, you shouldn't experience symptoms of hypoglycemia in that range.)

Blood Thinners

The dramatic change to your nutrition will affect the viscosity of your blood. The effect is even greater if you supplement with fish oil or increase your intake of fatty fish, flax oil, or other omega-3-rich supplements and foods. (Think of fish oil as a natural blood thinner.) A slight natural thinning of the blood might also occur due to much less glycation of the blood and blood vessels. If your blood is less "sticky" and the vessels are more forgiving, your blood will flow more smoothly and fluidly. If you are on a pharmaceutical drug to thin your blood or prevent clotting (such as Coumadin, Warfarin, Plavix, or even a baby aspirin), please work with your physician to monitor your health and evaluate whether it is advised that you keep taking it or discontinue it.

Prescription or Over-the-Counter Antacids

Long-term use of drugs that block or suppress secretion of stomach acid such as proton pump inhibitors (PPIs), H2 receptor antagonists, Pepcid, Rolaids, Tagamet, Tums, and Zantac will prevent you from properly digesting, absorbing, and assimilating the nutrients in your food. It does no good to choose health-promoting foods to heal your brain if your digestive capacity is compromised by drugs that are specifically designed to interfere with the digestive process. You might be surprised that this change in diet greatly reduces your need for these medications. Anecdotal reports from thousands of people who've adopted low-carb diets is that acid reflux and gastroesophageal reflux disease (GERD) disappear not long after they stop consuming grains—yes, even those "healthy whole grains." (We cover digestive function in detail in chapter 21.)

Cholesterol-Lowering Medication

Reducing the body's endogenous synthesis of cholesterol is in direct conflict with trying to increase the amount of nourishing, brain-boosting cholesterol we want to make available. Recall that cholesterol is absolutely essential for a healthy brain. If you are on a cholesterol-lowering medication, such as a statin (also known as HMG Co-A reductase inhibitors), speak with your doctor about titrating down your dose or possibly getting off the medication altogether. It is an obstacle to restoring healthy cognitive function. Other types of medication that reduce cholesterol levels (such as cholestyramine and other bile acid sequestrants) work via a different biochemical mechanism and do not have the devastating side effects that statins do.

Glucocorticoids and Steroid Drugs

Glucocorticoid and corticosteroid drugs are types of synthetic cortisols, often prescribed as pain relievers and anti-inflammatories. (Common names for these drugs include cortisone, prednisone, and dexamethasone.) They are particularly common among arthritis and rheumatoid arthritis patients—a population group with a large overlap into the Alzheimer's and cognitive impairment patient population. Like the body's own cortisol hormone, corticosteroids can elevate blood glucose, which is directly antagonistic to trying to keep insulin levels low and facilitating ketone production in order to nourish struggling neurons. The good news is, low-carbohydrate diets are wonderful for naturally reducing joint pain and inflammation (there's nothing more inflammatory than chronically high blood sugar and insulin, especially when combined with lots of omega-6-heavy vegetable oils), so you might find that after your body has transitioned to running on fat, your need for these medications is greatly reduced. If, over time, you find this is not the case, consider speaking with your physician about switching from glucocorticoids to targeted anti-inflammatory nutritional supplements (such as omega-3s and curcumin), which will not interfere with blood sugar and insulin.

Is There Anyone Who Should Not Follow a Low-Carb Diet?

The low-carbohydrate dietary strategy outlined in this book has been used safely to treat everything from epilepsy to diabetes (both type 1 and type 2) to heart disease. It is a health-supporting and health-restoring diet. That being said, there are some people for whom this diet is not appropriate, or who will require close monitoring by a physician. The following is a list of conditions for which a ketogenic diet is absolutely contraindicated:[3]*

- Carnitine deficiency (primary)
- Carnitine palmitoyltransferase (CPT) I or II deficiency
- Carnitine translocase deficiency
- Beta-oxidation defects

---

* Note: Most of these conditions are identified early in life, although porphyria can develop at any time.

- Mitochondrial 3-hydroxy-3-methylglutaryl-CoA synthase (mHMGS) deficiency
- Medium-chain acyl dehydrogenase deficiency (MCAD)
- Long-chain acyl dehydrogenase deficiency (LCAD)
- Short-chain acyl dehydrogenase deficiency (SCAD)
- Long-chain 3-hydroxyacyl-CoA deficiency
- Medium-chain 3-hydroxyacyl-CoA deficiency
- Pyruvate carboxylase deficiency
- Porphyria

Other conditions might not mean a ketogenic diet is out of the question, but if you have any of the following, work with your physician to determine if this way of eating is suitable for you:

- Reduced liver function
- Reduced kidney function
- Obstruction of the bile duct or hepatic duct

Although this diet is not a "high-protein" diet, it may contain more protein than you are used to eating. Higher amounts of protein are not problematic for healthy people, and research has proven that higher protein intakes do not cause liver or kidney damage.[4] However, if you have preexisting liver or kidney function compromise, you should exercise extra caution if you choose to implement this diet and work with your physician to regularly monitor pertinent lab values.

What if I've had my gallbladder removed?
You can absolutely follow this diet if you do not have a gallbladder, even if your doctor has advised a low-fat diet (as is common after gallbladder removal). For information regarding how to support your digestive function—especially the gallbladder and digestion of fats, refer to chapter 21.

Can I follow this diet if I keep kosher, observe the laws of halāl, or avoid specific foods for other religious reasons?
Yes, absolutely. Simply avoid the foods that are proscribed by your faith, and partake of the others. There is no single food that is

"required" on this diet, so avoiding pork, shellfish, beef, or whichever specific foods the tenets of your faith dictate is not a problem.
Whatever the particular foods you do consume, the important thing
is to keep carbohydrates very low, protein adequate, and fat high.

Can I follow this diet if I am a vegetarian or vegan?

Yes, but . . .

This diet emphasizes fat and protein from animal sources. If you
are a lacto-ovo vegetarian (someone who consumes dairy products
and eggs), you can absolutely still reap the benefits of this diet, as
you can obtain a fair number of calories and nutrients from cheese,
eggs (especially the yolks), butter, cottage cheese, and so on. You
can also get complete protein from eggs and dairy products, but if
you find yourself with a slight shortfall on protein, you might want
to consider a protein supplement (such as whey), because one of the
main sources of protein on a vegetarian diet—beans and legumes—
must be limited due to their carbohydrate content. In order to reap
the maximum benefit from this dietary strategy, I encourage you
to consider adding seafood to your diet—start with bivalves and
mollusks (oysters, clams, mussels, scallops) if you prefer to ease
your way back into consuming marine animal flesh. These are
particularly rich in some of the vitamins and minerals a struggling
brain needs most (including B_{12}, zinc, and selenium). If you prefer
to get the majority of your fat from plant sources, such as olive oil,
avocado, nuts, and seeds, that's fine, but do remember the critical
importance of the nutrients that are more bioavailable from animal
sources than from plants.

This diet will be much more difficult to follow as a vegan. However,
there are ways to implement at least some of the guidelines of this
diet while still completely avoiding any and all animal-sourced
foods if you insist on doing so. You will do your brain a wonderful
service by reducing your sugar and grain consumption as much as
possible, and getting the bulk of your calories from healthy fats (such
as avocados, olive oil, coconut products, and nuts and seeds) and
low-glycemic vegetables and fruits. Due to the restriction of beans,
you will likely need a supplemental protein source. For plant-sourced
proteins, consider pea, hemp, or rice proteins. I do not recommend

soy protein. If you wish to still get some of your protein and nutrients from legumes or pulses, many people find that lentils have a relatively low glycemic impact, and they are nutrient rich.

As I mentioned earlier in this book, I am not suggesting that beans and starchy vegetables are "bad" for health, nor that they are not nutritious. They are wholesome foods that have nourished healthy and robust populations for centuries. However, keep in mind that the dietary strategy outlined in this book is specifically intended to induce a metabolic shift in the body away from glucose as the predominant fuel source. So while a higher carbohydrate diet might be perfectly fine for young, healthy, fit individuals, a different approach is warranted for older people who are already experiencing signs and symptoms of metabolic derangement and cognitive impairment. Nevertheless, a vegan diet that emphasizes healthy fats, contains no grain or refined sugar, and is relatively low in starch might go a long way toward improving insulin sensitivity and overall metabolic health.

Certain nutrients that are critical for healthy cognition and mitochondrial function either are available only from animal foods or are more bioavailable from animal sources than from plants, such as pre-formed DHA and EPA (the long-chain omega-3 fats, as opposed to the ALA found in plants), zinc, iron, and B_{12}. If you are a vegan, I encourage you to reconsider your convictions regarding the consumption of animal foods that have been in the hominid food supply for millennia. Reintroducing these foods might quite literally save your life. If nothing else, consider reintroducing them for sixty to ninety days. If you notice no change at all in your cognitive function or overall health, then return to your previous plant-only way of eating. If you have been a lacto-ovo vegetarian or vegan for a significant length of time and you decide to reintroduce animal muscle or organ meats into your diet, you might find that supplemental digestive support, as outlined in chapter 21, helps your body readjust.

You will be pleasantly surprised at how many vegetarian recipes you'll find in low-carb cookbooks. Since low-carb diets typically exclude grains, beans, and starchy vegetables, low-carbers are seasoned veterans when it comes to making creative dishes using nonstarchy vegetables. Contrary to media stereotypes, low-carb diets are a far cry from being all about bunless bacon cheeseburgers. You certainly need not abandon the rainbow of delicious vegetables and lower sugar fruits you have come to enjoy; simply avoid the ones that are high in carbohydrate.

Beware of the Low-Carb "Flu"

Remember that you are making a dramatic change in your diet. The transition from running on carbohydrate to running on fat will be a shock to your body. There will be an adjustment period, and it's important to know how to make the switch as easily and comfortably as possible. For the first few days, you might experience flulike symptoms and actually feel a little worse before you feel better. Be aware of this, and be ready for it. It is completely normal, and it will pass. You are literally going through withdrawal from a drug—sugar—and it's only natural that you might experience some unpleasantness at the beginning.

Some of the things you might experience while your body learns to make the switch from burning sugar to burning fat are:

- Headaches (might be severe)
- Nausea
- Dizziness
- Irritability
- Low energy
- Hypoglycemia
- Reduced appetite (at first)

Please do not be alarmed or discouraged. You will get through it, and once you do, you'll likely feel much better. The difficult, temporary transition is a small price to pay for giving your brain a chance to heal. The worst will pass in just a few days. But to help ease you through it, here are some of the things you might notice and how to manage them:

Dehydration

Drink water. A lot of it. You might feel dehydrated because of the large amount of water your body will let go of in the first few days. This happens because you will be getting rid of the stored carbohydrate (glycogen) in your body. Along with glycogen, our bodies store water. In fact, for every gram of glycogen we store, we carry almost two and a half times as much water. So during the first few days of carbohydrate reduction, as your body burns through that glycogen, you'll lose a fair bit of water along with it.

Consider adding trace mineral drops to your water. Some of the symptoms listed above are the result of electrolyte imbalances due to changes in the way your body holds onto water and minerals in the context of a low starch intake. Don't wait until you're thirsty to drink. If possible, keep water near you, and drink from it throughout the day. It is recommended that you drink at least half your body weight in ounces of water per day. (For example, if you weigh 140 pounds, you should drink no less than 70 ounces, but you can count tea and coffee toward this amount.)

Leg or Muscle Cramps

With all the water you'll lose at first, you'll lose some minerals, too. (Think of them as being flushed out with the water.) Certain minerals and electrolytes are important for muscle contraction and relaxation, and leg cramps or other muscle pain sometimes result from imbalances in these minerals. Leg cramps usually respond to extra potassium and magnesium, via supplements. You might be especially low on sodium, since your salt intake will decrease dramatically when you eliminate packaged, carbohydrate-rich foods that are loaded with salt as a preservative. Don't be afraid to salt your food. Natural, whole, unprocessed foods tend to be very low in sodium, and it's okay to add some during cooking or at the table. Sodium is an essential nutrient, and it is especially important on a low-carb diet. (I recommend an unrefined salt, like Redmond Real Salt or Celtic Sea Salt, but regular table salt you can find at the supermarket is just fine. No need to search for fancy and expensive pink, red, or black salts from exotic locations!) If you experience fatigue or muscle cramps, consider drinking a cup or two of broth made with bouillon cubes.

Bad Breath

If you notice a metallic or just plain bad taste in your mouth (or a brave spouse or loved one points it out to you), this is a sure sign you've made the switch to running on fat. In the early stages of dramatically reducing your carbohydrate intake, you'll break down fat at such a high rate that the ketone by-products overwhelm your body's ability to metabolize them all, and some of them get released via your breath, sweat, and urine. When they come out in the breath, they taste and smell like acetone. (In fact, acetone is exactly what the breath ketones are.) The best remedy for this "keto breath" is to stay hydrated by drinking plenty of water. An occasional sugar-free breath mint or piece of sugar-free gum is permitted, and chewing on fresh mint leaves or raw parsley is a good, natural way to freshen breath.

Reduced Appetite

When your body transitions to running on fat, you might find that your appetite isn't what it used to be. This is because, on a cellular level, your body is *already* eating—it's "eating" its own fat stores, and since even a lean person has a relatively solid supply of body fat to draw on, you might not feel hungry as much or as often as you're accustomed to. Don't force yourself to eat. It's okay to skip meals or eat less than you're used to eating. However, if low appetite persists for several days and you find yourself feeling lethargic (low energy), try to eat some fat and protein. A sustained lack of appetite might cause you to go too long without sufficient calories, and the low energy might simply mean you need to get some fuel in. This is especially important if you or the person you care for are underweight. (Many older people are, and it's important that they eat sufficient food.) Coconut milk is an excellent and easy way to get in a large amount of calories from fat, with the added brain boost from the medium-chain triglycerides.

Constipation

In some people, this dramatic change in diet will result in a change to usual bowel habits. This is due in part to how the body holds on to water, and also to the overall reduction in fiber from whole grains and even from vegetables. A relatively lower potassium intake might also play a role, so supplemental potassium might be warranted. You will be consuming plenty of fibrous vegetables, but you will have eliminated bran cereal, fiber bars, prune juice, and other things you might have relied on in the past to help keep you regular. If you find that constipation is an issue for you, I recommend herbal laxative teas. Two good ones are Smooth Move from Traditional Medicinals and Get Regular from the Yogi brand. You can find these at most health food stores, at well-stocked regular supermarkets, and online. You can also find psyllium husk online or at health food stores. This is a good fiber supplement. An additional method for easing constipation is supplementing with magnesium citrate. A popular way to do this is by using a magnesium citrate powder, adding it to warm or cold water in the evening, before bed. A brand of magnesium citrate powder you can find at health food stores and online is Natural Calm. It's available in a variety of delicious flavors, all sweetened with stevia. It's fine to drink this magnesium powder earlier in the day, but it's recommended in the evening because in addition to its laxative effects, magnesium is a natural muscle relaxer, and some people find it helps them fall asleep.

Your bowel habits aren't the only thing that might change because of the shift in your diet. Because you'll be avoiding many of the foods that were likely dietary staples for you, and you might also be introducing foods that are new to you, it's important to make sure your digestive system is up to the task. Many older people struggle with healthy digestion. Ensuring good digestive function is the subject of the next chapter.

CHAPTER 21

Support for Healthy Digestive Function

The dramatic change in diet you will be undertaking requires good digestive function. You will likely be eating more fat and protein than you were previously, so it's important that you have adequate production of stomach acid, bile, and pancreatic digestive enzymes in order to break down and absorb all of the wonderful nutrients in these foods. It does no good to eat brain-nourishing foods if your digestive function is compromised.

Unfortunately, digestive fire naturally declines with age. Production of stomach acid, bile, and digestive enzymes in older age is often not what it was in youth. Additional complicating factors affecting digestion in older individuals include ill-fitting dentures, weakened jaw muscles, dental decay, and other issues in the oral cavity that might result in difficulty chewing or swallowing. There are reasons many older people prefer a bowl of noodles or a few slices of bread for dinner rather than a pork chop. (Also, high-carbohydrate foods seem easier to prepare. For someone in their eighties living alone, boiling macaroni or microwaving a bowl of oatmeal is a less burdensome task than grilling a steak.) These issues need not interfere with implementing a low-carb, high-fat diet. Easy modifications can be made so that your loved one can easily and comfortably enjoy suitable foods. But first, let's have a short lesson in basic digestion.

Stomach acid production declines with age, so there is a chance that you or the person you care for do not produce robust amounts of it. Some signs of reduced stomach acid production are bloating, gas, excessive fullness after meals (feeling like your food is sitting there like a brick), and, ironically, heartburn or acid reflux. Yes, it's true: Acid reflux is often the result of too *little* stomach acid, rather than too much. There's even a fascinating book about this written by a medical doctor, Jonathan Wright, along with Lane Lenard, PhD, called *Why Stomach Acid Is Good for You.*[1]

In a nutshell, the stomach is supposed to be acidic. The pH of stomach acid (hydrochloric acid, or HCl) is approximately 1–3 when empty (3–5 when full)—this is a very strong acid! (On the pH scale, which measures acidity and alkalinity, 7.0 is neutral. Lower numbers are acidic; higher numbers are alkaline. It's a logarithmic scale, so pH 6 is ten times more acidic than pH 7, and pH 5 is a hundred times more acidic than pH 7. So you can see that stomach acid is an extremely strong acid.) The stomach needs to be highly acidic because the acidity helps to prepare proteins to be broken down and digested farther along in the gastrointestinal tract, and there are digestive enzymes released in the stomach that function optimally only in a very acidic environment. Moreover, the acidity of the stomach contents as they hit the first part of the small intestine is what triggers the secretion of subsequent digestive enzymes from the pancreas, which help break down proteins, fats, and carbohydrates. So if the stomach is less acidic than it's supposed to be, the entire digestive cascade will be compromised.

One of the reasons heartburn and acid reflux are associated with low stomach acid is that if there isn't enough acid to start the breakdown of food as quickly and efficiently as is supposed to occur, then foods remain in the stomach longer than they should. They begin to ferment and putrefy, and it is this bubbling gas that "refluxes" back into the esophagus, causing the familiar burning and irritation you might experience as heartburn. So you see, in many cases, when you suffer from indigestion, it is *more* stomach acid you need, rather than less, and over-the-counter or prescription antacids will actually make the problem worse. In the short-term, they will provide relief from the immediate symptoms you feel, but they do nothing to address the underlying cause of the problem for the long term.

If you or the person you care for are currently taking a prescription antacid, please be aware that this will absolutely compromise your ability to digest your food and absorb and assimilate the nutrients it contains—nutrients the struggling, starving Alzheimer's brain is desperate for. Work with your physician to see if you can titrate down to a lower dose, or perhaps, in time, get off the drug(s) entirely.

If you take over-the-counter antacids for occasional heartburn and indigestion, consider weaning yourself off them and boosting your stomach's acidity naturally. Remember—very often, it is more acidity you need, not less. Here are several ways to naturally boost stomach acidity and help support healthy digestion:

- Consider taking 2–3 tablespoons of apple cider vinegar 10–15 minutes before your meal. (You can dilute this with a small amount of water.) Any type of vinegar will aid digestion, so consider using homemade vinaigrettes on salads and steamed or roasted vegetables. Many mustards and hot sauces also contain vinegar, so use them liberally as condiments. It is not a coincidence that many cultures around the world include some type of acidic or lacto-fermented foods (containing lactic acid) with their meals to ease digestion. In Eastern Europe, they take sauerkraut or pickles with meat meals; in Asia, there's kimchi, pickled radishes, or pick-led ginger with meat and fish. In Greece and the Balkans, yogurt sauce is customarily served alongside lamb, and yogurt is also often included alongside Indian cuisine. These culinary traditions have persisted through the ages for good reason. Moreover, vinegar has some surprising and fascinating beneficial effects for lowering blood sugar and insulin after meals, so that's even more of a reason to incorporate vinegar into meals.[2]
- Eat slowly and calmly. If your body is engaged in the fight-or-flight response because you are stressed out, anxious, worried, or wolfing down your food in a hurry, then the rest-and-digest part of your nervous system will have trouble kicking into gear.
- Avoid drinking large amounts of liquid with your meals—cold liquids, in particular. Large amounts of beverages will dilute what-ever little stomach acid you do produce. We don't want that! Stick with sipping from a small glass of cool or room temperature water, or at least water that isn't ice cold from the refrigerator. You should not need to drink large amounts of beverages with meals. You should be drinking enough water throughout the day that you are not overly thirsty come mealtime. If you are accustomed to using liquids to "wash your food down," the solution for this is simple: Chew more thoroughly! If you find that you need liquid to wash your food down, you are likely trying to swallow boluses that are too large. Just chew more thoroughly and break your food down

into smaller pieces. Sipping warm or room temperature water with fresh lemon juice is another good way to have a small amount of liquid and aid digestion.

- Always chew thoroughly. The more your food is broken down by chewing, the greater the amount of surface area your stomach acid and digestive enzymes have to do their work. When you think you're ready to swallow, stop and chew ten more times!
- Consider using supplemental HCl or digestive enzymes.

If You've Had Your Gallbladder Removed

Special consideration should be given if you have had your gallbladder removed (cholecystectomy). You can absolutely still follow and benefit from this high-fat, low-carbohydrate diet, but you might require some supplemental digestive support, specifically in the form of ox bile.

The gallbladder is a small sack that sits under and behind the liver, and it stores bile. (The liver produces bile; think of the gallbladder as its holding tank.) So what is bile? Bile does to fats what laundry detergent does to dirt: it's an emulsifier. It breaks down fats into tiny droplets, which gives fat-digesting enzymes more surface area upon which to do their work. Bile doesn't actually digest anything itself; its job is to help the enzymes that *do* digest fats work better. What triggers the release of bile at the proper time is the presence of fat in the small intestine. According to Dr. David Williams:

> With a healthy gallbladder, proper amounts of bile are released into the digestive tract as needed. Without a gallbladder, there is a continuous trickle of bile into your system regardless of the presence or absence of fat. The failure to match bile output to fat presence jeopardizes one's ability to properly digest fat and, eventually, leads to deficiencies in fat-soluble vitamins and essential fatty acids, poor cholesterol metabolism, and the absorption of improperly digested fat globules.[3]

So you see, even without a gallbladder, your body still produces bile. The difference is, it gets released constantly (albeit in small amounts), whether you've consumed any dietary fat or not, because your gallbladder is no longer there to receive the physiological signals that regulate the properly timed release of bile. And when you ingest dietary fat, the amount of bile that gets released might not match up with the amount of fat waiting to be digested. So even though the liver actually makes bile and the gallbladder simply stores it and sends it out, many people who've had their gallbladder removed find that their digestion of fats is improved with ox bile supplements. Even if you do have a functioning gallbladder, you might find you cannot "tolerate" a high-fat diet without supplemental biliary support—at least, at first. Over time, as your body gets accustomed to the higher fat intake, your own bile production might adjust and catch up. During the early stages, signs that you are not digesting your fats well (and therefore are not getting the nutritional benefits of the fat itself nor the fat-soluble vitamins) include stomachache, loose stools, and fatty or greasy stools.

A Note about HCl and Digestive Enzyme Supplements

There are many avenues available for supplements designed to stoke digestive fire. These are available over the counter and can be found at most health food stores and online. Work with your qualified health care practitioner in order to determine if any of these might help you make sure you're getting the most out of your brain-nourishing high-fat diet, and to determine appropriate dosing.

- HCl-only supplements: Supplemental stomach acid, usually sold as betaine HCl.
- Gallbladder support: At well-stocked health food stores, you can find ox bile supplements or digestive blends that include ox bile and other ingredients intended to support the digestion of fats. (Beet juice and taurine are often included for this purpose.)
- Broad-spectrum digestive support formulas: These are blends that contain several compounds intended to improve digestion. They typically include HCl, pancreatic enzymes, lipases, amylases, and proteases (enzymes that digest fats, starches, and proteins, respectively), pepsin, ox bile, taurine, beet juice, and bromelain or papain. (Bromelain and papain are plant-sourced enzymes that help break down proteins.)

Be aware that many signs and symptoms of reduced digestive function—gas, bloating, belching, heartburn, and feeling overly full after a small amount of food—often go away on their own upon adoption of a low-carb diet. These symptoms are frequently the result of poor digestion of grains, so removing them from your diet will likely help a great deal. Reduced need for antacids—and often, no need at all—is a common beneficial effect of low-carb diets. You might wish to start the diet and see how you feel for a while without supplemental digestive aids, and add them in later on only if you feel you need them.

Modifications for Impaired Chewing and Digestion

As I mentioned earlier, many elderly individuals aren't able to chew, swallow, and digest as heartily as they did in their youth. This need not be an obstacle to following this type of diet. There are myriad recipes for low-carb, high-fat soups, stews, curries, chili, and other dishes that are soft and easily chewed. Rather than tough cuts of meat, people with difficulty chewing can enjoy ground beef, lamb, pork, chicken, or turkey. Tough cuts of meat can be made amazingly tender by cooking them in a slow cooker at a low temperature for a longer amount of time. "Low and slow" is an excellent way to create meals from cuts of meat that are inexpensive and extremely nourishing for the body and brain, such as oxtails, beef or lamb shanks, and, of course, a good stock or broth made with gelatinous bones and joints. For those who have difficulty consuming enough calories (many elderly people have a low appetite), soup is a great vehicle for added fat, such as coconut milk, butter, tallow, or any other fat that would lend flavor and calories.

Vegetables can be roasted or steamed until soft, and then puréed in a blender or food processor. Once puréed, they're an additional vehicle for butter, coconut oil, olive oil, or another delicious fat that can be either blended right in or drizzled on liberally as a finishing garnish. This is a simple way to get vegetables into people who might otherwise have a hard time eating them. Puréeing is not required, of course. Even foods as tough in their raw state as broccoli, cauliflower, and brussels sprouts become very tender when steamed or roasted, and they can be eaten as is. For steaming vegetables, I recommend using a metal stove-top steamer basket rather than boiling directly in water, as some of the minerals might leach into the cooking water.

I don't typically recommend the use of "liquid food," but for individuals with very compromised ability to chew, and also those with low appetite, high-fat smoothies are a good way to provide a substantial amount of calories in a way that doesn't need to be chewed at all. Using coconut milk as the base for these is a good way to get brain-boosting MCTs into your loved one. For those who dislike the taste of coconut, unsweetened almond, hemp, or other nut or seed milks may be used, and consider adding pure MCT oil for the potential rise in ketones.

—CHAPTER 22—

Not by Diet Alone: Effective Nutritional Supplements

B ecause the damage observed in AD brains is complex and multifactorial, any intervention intended to delay or possibly reverse this damage should be a multipronged strategy designed to address as many of the individual contributing factors as possible. As emphasized throughout this book, the foundation of what might be considered an "anti-Alzheimer's" strategy is a ketone-producing, low-carbohydrate diet. We have also explored lifestyle practices that can improve insulin sensitivity and support healthy cognition by inducing brain mitochondrial biogenesis and increasing synaptic plasticity. In addition to these interventions, there are numerous nutritional supplements that could be effective based on their biochemical functions.

Your intake of some of these nutrients will increase naturally as a result of the change in your diet, but you might find benefit in including some of them in amounts above and beyond what you would typically get from food. Please work with a qualified health care practitioner to determine which of these—if any—might be appropriate for you or your loved one. Additionally, please keep in mind that supplements are just that: supplements, not substitutes. Dietary supplements are *supplemental* to the nutrients you get from your diet. They aren't magic pills, and they don't exert their effects in a vacuum. Supplements can help, but since they do relatively little to alter the underlying metabolic aberrations most likely causing cognitive impairment in the first place, they should be used in conjunction with the diet and lifestyle interventions that do more strongly impact metabolism and insulin sensitivity. They are an adjunct to, not a substitute for, the more powerful factors.

That being said, some of these nutrients and compounds are required for healthy insulin signaling, blood glucose management, and mitochondrial efficiency, so if you or your loved one has subclinical or outright deficiencies of them, then restoring your body to adequate levels could have a significant beneficial impact on cognitive function and overall health. With that in mind, here is a selection of supplements that might be of benefit:

Zinc

Insulin-degrading enzyme, which breaks down amyloid plaques in the brain, requires zinc as a cofactor.[1] Interestingly, zinc deficiency is known to cause reduced senses of taste and smell (olfaction), and many Alzheimer's patients have impaired olfactory senses.[2] In fact, worsening of olfaction has been used as a marker for disease progression.[3] Suboptimal zinc status could be contributing to Alzheimer's pathology on multiple levels. (Red meat, liver, and shellfish—oysters, in particular—are good low-carb sources of zinc.)

Chromium Picolinate

The mineral chromium is part of what is called the "glucose tolerance factor" and has been proven to aid in glucoregulation and insulin sensitivity.[4] Any condition involving insulin resistance and disordered carbohydrate metabolism might benefit from supplemental chromium.

Alpha-Lipoic Acid

Alpha-lipoic acid is a powerful antioxidant.[5] It can actually help the body "recycle" other antioxidants, such as glutathione and vitamins C and E, leading some researchers to call it "an antioxidant of antioxidants."[6] Considering the role of mitochondrial oxidative stress in the etiology and progression of MCI and Alzheimer's disease, this could be a helpful intervention. Additionally, alpha-lipoic acid has been shown to aid in glucoregulation, largely by enhancing insulin secretion and sensitivity,[7] so supplementation could be effective via multiple mechanisms that might be beneficial to someone with cognitive impairment or Alzheimer's disease stemming from insulin resistance or poor glycemic control.[8] Lipoic acid might increase the need for biotin (a B-vitamin), so biotin should be included in the supplement regimen of individuals taking alpha-lipoic acid.[9]

High-Quality Fish Oil, Krill Oil, Cod Liver Oil, or Other Omega-3 Supplements

These supplements balance the omega-6 to omega-3 ratio and decrease inflammation. As discussed in chapter 13, high consumption of oils rich in omega-6 fatty acids (such as soybean, corn, cottonseed, and sunflower) contribute to chronic inflammation in the body, while n-3-rich oils generally stimulate anti-inflammatory pathways. Omega-3 and omega-6 fats are both "essential fatty acids," and we do require some omega-6 in our diet. The problem arises when we consume far too much omega-6 relative to omega-3, as is the case in the typical modern American diet.[10] And don't forget, neuronal cell membranes require lots of omega-3s, especially DHA. Fatty fish is the best source of omega-3s, but if you don't consume this on a regular basis, fish, krill, or cod liver oil supplementation might be beneficial.

Coenzyme Q$_{10}$

CoQ$_{10}$ is a critical component of the mitochondrial electron transport system, which is what produces energy in our bodies. It is also a potent antioxidant. With the Alzheimer's brain struggling to produce energy and under great oxidative stress, CoQ$_{10}$ could be a powerful adjunct. Supplemental CoQ$_{10}$ might be especially important for people taking statin drugs. (Recall from chapter 9 that statin drugs impair the body's ability to generate CoQ$_{10}$, and memory loss, fuzzy thinking, and problems with cognition are frequently reported side effects of statin use.) Animal models of neurodegenerative disease show that CoQ$_{10}$ supplementation increases brain mitochondrial content and might help these conditions, many of which stem from impaired mitochondrial function.[11] There haven't been many trials looking at CoQ$_{10}$ in human Alzheimer's patients, but it has shown a lot of promise in reducing the amyloid plaque burden and improving symptoms in mouse models of the condition.[12] It's possible that CoQ$_{10}$ supplementation could be particularly beneficial for vegetarians following a low-carb or ketogenic diet, since the richest food sources of this compound are animal proteins. Moderate amounts occur in nuts and seeds, and small amounts in some vegetables and fruits.[13] Among animal sources of CoQ_{10}, the highest concentrations are found in hardworking tissue, such as heart, liver, and kidney.[14]

L-carnitine

Carnitine is an amino acid required to burn fats at a cellular level. When we transition the body from running on carbohydrates to running on fats, we need to make sure the "metabolic machinery" is in place to handle the fats. As discussed in chapter 5, the furnaces where fats are broken down for fuel are inside the mitochondria, the tiny power plants inside our cells. Carnitine helps transport fats into the mitochondria, so someone on a reduced carbohydrate diet with the specific intention of ramping up ketone production and energy generation from fatty acids might benefit from supplemental carnitine.[15] The human body synthesizes carnitine, so it's not technically an "essential" nutrient, but supplemental amounts could potentially be helpful. The richest food sources are animal proteins and dairy products, and L-carnitine is absorbed better from foods than from supplements.[16] Data has been mixed regarding the efficacy of L-carnitine specifically for Alzheimer's, with some studies showing promise for delaying progression, and others showing no effect.[17] It would be fascinating to see a clinical trial comparing the effects of carnitine supplementation versus no supplementation in AD patients following a ketogenic diet, as most studies are typically done in people following their habitual high-carb diets.

Berberine

Berberine is an alkaloid compound found in the roots, rhizomes, stems, and bark of several plants commonly used in botanical and Chinese medicine, such as goldenseal, Oregon grape, and barberry. It is widely regarded for its pharmacological effects on insulin levels and blood glucose management. Berberine has been shown to be as effective as the commonly prescribed diabetes drug, metformin, in lowering fasting insulin, blood glucose, hemoglobin A1c, triglycerides, and HOMA-IR (a measure of insulin resistance), with these effects occurring in as little as five weeks.[18] One of the ways berberine might influence conditions related to insulin resistance—such as Alzheimer's—is by increasing the expression of cellular insulin receptors.[19] Berberine also inhibits the activity of some of the carbohydrate-digesting enzymes in the small intestine, which could potentially lower the glycemic and insulin impact of carbohydrate-dense foods.[20] (This is one of the mechanisms by which vinegar helps mitigate the glycemic response to meals.)

As for Alzheimer's disease, specifically, berberine is an inhibitor of the enzyme acetylcholinesterase (AChE).[21] Acetylcholine is a neurotransmitter important for learning, memory, and cognition, and the acetylcholinesterase enzyme helps to break down acetylcholine. By inhibiting this enzyme, acetylcholine stays active in the neuronal synapse for a longer period of time, which might help facilitate better cognitive function. (Some of the pharmaceutical drugs aimed at AD have acetylcholinesterase-inhibiting effects.) Berberine is also an antioxidant, and these two combined effects led researchers to suggest berberine and related compounds "would clearly have beneficial uses in the development of therapeutic and preventive agents for AD and oxidative stress-related disease."[22] Owing to its influence on lowering insulin and blood glucose levels, combined with its antioxidant properties and AChE inhibition, one study's authors wrote that berberine has "potential to act as a multipotent agent to treat AD."[23] Beyond these impressive effects that directly target one of the fundamental issues in AD—hyperinsulinemia—berberine has also been shown to reduce the buildup of Aβ proteins and inhibit the glycogen synthase kinase-3 enzyme, whose activity contributes to the neurofibrillary tangles that alter the neuronal cytoskeleton and are another hallmark of AD.[24]

Huperzine A (HupA)

HupA is a compound found in the Chinese herb *Huperzia serrata*. Physiologically, it acts as an acetylcholinesterase inhibitor, just as berberine does. Compared to pharmaceutical cholinesterase-inhibiting agents, such as tacrine and donepezil, HupA has greater oral bioavailability, more effectively penetrates the blood-brain barrier, and its inhibitory action on acetylcholinesterase lasts longer.[25] HupA has properties in addition to AChE inhibition that might make it especially helpful for Alzheimer's, such as being anti-inflammatory and protecting against mitochondrial oxidative stress and apoptosis.[26] Small studies of relatively short duration (eight to twelve weeks) indicate that HupA does show promise for improving cognition, including improvement—albeit very modest—in scores on the commonly used Mini-Mental State Examination (MMSE).[27] To be fair, a meta-analysis of studies investigating the role of HupA as an intervention for AD found that most studies were of poor methodological quality. However, these studies of eight to twelve weeks among AD patients could be considered short; after all, AD does not develop overnight. The pathology accumulates over time, until the brain's compensatory mechanisms begin to fail and observable signs and symptoms begin to manifest. It might be that more time is needed to have a greater impact upon a condition that has likely been building for years, potentially decades. Nevertheless, the meta-analysis concluded that HupA does have beneficial effects for improving general cognitive function, behavioral disturbance, and functional performance.[28] Similar findings have been published more recently in another meta-analysis: Individual studies have shortcomings in design and quality, but overall, the data indicate a role for HupA in improving cognitive function, performance of daily living tasks, and global clinical assessment.[29] Results from other trials are mixed but promising.[30] Certainly, HupA is not a miracle worker, but as with any of these supplements, it would be interesting to see the effects of HupA in combination with a ketogenic diet. Additionally, considering the drastic toll dementia takes on its victims and their caregivers, even modest and temporary symptom improvement would ease the burden slightly and be most welcome.

Pyrroloquinoline Quinone (PQQ)

Much of the research on PQQ to date has been conducted in animals, but there is a small body of work supporting its use in humans, particularly as an influencer of mitochondrial biogenesis and healthy mitochondrial function.[31] Researchers had hypothesized in the past that PQQ might be an essential vitamin, but more recent research has disproven this. Nevertheless, PQQ, which is instead considered a "bioactive compound" (along the lines of quercetin and resveratrol, which are found in red wine, grapes, apples, and red onions, among other foods), seems to play an important role in supporting neuronal health, largely by reducing oxidative stress and supporting healthy mitochondria.[32]

Medium-Chain Triglycerides (MCTs)

As discussed throughout this book, these special saturated fatty acids, found mostly in coconut and palm kernel oils, are metabolized differently from others and are more prone to being converted into ketones, rather than stored as body fat. This means that even in the absence of carbohydrate restriction, MCTs can serve as a rich source of ketones. I will emphasize again that this should not be taken to mean that MCTs alone can be effective in combating Alzheimer's. They can help boost cognition in the acute sense, which is, of course, a huge boon to AD sufferers and their caregivers, but this does nothing to address the underlying metabolic abnormalities that are driving disease progression. A significant body of evidence is mounting that coconut oil and other MCT-rich coconut products might have a role to play in boosting cognition in Alzheimer's patients.[33] Coconut oil is only one source of MCTs. Purified medium-chain triglyceride oils are now available at health food stores and online. They have no coconut odor or flavor, so they might be helpful for individuals who have taste aversions to coconut. Moreover, only about 15 percent of the total fatty acids in coconut are MCTs. (The rest are short or long-chain fats.) Purified MCT oil is closer to 100 percent MCTs and might be more effective at improving cognition—at least temporarily.

—CHAPTER 23—

Don't Go It Alone: Moral Support and Other Support Strategies for a Low-Carb Diet

Having come this far, you've gathered by now that the diet I advocate to nourish the brain is quite different from what most people in the industrialized world—the United States, especially—are accustomed to eating. It requires largely abandoning the foods that make up the vast majority of what people consider "normal" meals. While a low-carb diet certainly allows and encourages people to consume a wide variety of delicious meats, seafood, dairy products, vegetables, nuts, and small amounts of fruit, the carbohydrate-dense foods that are limited can, for some people, make this diet difficult to stick to.

For this reason, it might help you or your loved one to have a "diet buddy"— someone who will join you in following the nutritional plan. This will provide much needed moral support when discipline, interest in, or dedication to the diet is flagging. It will also provide direct support at the dinner table or out at restaurants when someone in your party is ordering and eating similarly to the individual afflicted with dementia. They are less likely to feel deprived or feel like the odd one out if someone else is eating the same way.

I highly encourage having someone close to you or your loved one accompany you along this nutritional journey. Sometimes you might need a friend or relative who can be at the other end of the line for that late-night phone call when you want to dive headfirst into a dozen donuts. They can keep you on the straight and narrow and remind you how important it is that you don't stray from the appropriate foods.

But No One Else I Know Has Alzheimer's
or Needs to Lose Weight . . .

Apart from fueling the brain, the purpose you are probably most familiar with people using low-carb diets for is fat loss. And while carbohydrate restriction can most certainly be effective for this, the benefits of this nutritional strategy don't stop there. In fact, compared to the myriad other health benefits that result from carbohydrate reduction and the lowering of insulin and blood glucose levels, fat loss is probably the least impressive and important.

The goal of a low-carbohydrate diet for an Alzheimer's or MCI sufferer is to provide the brain with a fuel it can use, while simultaneously decreasing accumulated inflammation and oxidative damage. However, beyond these most important aspects of the diet, there are a number of other beneficial side effects you (and your loved ones who join you) might notice that can be attributed directly and indirectly to this nutritional approach:

Steady Blood Sugar

If you have experienced hypoglycemia or irritability when meals are delayed or skipped, or felt other symptoms related to fluctuations in blood sugar, low-carb diets largely prevent these, as most of your body's processes will be fueled by fat, rather than glucose. You will no longer be riding the "blood sugar roller coaster," and your energy levels will remain relatively stable throughout the day. You will be able to go several hours without food very comfortably and not be overwhelmed by the immediate and urgent need to eat. (You will avoid feeling "hangry"—the combination of hungry and angry—when it's been a while since you've eaten, and you're so hungry you think you might start gnawing on your own arm if you don't get fed soon!)

Stable Moods

Another beneficial effect of low-carb diets is often an improvement in mood swings, anxiety, and other psychological disturbances. Not surprisingly, these are common results of blood sugar dysregulation. Adequate protein intake also ensures a sufficient supply of the amino acids that serve as building blocks for neurotransmitters—chemicals the brain uses to regulate mood and emotions, energy levels, and sleep cycles (for example, serotonin, dopamine, epinephrine, norepinephrine, and melatonin).

Increased Energy

You might notice that you have more energy throughout the day. This is because fat is a more efficient fuel than carbohydrate. A sudden increase in energy levels is one of the quickest and most often reported effects of a low-carb diet. (After the low-carb flu passes, that is!) The main reason for this is lowered insulin levels. Think of your body as a car: When insulin levels are high, it's as if all your fuel were sitting in gallon jugs on the backseat, instead of in the gas tank, where it can be shuttled toward the engine to make the car run. When we lower insulin levels (primarily via reducing carbohydrate intake), all that fuel gets moved from the backseat into the tank, and now the engine can access it and use it. In this analogy, the gas is fat—both stored body fat and dietary fat from the foods you eat. Previously, you were running on an inefficient fuel (glucose), and because your insulin levels were chronically high, you were unable to switch over to using fat. (Insulin inhibits lipolysis, the breakdown of triglycerides into fatty acids, which can then be used as fuel.) But now, because insulin is lower, you'll be running on fat all the time. And because even relatively lean people still have large reserves of body fat, all bodies can run on stored body fat, thus avoiding the "energy crash" that would inevitably result from low blood glucose for those running on carbohydrates.

Lowered Blood Pressure

One of the quickest effects of a low-carb diet is a reduction in blood pressure. (If your blood pressure is already normal, the diet will not cause it to lower to dangerous levels; however, if it is high [if you have hypertension], this will likely lower it quickly. Please be cognizant of this and work closely with your physician if you are taking drugs or supplements to help control your blood pressure. You might find that very soon after adopting a low-carbohydrate diet, your need for medication is reduced. See chapter 20 for more information.) The role of chronically elevated blood glucose in affecting the viscosity of blood and the flexibility of blood vessels helps explain this, as does the role of insulin in regulating sodium and water retention. When blood glucose and insulin levels are restored to healthier levels, blood pressure decreases naturally, often within just days or weeks of adopting the diet.

Improved Memory and Clearer Thinking

Fuzzy headedness and foggy thinking ("brain fog") are usually the result of unstable blood sugar resulting in the brain's not being adequately fueled.

When you switch to running primarily on fat and ketones, the brain will have a steady source of nutrients and you won't experience gaps in cognition or memory as you might have in the past. Clearer thinking is one of the first things people report on low-carbohydrate, high-fat diets once the low-carb flu passes. It's like someone cleared out the cobwebs that had accumulated in your head or like someone turned the lights on.

Beyond these somewhat generalized effects, a low-carbohydrate, high-fat diet has been shown to positively impact a number of health conditions. It is most famous and has the longest history of use for facilitating the management of otherwise intractable epilepsy (epilepsy that did not respond to drug treatment). Apart from this most obvious application, here are some of the other issues this type of nutritional therapy has proven effective for:

- Metabolic syndrome and type 2 diabetes[1]
- Type 1 diabetes[2]
- Cardiovascular health and blood lipids (cholesterol)[3]
- Obesity and overall metabolic function[4]
- Inflammation[5]
- Vascular function (related to blood vessel health)[6]
- Acid reflux; gastroesophageal reflux disease (GERD)[7]
- Polycystic ovarian syndrome (PCOS)[8]
- Bipolar disorder[9]

Clinical research in applying ketogenic diets for other issues is in its infancy, but based on the biochemical mechanisms by which carbohydrate restriction and ketogenic diets exert their effects, they might also hold promise for neurodegenerative and neuromuscular disorders (Parkinson's disease, multiple sclerosis, amyotrophic lateral sclerosis [ALS, aka Lou Gehrig's disease]),[10] head trauma and traumatic brain injury,[11] and as an adjuvant to conventional cancer therapies.[12]

Still, No One Will Do This with Me . . .

If no one in your immediate family or circle of friends is willing to be your partner on this dietary journey, they can still support you by going at least some of the way. Here are some ways the people close to you can set you up for success and create an environment that is conducive to your sticking to your brain-nourishing diet:

1. Cut back on their refined sugar and starch consumption. Regardless of whether someone needs to lose weight or has any nagging health issues they'd like to resolve, no one's health ever got *worse* when they reduced their intake of sugar and junk food.

2. Avoid consuming sugar in front of you. If your loved ones do not have the desire or psychological fortitude to adopt a low-carbohydrate diet with you, then the least they can do is try not to consume sweets and starches while you are present. If they want to snack on pretzels, chips, candy, soda, crackers, granola bars, and the like, they can do so in another room.

3. Clear pantry and counter space for you to stock appropriate foods. It will be easier to stick to your healthy low-carb diet if sugary and starchy foods are out of your sight and, as much as possible, out of your reach. It might help to have a kitchen cabinet or drawer that is exclusively for your use, in which you store only foods that are suitable for you. This will save you from having to rummage through packages of wheat and corn-based products embalmed with sugar, corn syrup, and vegetable oils, in order to get to your canned seafood, nuts, beef jerky, coconut oil, dark chocolate, and other nonperishables.

4. Consider giving up a favorite food or beverage. Even if someone won't go all the way in terms of joining you in your diet, they can provide important moral support by giving up just one or two of their favorite foods or drinks. If someone in your life has a six-pack of soda a day habit, perhaps they'd be willing to forgo just that one item. Or if someone claims they "can't live" without coffee, or bread, or whatever is their item of choice, maybe they'd consider going without it (even for just a month or two) as a gesture of support for you.

CHAPTER 24

Potential Prevention Strategies

A t this time, no one knows for certain what might prevent Alzheimer's disease and mild cognitive impairment—or, indeed, if they even can be prevented by deliberate measures. Perhaps there are concrete steps we can take to protect and ensure our neurological health and cognitive function as we age, or perhaps this fate is beyond our control. However, based on what we now believe to be the primary factors causing and exacerbating cognitive decline, I believe there are potential—and I emphasize the word potential—prevention strategies, most of which are completely within our power to implement.

Just because we aren't absolutely certain of everything doesn't mean we don't have at least *some* actionable information, all of it based on research that has been done and continues to be done by brilliant and talented people across a wide variety of disciplines. So no, we don't have a foolproof, ironclad, step-by-step procedure for guaranteeing we'll all be intellectual and physical ninjas until we drop dead from happiness as we reach the top of Mt. Everest at age 112. But what we do have are some strategies that might—*might*—go a long way toward keeping us firing on all cognitive cylinders for as long as possible.

Diet

Considering the focus on low-carbohydrate nutrition in this book, your first question might be whether a ketogenic or very low-carb diet is *required* in order to preserve long-term metabolic health and cognitive function. I don't believe it is.

An exponentially expanding body of research indicates that maintaining insulin sensitivity and keeping blood glucose levels in check are among the most powerful things we can do for our health.[1] Consuming a low-carbohydrate diet is one way to influence this. Some people will be perfectly content to eat fewer than 30–50 grams of carbohydrate per day for the rest of their lives, but others prefer some sweet potato fries now and then, a tantalizingly sweet ear of corn in high summer, some garlic bread and a bowl of spaghetti to accompany a few meatballs, and sure, a brownie, cookie, piece of cake, or candy bar once in a while. Are we jeopardizing our health and playing Russian roulette with our cognitive function if we indulge in a treat now and then or consume fruits and starchy vegetables that have been part of the human diet for millennia?

Unfortunately, no one can tell us the exact number of carbohydrate grams that each of us, as individuals, can consume with no adverse effects on long-term health. The overall takeaway point is to stay within whatever range of carbohydrate consumption preserves insulin sensitivity and keeps blood glucose at healthy levels. The complicating factor, of course, is that this amount will be different for each of us. What is the exact amount of carbohydrate that, when consumed over a day, a week, a year, or a lifetime, could potentially bring about impaired cognition? Would that amount be different for a small-framed librarian compared to a professional hockey player? How about a 120-pound sedentary office worker and a 230-pound Olympic powerlifter? The mere nature of these questions shows us how difficult it is to posit answers.

A strict ketogenic diet is likely not required in order to preserve cognitive function. Just because this type of dietary strategy seems to be effective in some conditions for which conventional pharmaceuticals have largely failed or even made things worse, it doesn't mean that each and every one of us needs to adopt this special diet to prevent these conditions from developing. It makes sense that people who are quite far gone would need a strict, no-nonsense dietary intervention as a therapy. They don't have the luxury to play around with dipping their toes in the water to test things out. They need to do a cannonball into the deep end. But this is what makes the most sense after the damage is already done and we're trying to reverse it, stop it, or at least slow it down a little. This does not automatically translate to this same dramatic protocol being required to prevent the damage from occurring in the first place.

As a helpful analogy, consider an insect infestation: Having an exterminator fumigate your house will get rid of the infestation, but that doesn't mean setting off toxic bug bombs in your house is required to prevent the infestation in the first place. There are other, less drastic measures you could take to ensure you don't need the more extreme solution later on. In the case of a bug infestation, these might include better insulation on doors and windows, and not leaving food out on the counter. For aging with our cognitive faculties intact, I believe maintaining insulin sensitivity and protecting against chronic hyperinsulinemia and hyperglycemia are of paramount importance. The question is, how do we determine the amount of carbohydrate that will start to tip the scale in a detrimental direction?

As mentioned earlier in this book, some individuals at risk for Alzheimer's show reduced cerebral glucose metabolism as early as their thirties and forties. But since most of us are not likely to seek a PET scan to measure our cerebral glucose usage—nor is an insurance company likely to pay for such a seemingly odd request—there are metabolic markers you and your physician can keep track of with periodic blood tests that will give you valuable information about whether your habitual way of eating is suitable for you. Obviously, they can't directly tell you how well your brain is metabolizing glucose, but they do provide helpful indicators as to your insulin sensitivity and overall health. They are influenced strongly by diet (including occult and subclinical nutrient insufficiencies), and they're also affected by low-level chronic infections, under- or overexercising, and poor sleep, and they might also be influenced by exposure to environmental toxins that adversely affect metabolic function. So keep in mind that while diet is a powerful driver here, it's not the only one. Many of the following values are provided in standard blood tests, but you might have to specifically request others:

- **Fasting blood glucose:** ideally less than 90 mg/dL[2] (5 mmol/L). Between 70–99 mg/dL (3.9–5.5 mmol/L) is acceptable; however, in individuals who have been following low-carb diets for a significant amount of time, fasting blood glucose might be slightly higher than this, and it is not considered a pathological development.[3]
- **Fasting insulin:** ideally less than 5 μIU/mL[4]
- **Hemoglobin A1c:** ideally less than 5.6 percent[5]
- **HOMA-IR:** less than 2.0; lower is better[6]
- **Triglycerides:** less than 150 mg/dL (1.7 mmol/L). Under 100 mg/dL (1.1 mmol/L) is preferred, and under 70 mg/dL (0.79 mmol/L) is even better.[7]

- **HDL:** above 40 mg/dL (1.0mmol/L) for males; above 50 mg/dL (1.3 mmol/L) for females. Above 60 mg/dL (1.6 mmol/L) is preferred for both sexes.[8]
- **Total cholesterol-to-HDL ratio:** less than 4.5[9]
- **Triglyceride-to-HDL ratio:** less than 3.5; ideally under 2[10]
- **Omega-3 index (red blood cell concentration of EPA + DHA):** greater than 8 percent[11]
- **C-reactive protein (*hs*-CRP):** ideally less than 1.0 mg/L[12]
- **Homocysteine:** less than 15 μmol/L.[13] Between 7 μmol/L and 9 μmol/L is optimal.[14]
- **ALT:** 7–55 units per liter (U/L);[15] the lower, the better[16]
- **AST:** 8–48 U/L;[17] the lower, the better [18]

We wouldn't go on a cross-country drive without occasionally glancing down at the gas and oil gauges. Why should we drive through our lives without checking the numbers once in a while? When we see fasting blood glucose, A1c, and triglycerides inching upward over the years, that could be a sign we're eating more carbohydrates than our body can handle appropriately. We don't have to wait for full-blown type 2 diabetes to come knocking on the door and we're all but forced into cutting carbohydrates— or worse, injecting insulin, along with all the detrimental effects that brings. (I am referring to people with type 2 diabetes, specifically, who are typically chronically hyperinsulinemic. The last thing they need is more insulin. I am not referring to type 1 diabetics, who will always require at least a small amount of insulin.) We can self-check now and then to see where we are and do modest repairs before the wheels completely fall off the wagon.

That's the good thing about these numbers: Unlike a smoke detector that only goes off when there's already smoke—and possibly a fire—some of the biomarkers we currently believe offer clues about our health start moving unfavorably long before we're diagnosed with anything. Overt symptoms sometimes take years to manifest, and they only show themselves when the problem has existed unchecked for so long and has become severe or widespread enough that the body can no longer compensate for or hide it. So keeping an eye on some of these markers over time can be a kind of metabolic GPS, telling us when we need a course correction.

But remember: These numbers are imperfect guides. If fasting blood glucose at 100 mg/dL makes someone "prediabetic," how different is that from someone at 99 mg/dL? Or what about HDL? Is a woman "fine" at 50 mg/dL, but at risk for cardiovascular disease at 49 mg/dL? It's important to keep in mind that your health is a mosaic—a larger entity composed of smaller pieces, and your overall health and metabolic status is not determined by single markers in isolation. Rather, it is the total picture that should be considered when assessing your risk for chronic illness. Ideally you will work with a physician who treats *people*, not numbers; one who respects the whole person and does not ignore obvious dietary and lifestyle issues in favor of monotherapy (using single pharmaceutical drugs to target single biomarkers without addressing underlying causes that are likely affecting multiple organs and tissues simultaneously).

In addition to the markers indicated above, you might also wish to monitor your vitamin D levels, thyroid gland function, and levels of sex hormones (estrogen fractions, progesterone, testosterone). However, reference ranges and what is considered optimal for these measurements vary widely. Work with your physician to determine the levels that are right for you and at which you feel your best. As discussed in chapter 3 with regard to vitamin B_{12}, keep in mind that many metabolic and hormonal markers have broad ranges of what is considered "normal." Just because you fall within the normal range doesn't automatically mean you will feel your best. You might feel okay at one level, but it's possible you'd feel worlds better a bit higher (or lower), which would still have you within that large range of normal. Do your homework, and be an active participant in your health future, rather than an idle observer. It is your physician's job to help you stay well, but make no mistake: No one should be more invested in your health than you are.

As for specific dietary recommendations geared toward prevention of cognitive decline, for reasons discussed throughout this book, limiting intake of refined carbohydrates and omega-6-heavy vegetable oils would likely be helpful, as would ensuring adequate intake of omega-3 fats, complete proteins, and essential micronutrients (vitamins and minerals). For those who prefer a higher carbohydrate intake, those carbohydrates might be better coming from sources that are higher in fiber and micronutrients, such as fruit, legumes, pulses, and starchy tubers, rather than refined grains and simple sugars. For example, potatoes, beets, yams, yucca, beans, and lentils, as opposed to breakfast cereals, toaster pastries, crackers, and sugar-sweetened sodas or large amounts of fruit juice. Even products made with "whole-grain" flour and with dietary fiber added (such as in the form of wheat bran or oat bran) should be considered refined, as the grains have been pulverized into flour and might have quite different effects on insulin and blood glucose than the same foods consumed in a less refined state. (For example, a rice pilaf as opposed to crackers made from rice flour, or a wheatberry salad compared to cereal made with puffed or extruded wheat flakes.)

Exercise

What's good for the body is good for the brain. The human animal is designed to move. But we're designed to move a reasonable amount. Too much can be as harmful as too little. In the modern industrialized world, we tend to think that if a little of something is good, then more is better, and more still is even better than that. If a moderate amount of physical activity is beneficial, then we should all run marathons and do triathlons as often as possible, right?!

Not exactly. (We talked a little bit about this in chapter 17.)

If you enjoy engaging in those activities, then by all means, keep doing so. Doing what we love brings us joy and can provide a great relief from psychological stress—a win for a healthy brain. But exercise is a physical stress, and overdoing it—chronically, for years—can have unintended and harmful consequences. Whatever physical activity you enjoy, engage in it intelligently. Be sure to inject appropriate rest periods and replenish nutrient stores that might be depleted or that can support growth and maintenance of healthy muscles, bones, and connective tissue. Working hard is great, but don't forget to rest hard, too.

Incorporating more physical activity doesn't have to mean getting a gym membership or signing up for the next local 10K race. I emphasize the phrase "physical activity," rather than exercise, because there are all kinds of very easy ways to incorporate more physical activity—that is, just plain movement—into our daily lives. Deliberate exercise has its benefits, especially muscle-building and muscle-strengthening activities, but maintaining a baseline of being active in general is important.

It's also important to move our bodies in diverse ways. Biomechanist Katy Bowman calls this "nutritious movement." Just as we need a variety of nutrients in order to stay healthy, our bodies expect a variety of different types of movement in order to maintain strength, mobility, and flexibility as we age.[19] (These three things are key to maintaining our independence, too.) To borrow Ms. Bowman's analogy, we can't live by vitamin C alone. We need B vitamins, zinc, folate, magnesium, and on and on. In the same way, while walking is a wonderful way to move our bodies, and perhaps the most natural way of all to move them, we might do well to interject occasional sprints or lifting things (be they weights or our own body weight) through some form of pushing and pulling, in both horizontal and vertical planes. We can't maintain mobility and strength solely through jogging, or a bench press, or sit-ups. Just as we require lots of different vitamins and minerals, we require lots of different types of movement.

Here are some easy places to start:

- Take the stairs when possible instead of an elevator or escalator.
- Intentionally choose a parking space farther away from your destination.
- Walk or ride a bicycle to run errands in your neighborhood (if it's safe to do so). Bonus points for having to carry grocery bags or other parcels on the way back.
- If you use public transportation, exit the bus or train a stop or two early and walk the rest of the way.
- Do push-ups, sit-ups, planks, air squats, or other body-weight exercises while watching TV or movies. No special equipment required!
- If you're an office worker, consider "walking meetings"—instead of sitting around a conference table (often laden with pastries), conduct meetings while walking inside or outside the building, weather permitting.
- Take breaks—if your work is largely sedentary, set an alert on your phone or computer to remind you to get up and move around several times throughout the day. Or do "cubicle calisthenics."[20] Your coworkers might look at you funny, but they won't be laughing so hard when they're hitting the vending machine at 3 p.m. looking for a sugary energy boost, and you're getting yours from jumping jacks.

- Above all: Look for ways to deliberately inject more physical activity into your everyday life through the course of your normal routine. Just as intermittent fasting is a way to (beneficially) introduce periods of food scarcity into an environment where we're surrounded by food, intentionally making activities slightly less convenient (by walking instead of driving, carrying heavy bags instead of using a cart, and so on) is a way to increase physical activity without causing much disruption to what you were already doing.

Stress and Sleep

In a word—or three—go to sleep!

In the age of social media, smartphones, tablets, doodads, gadgets, and gizmos, there are endless things competing for our time and attention, especially late at night, after we've already dealt with the other demands on our time and attention. We explored the detrimental effects of chronic stress and long-term sleep debt earlier; we need not reiterate the details here. To put it simply, don't underestimate the power of these issues to influence your physical, emotional, and cognitive health. We like to pride ourselves on being tough and resilient, and while there's nothing wrong with these qualities, we ignore the need for relaxation, unplugging, and indulging in downtime at our peril. Work hard, but let yourself relax hard, too. No one on their deathbed ever said, "I wish I'd spent more time at work."

With all the above in mind, here's the quick-and-dirty list of things that are likely to facilitate healthy aging for body and mind:

- A diet of primarily whole, nutrient-dense foods—that is, single-ingredient foods that do not come in bags or boxes with tongue-twisting ingredient lists
- Low intake of added sugars and refined carbohydrates
- Generous intake of omega-3 fatty acids (especially DHA) and naturally occurring fats
- Emphasis on low-glycemic vegetables and fruits
- Avoidance of easily oxidized vegetable and seed oils
- Regular physical activity via a diverse array of movement patterns, aerobic exercise, and muscle-building activities

- Occasional fasting
- Stress reduction
- Adequate sleep
- Joy—don't forget to be happy!

Why Alzheimer's Is on the Rise and How to Repair a Broken Brain

N ow that you understand more about the etiology of Alzheimer's disease and the pathological influence of our modern diet—high in refined carbohydrates, heavy in fragile and easily oxidized vegetable and seed oils, and low in fresh, micronutrient-rich colored vegetables—combine that with our stressful and sedentary lifestyles as well as insufficient sleep and disrupted circadian rhythms, toss in strong antacid drugs and cholesterol-reducing medications, and you have nothing less than a blueprint for dementia in older age.

If someone were to ask me how to damage the human brain, here is what I would say about attacking on the dietary front:

- Deprive it of cholesterol
- Deprive it of omega-3 fats
- Load it up with oxidized vegetable oils
- Avoid animal fats that have nourished robust humans for thousands of years
- Load it up with carbohydrates to the point where it can no longer metabolize them and, in fact, as a protective measure, actively shuts down the use of glucose
- Emphasize that a "healthy diet" is one that is very low in animal foods—especially animal fat—and that high-glycemic grains should be the foundation of the diet

And if I wanted to make things even worse and absolutely ensure the brain would not get the critical nutrients it needs, I would attack it on a pharmacological front, too:

- Take a statin drug or other medication to lower cholesterol
- Take a stomach acid–blocking drug or use other prescription or over-the-counter antacids long-term

And to wipe out any remaining semblance of brain health that had managed to survive all of the above, I would engage in the following lifestyle practices:

- Remain sedentary
- Avoid long, slow, therapeutic walks in the outdoors—anywhere outdoors, but preferably in a green space surrounded by fresh, clean air and the natural sights and sounds my brain and nervous system have come to expect: birds chirping, insects calling, a breeze rustling the leaves, green plants all around
- Avoid challenging myself physically, such as by lifting weights or even just riding a bike or going for a hike
- Stay out of the sun, and fear exposing my skin to natural daylight and the potential for vitamin D synthesis
- Deprive myself of sufficient sleep for years, possibly decades
- Deprive myself of darkness at appropriate times, such as when I am falling asleep and while I am asleep
- Overwork myself physically or psychologically to the point where stress is impacting my health

When you put all of these factors together and consider the combined burden of damage inflicted, it's no wonder Alzheimer's is on the rise. As you can see, the modern diet and lifestyle are a potent combination for creating Alzheimer's disease. The evidence linking chronically elevated insulin, glucose dysregulation, uncontrolled oxidative stress, and inflammation—all resulting from diets high in refined carbohydrates and vegetable and seed oils rich in omega-6 polyunsaturated fats and low in antioxidants and micronutrients—to Alzheimer's disease suggests that the time has come for an unbiased reevaluation of conventional dietary guidelines that emphasize grains and starches as primary sources of energy and demonize consumption of animal fats and saturated fats from plants. Combined with stressful, sedentary lifestyles, and particularly when complicated by zealously overprescribed medications such as antacids and statin drugs, which interfere with the body's normal physiological and metabolic processes, this outdated advice equates to nothing less than a road map for arriving at Alzheimer's disease.

Even in the face of this seemingly insurmountable onslaught, there is reason to remain hopeful. Yes, hopeful! If I were not convinced that there is something we can do to help individuals with dementia, I would not have written this book. And if cognitive impairment and Alzheimer's were not reversible at all, then physicians would not have reported on cases where exactly this has happened. With this in mind . . .

How Soon Will I Notice an Improvement in My or My Loved One's Cognition?

Because Alzheimer's disease is a complex and multifactorial illness, and each sufferer experiences the signs and symptoms in a unique way, it is impossible to speculate as to when you or your loved one might begin to notice improvements in cognitive function after following the guidelines in this book. The amount of time needed to improve insulin sensitivity, reduce inflammation and glycation in the brain, and provide a continuous supply of ketones to fuel struggling neurons will differ from person to person. The degree and rate of improvement will likely be tied to disease severity and duration. The longer you or your loved one have been experiencing impaired cognition, and the more severe the damage and incapacitation, the longer it will likely be before improvements are noticeable upon implementation of a low-carbohydrate diet and other lifestyle interventions.

That being said, if you are disciplined in sticking with a strict low-carbohydrate diet (perhaps fewer than 30–40 grams of carbs per day to start), it generally only takes 48–72 hours for the body's stockpile of glycogen to dwindle down to the point where the body makes the switch to running on fats. It will take a little more time beyond this, however, before the body ramps up ketone production to the levels that might begin to have a positive impact upon memory and cognition.

If it has been a full two months of strictly limiting carbohydrates and you do not observe any improvements, don't give up hope. My recommendation is to persevere and continue on for several more weeks. In some people, the damage will be so widespread and longstanding that it just takes more time before the beneficial effects of elevated ketones start making a dent and changes become noticeable. I would be faithful to strictly following the diet for a minimum of three months before assessing whether it is appropriate to continue. My hope is that during that time there would be at least some hint of improvement—however small—that would provide motivation to keep going and redouble your efforts. Remember: The damage that causes Alzheimer's disease starts accruing decades before overt signs and symptoms begin to manifest. It is unreasonable, therefore, to expect this damage to be repaired in a matter of days or weeks, particularly among older individuals, whose bodies naturally have a reduced capacity for repair and regeneration compared to younger people.

The younger Alzheimer's or MCI sufferers are when they adopt a low-carbohydrate diet (and the milder the condition), the greater their probability for cognitive improvement. However, don't let this discourage you from helping a parent or grandparent of very advanced age implement this diet. The human body is nothing if not stunning in its ability to awe and surprise us. No matter how advanced the disease, nor how "seasoned" or "senior" the Alzheimer's patient, there is no reason not to attempt this diet and provide their brain with nourishing fuel. There is no one so far gone that their brain health should be considered "a lost cause." The human body constantly surprises us with feats we didn't know it was capable of—and nowhere is this more true than in the brain.

Of course, I must also emphasize that the use of low-carbohydrate and ketogenic diets for Alzheimer's disease is a small but growing field. Scientific studies employing ketogenic diets, exogenous ketones, and the lifestyle strategies discussed in this book are in their infancy, so there is not yet a lot of data indicating that this approach can or will be effective for everyone. That being said, based on the etiology of Alzheimer's disease as a metabolic condition, strict carbohydrate reduction and lowering of insulin levels is the most logical and scientifically sound method to ameliorate, delay, and possibly even reverse the signs of this condition, particularly when compared to medications that have proven to be as ineffective as they are expensive.

I will say again that the use of ketogenic diets and exogenous ketones as therapy for Alzheimer's disease is in its infancy. For those of very advanced age, and with extremely severe and long-standing dementia, the disease might have progressed to a point where the damage is irreversible. As Dr. Bredesen has said, "AD is not a mysterious, untreatable brain disease—it is a reversible, metabolic/toxic, usually systemic illness with a relatively large window for treatment."[1] The window for treatment is "large," but it is likely not infinite. There might well be a point of no return, where the physical structure of the brain has been so compromised for so long that even adoption of all the recommendations in this book will fail to have a positive impact. If this appears to be the situation with your loved one, I would refer you back to the discussion of brain fuel metabolism in chapter 2. According to prominent AD researcher Samuel Henderson, "By the time clinical dementia is diagnosed, irreparable damage may have occurred and reversal will be difficult. One strategy that might be effective is [direct elevation of acetyl-CoA levels] using ketone bodies."[2] For individuals who are unable or unwilling to change their diet and lifestyle, it's possible that liberal intake of coconut oil, MCT oil, and use of exogenous ketones might improve quality of life in the time they have left and might also slightly ease the emotional burden on caregivers.

In order to stop, slow, or potentially reverse the damage that has been done to the brain, it follows logically that we should endeavor to adopt the opposite of the behaviors theorized to have caused it; hence, the low-carbohydrate, high-fat, high-cholesterol nutritional strategy and lifestyle recommendations presented in this book.

My goal in writing this was to deliver this critical information to you, the individuals afflicted with Alzheimer's disease or mild cognitive impairment, and your loved ones and caregivers.

You are *not* powerless in this battle.

There *is* something you can do.

There are *many things* you can do.

There is hope.

My sincerest wish is that, through implementing the brain-healing strategy I've outlined—or as many parts of it as you are capable of—the coherent, vibrant, lively individual that is still inside you or your loved one shines through once again.

NOTES

Chapter 1: The Origins of Alzheimer's and a Strategy to Fight It

1. Alzheimer's Association, "2016 Alzheimer's Disease Facts and Figures," Alzheimer's Association, http://www.alz.org/facts/overview.asp (August 30, 2016).
2. Ely Lilly and Company, "Lilly Halts Development of Semagacestat for Alzheimer's Disease Based on Preliminary Results of Phase III Clinical Trials," Eli Lilly and Company, https://investor.lilly.com/releasedetail.cfm?releaseid=499794 (September 12, 2016).
3. Zina Kroner, "The Relationship Between Alzheimer's Disease and Diabetes: Type 3 Diabetes?" *Alternative Medicine Review* 14, no. 4 (2009): 373–79; and Suzanne M. de la Monte, "Type 3 Diabetes is Sporadic Alzheimer's disease: Mini-Review," *European Neuropsychopharmacology* 24, no. 12 (2014): 1954–60, doi:10.1016/j .euroneuro.2014.06.008.
4. Loren Cordain, S. Boyd Eaton, Anthony Sebastian, Neil Mann, Staffan Lindeberg, Bruce A. Watkins, James H. O'Keefe, et al., "Origins and Evolution of the Western Diet: Health Implications for the 21st Century," *American Journal of Clinical Nutrition* 81 (2005): 341–54; and Loren Cordain and Boyd Eaton, "Evolutionary Aspects of Diet: Old Genes, New Fuels," *World Review of Nutrition and Dietetics* 81 (1997): 26–37.
5. Glen D. Lawrence, "Dietary Fats and Health: Dietary Recommendations in the Context of Scientific Evidence," *Advances in Nutrition* 4, no. 3 (2013): 294–302.
6. Loren Cordain, Michael R. Eades, and Mary Dan Eades, "Hyperinsulinemic Diseases of Civilization: More Than Just Syndrome X," *Comparative Biochemistry and Physiology. Part A, Molecular & Integrative Physiology* 136, no. 1 (2003): 95–112; Ian Spreadbury, "Comparison with Ancestral Diets Suggests Dense Acellular Carbohydrates Promote an Inflammatory Microbiota, and May Be the Primary Dietary Cause of Leptin Resistance and Obesity," *Diabetes, Metabolic Syndrome and Obesity: Targets and Therapy* 5 (2012): 175–89, doi:10.2147/DMSO.S33473; and Colin E. Champ, Jeff S. Volek, Joshua Siglin, Lianjin Jin, and Nicole L. Simone, "Weight Gain, Metabolic Syndrome, and Breast Cancer Recurrence: Are Dietary Recommendations Supported by the Data?" *International Journal of Breast Cancer* 2012 (2012): 506868.
7. Gerard J. Tortora and Bryan H. Derrickson, eds., *Principles of Anatomy and Physiology 11th Edition* (Hoboken, NJ: John Wiley & Sons, 2006): 477.

8. Jeff S. Volek and Richard D. Feinman, "Carbohydrate Restriction Improves the Features of Metabolic Syndrome. Metabolic Syndrome May Be Defined by the Response to Carbohydrate Restriction," *Nutrition and Metabolism* 2 (2005): 31, doi:10.1186/1743-7075-2-31.

9. P. Reaven, "Metabolic syndrome," *Journal of Insurance Medicine* 36, no. 2 (2004): 132–42.

10. Volek and Feinman, "Carbohydrate Restriction Improves the Features of Metabolic Syndrome"; Anthony Accurso, Richard K. Bernstein, Annika Dahlqvist, Boris Draznin, Richard D. Feinman, Eugene Fine, Amy Gleed, et al., "Dietary Carbohydrate Restriction in Type 2 Diabetes Mellitus and Metabolic Syndrome: Time for a Critical Appraisal," *Nutrition & Metabolism* 5 (2008): 9; and Richard D. Feinman and Jeff S. Volek, "Carbohydrate Restriction as the Default Treatment for Type 2 Diabetes and Metabolic Syndrome," *Scandinavian Cardiovascular Journal* 42, no. 4 (2008): 256–63, doi:10.1080/14017430802014838.

11. Hidenao Fukuyama, Masafumi Ogawa, Hiroshi Yamauchi, Shinya Yamaguchi, Jun Kimura, Yoshiaru Yonekura, and Junji Konishi, "Altered Cerebral Energy Metabolism in Alzheimer's Disease: A PET Study," *Journal of Nuclear Medicine* 35, no. 1 (1994): 1–6.

12. David G. Cook, James B. Leverenz, Pamela J. McMillan, J. Jacob Kulstad, Sasha Ericksen, Richard A. Roth, Gerard D. Schellenberg, et al., "Reduced Hippocampal Insulin-Degrading Enzyme in Late-Onset Alzheimer's Disease Is Associated with the Apolipoprotein E-ε4 Allele," *American Journal of Pathology* 162, no. 1 (2003): 313–19.

13. Ling Xie, Erik Helmerhorst, Kevin Taddei, Brian Plewright, Wilhelm Van Bronswijk, and R. Martins, "Alzheimer's β-amyloid Peptides Compete with Insulin for Binding to the Insulin Receptor," *Journal of Neuroscience* 22, no. 10 (2002): RC221.

14. Wei Qiao Qiu, Dominic M. Walsh, Zhen Ye, Konstantinos Vekrellis, Jimin Zhang, Marcia B. Podlisny, Marsha Rich Rosner, et al., "Insulin-Degrading Enzyme Regulates Extracellular Levels of Amyloid β-Protein by Degradation," *Journal of Biological Chemistry* 273, no. 49 (1998): 32730–8.

15. A. Ott, R. P. Stolk, F. van Harskamp, H. A. P. Pols, A. Hofman, and M. M. B. Breteler, "Diabetes Mellitus and the Risk of Dementia: The Rotterdam Study," *Neurology* 53, no. 9 (1999): 1937–42.

16. George F. Cahill and Richard L. Veech, "Ketoacids? Good medicine?" *Transactions of the American Clinical and Climatological Association*, 114 (2003): 149–63; and Theodore B. VanItallie and Thomas H. Nufert, "Ketones: Metabolism's Ugly Duckling," *Nutrition Reviews* 61, no. 10 (2003): 327–41, doi:10.1301/nr.2003.oct.327-341.

17. Ibid.; and Sami A. Hashim and Theodore B. VanItallie, "Ketone Body Therapy: From the Ketogenic Diet to the Oral Administration of Ketone Ester," *Journal of Lipid Research* 55, no. 9 (2014): 1818–26, doi:10.1194/jlr.R046599.

18. Thomas M. Devlin, ed., *Textbook of Biochemistry with Clinical Correlations* (Hoboken, NJ: John Wiley & Sons, 2011): 699, 700.

19. Samuel T. Henderson, "Ketone Bodies as a Therapeutic for Alzheimer's Disease," *Neurotherapeutics* 5, no. 3 (2008): 470–80.

20. Carl E. Stafstrom and Jong M. Rho, "The Ketogenic Diet as a Treatment Paradigm for Diverse Neurological Disorders," *Frontiers in Pharmacology* 3 (2012): 59, doi:10.3389/fphar.2012.00059; and Maciej Gasior, Michael A. Rogawski, and Adam L. Hartman, "Neuroprotective and Disease-Modifying Effects of the Ketogenic Diet," *Behavioural Pharmacology* 17, no. 5-6 (2006): 431–39.

21. Samuel T. Henderson, Janet L. Vogel, Linda J. Barr, Fiona Garvin, Julie J. Jones, and Lauren C. Costanti, "Study of the Ketogenic Agent AC-1202 in Mild to Moderate Alzheimer's Disease: A Randomized, Double-Blind, Placebo-Controlled, Multicenter Trial," *Nutrition and Metabolism* (London) 6 (2009): 31, doi:10.1186/1743-7075-6-31; and Mark A. Reger, Samuel T. Henderson, Cathy Hale, Brenna Cholerton, Laura D. Baker, G. S. Watson, Karen Hyde, et al., "Effects of Beta-Hydroxybutyrate on Cognition in Memory-Impaired Adults," *Neurobiology of Aging* 25, no. 3 (2004): 311–14, doi:10.1016/S0197 -4580(03)00087-3.

22. Robert Krikorian, Marcelle D. Shidler, Krista Dangelo, Sarah C. Couch, Stephen C. Benoit, and Deborah J. Clegg, "Dietary Ketosis Enhances Memory in Mild Cognitive Impairment," *Neurobiology of Aging* 33, no. 425 (2012): e19–e27.

23. Loren Cordain, "The Nutritional Characteristics of a Contemporary Diet Based on Paleolithic Food Groups," *Journal of the American Nutraceutical Association* 5 (2002): 15–24.

24. Patty W. Siri-Tarino, Qi Sun, Frank B. Hu, and Ronald M. Krauss, "Meta-Analysis of Prospective Cohort Studies Evaluating the Association of Saturated Fat with Cardiovascular Disease," *American Journal of Clinical Nutrition* 91, no. 3 (2010): 535–46, doi:10.3945/ajcn.2009.27725; Jeff S. Volek, Maria Luz Fernandez, Richard D. Feinman, and Stephen Phinney, "Dietary Carbohydrate Restriction Induces a Unique Metabolic State Positively Affecting Atherogenic Dyslipidemia, Fatty Acid Partitioning, and Metabolic Syndrome," *Progress in Lipid Research* 47, no. 5 (2008): 307–18, doi:10.1016/j.plipres.2008.02.003; Jeff S. Volek and Cassandra E. Forsythe, "The Case for Not Restricting Saturated Fat on a Low Carbohydrate Diet," *Nutrition & Metabolism* 2 (2005): 21, doi:10.1186/1743-7075-2-21; Cassandra Forsythe, Stephen D. Phinney, Richard D. Feinman, Brittanie M. Volk, Daniel Freidenreich, Erin Quann, Kevin Ballard et al., "Limited Effect of Dietary Saturated Fat on Plasma Saturated Fat in the Context of a Low Carbohydrate Diet," *Lipids* 45, no. 10 (2010): 947–62, doi:10.1007/s11745-010-3467-3; and Brittanie M. Volk, Laura J. Kunces, Daniel J. Freidenreich, Brian R. Kupchak, Catherine Saenz, Juan C. Artistizabal, Maria Luz Fernandez, et al., "Effects of Step-Wise Increases in Dietary Carbohydrate on Circulating Saturated Fatty Acids and Palmitoleic Acid in Adults with Metabolic Syndrome," PLoS ONE 9, no. 11 (2014): e113605, doi:10.1371 /journal.pone.0113605.

25. Dale E. Bredesen, *Cognitive Health: Dawn of the Era of Treatable Alzheimer's Disease*, film, 56:21, August 4, 2016, https://vimeo.com/173061978.

26. Dale E. Bredesen, "Reversal of Cognitive Decline: A Novel Therapeutic Program,"
    Aging 6, 9 (2014): 707–17.

Chapter 2: Brain Fuel Metabolism: Key to Understanding Alzheimer's Disease

1. Giulia Accardi, Calogero Caruso, Giuseppina Colonna-Romano, Cecilia
   Camarda, Roberto Monastero, and Giuseppina Candore, "Can Alzheimer Disease
   Be a Form of Type 3 Diabetes?" *Rejuvenation Research* 15, no. 2 (2012): 217–21,
   doi:10.1089/rej.2011.1289; Vincenza Frisardi, Vincenzo Solfrizzi, Davide Seripa,
   Cristiano Capurso, Andrea Santamato, Daniele Sancarlo, Gianluigi Vendemiale,
   et al., "Metabolic-Cognitive Syndrome: A Cross-Talk Between Metabolic
   Syndrome and Alzheimer's Disease," *Ageing Research Reviews* 9, no. 4 (2010):
   399–417, doi:10.1016/j.arr.2010.04.007; and Vincenza Frisardi, Vincenzo Solfrizzi,
   Cristiano Capurso, Bruno P. Imbimbo, Gianluigi Vendemiale, Davide Seripa,
   Alberto Pilotto, et al., "Is Insulin Resistant Brain State a Central Feature of the
   Metabolic-Cognitive Syndrome?" *Journal of Alzheimer's Disease* 21, no. 1 (2010):
   57–63, doi:10.3233/JAD-2010-100015.
2. Bhumsoo Kim and Eva L. Feldman, "Insulin Resistance as a Key Link for the
   Increased Risk of Cognitive Impairment in the Metabolic Syndrome," *Experimental
   & Molecular Medicine* 47, no. 3 (2015): e149, doi:10.1038/emm.2015.3.
3. American Diabetes Association, "Diagnosis and Classification of Diabetes
   Mellitus," *Diabetes Care* 33, Suppl 1 (2010): S62–S69, doi:10.2337/dc10-S062.
4. Ibid.
5. Joseph Kraft, *Diabetes Epidemic & You* (Bloomington, IN: Trafford
   Publishing, 2011).
6. Ibid.
7. Stephen C. Cunnane, Scott Nugent, Maggie Roy, Alexandre Courchesne-Loyer,
   Etienne Croteau, Sébastien Tremblay, Alex Castellano, et al., "Brain Fuel
   Metabolism, Aging and Alzheimer's Disease," *Nutrition* 27, no. 1 (2011): 3–20,
   doi:10.1016/j.nut.2010.07.021.
8. G. Stennis Watson and Suzanne Craft, "The Role of Insulin Resistance in the
   Pathogenesis of Alzheimer's Disease: Implications for Treatment," *CNS Drugs* 17,
   no. 1 (2003): 27–45.
9. Sara E. Young, Arch G. Mainous 3rd, and Mark Carnemolla, "Hyperinsulinemia
   and Cognitive Decline in a Middle-Aged Cohort," *Diabetes Care* 29, no. 12 (2006):
   2688–93, doi:10.2337/dc06-0915.
10. Jose A. Luchsinger, Ming-Xin Tang, Steven Shea, and Richard Mayeux,
    "Hyperinsulinemia and Risk of Alzheimer Disease," *Neurology* 63, no. 7
    (2004): 1187–92.
11. Kraft, *Diabetes Epidemic*.
12. Abel Romero-Corral, Virend K. Somers, Justo Sierra-Johnson, Yoel Korenfeld,
    Simona Boarin, Josef Korinek, Michael D. Jensen, et al., "Normal Weight Obesity:
    A Risk Factor for Cardiometabolic Dysregulation and Cardiovascular Mortality,"
    European Heart Journal 31, no. 6 (2010): 737–746, doi:10.1093/eurheartj/ehp487;
    and Estefania Oliveros, Virend K. Somers, Ondrej Sochor, Kashish Goel, and

Francisco Lopez-Jimenez, "The Concept of Normal Weight Obesity," *Progress in Cardiovascular Diseases* 56, no. 4 (2014): 426–33, doi:10.1016/j.pcad.2013.10.003.

13. Christina Voulgari, Nicholas Tentolouris, Polychronis Dilaveris, Dimitris Tousoulis, Nicholas Katsilambros, and Christodoulos Stefanadis, "Increased Heart Failure Risk in Normal-Weight People with Metabolic Syndrome Compared with Metabolically Healthy Obese Individuals," *Journal of the American College of Cardiology* 58, no. 13 (2011): 1343–50, doi:10.1016/j.jacc.2011.04.047; and Minjoo Kim, Jean Kyung Paik, Ryungwoo Kang, Soo Young Kim, Sang-Hyun Lee, and Jong Ho Lee, "Increased Oxidative Stress in Normal-Weight Postmenopausal Women with Metabolic Syndrome Compared with Metabolically Healthy Overweight/Obese Individuals," *Metabolism* 62, no. 4 (2013): 554–60, doi:10.1016/j.metabol.2012.10.006.

14. Catherine M. Phillips, Christina Dillon, Janas M. Harrington, Ver J. C. McCarthy, Patricia M. Kearney, Anthony P. Fitzgerald, and Ivan J. Perry, "Defining Metabolically Healthy Obesity: Role of Dietary and Lifestyle Factors," *PLoS ONE* 8, no. 10 (2013): e76188, doi:10.1371/journal.pone.0076188.

15. Catherine Crofts, Caryn Zinn, Mark Wheldon, and Grant Schofield, "Hyperinsulinemia: A Unifying Theory of Chronic Disease?" *Diabesity* 1, no. 4 (2015): 34–43, doi:10.15562/diabesity.2015.19; Loren Cordain, Michael R. Eades, and Mary Dan Eades, "Hyperinsulinemic Diseases of Civilization: More Than Just Syndrome X," *Comparative Biochemistry and Physiology. Part A, Molecular & Integrative Physiology* 136 no. 1 (2003): 95–112; Joseph R. Kraft, "Hyperinsulinemia: The Common Denominator of Subjective Idiopathic Tinnitus and Other Idiopathic Central and Peripheral Neurootologic Disorders," *International Tinnitus Journal* 1, no. 1 (1995): 46–53; H. Kaźmierczak and G. Doroszewska, "Metabolic Disorders in Vertigo, Tinnitus, and Hearing Loss," *The International Tinnitus Journal* 7, no. 1 (2001): 54–8, http://www.ncbi.nlm.nih.gov /pubmed/14964957; and P. L. Mangabeira Albernaz and Y. Fukuda, "Glucose, Insulin and Inner Ear Pathology," *Acta Otolaryngologica* 97, no. 5–6 (1984): 496–501, http://www.ncbi.nlm.nih.gov/pubmed/6380207.

16. G. J. Biessels, L. J. Kappelle, and Utrecht Diabetic Encephalopathy Study Group, "Increased Risk of Alzheimer's Disease in Type II Diabetes: Insulin Resistance of the Brain or Insulin-Induced Amyloid Pathology?," *Biochemical Society Transactions* 33, no. 5 (2005): 1041–4, doi:10.1042/BST20051041; and Rachel A. Whitmer, "Type 2 Diabetes and Risk of Cognitive Impairment and Dementia," *Current Neurology and Neuroscience Reports.*7, no. 5 (2007): 373–80.

17. Suzanne M. de la Monte, "Contributions of Brain Insulin Resistance and Deficiency in Amyloid-Related Neurodegeneration in Alzheimer's Disease," *Drugs* 72 no. 1 (2012): 49–66, doi:10.2165/11597760-000000000-00000; Melita Salkovic-Petrisic, Jelena Osmanovic, Edna Grünblatt, Peter Riederer, and Siegfried Hoyer, "Modeling Sporadic Alzheimer's Disease: The Insulin Resistant Brain State Generates Multiple Long-Term Morphobiological Abnormalities Including Hyperphosphorylated Tau Protein and Amyloid-Beta," *Journal of Alzheimer's Disease* 18, no. 4 (2009): 729–50, doi:10.3233/JAD-2009-1184; Siegfried Hoyer, "Glucose Metabolism and

Insulin Receptor Signal Transduction in Alzheimer Disease," *European Journal of Pharmacology* 490, no. 1–3 (2004): 115–25, doi:10.1016/j.ejphar.2004.02.049; Siegfried Hoyer, "The Aging Brain. Changes in the Neuronal Insulin/Insulin Receptor Signal Transduction Cascade Trigger Late-Onset Sporadic Alzheimer Disease (SAD). A Mini-Review," *Journal of Neural Transmission (Vienna)* 109, no. 7-8 (2002): 991–1002, doi:10.1007/s007020200082; and G. Stennis Watson and Suzanne Craft, "Modulation of Memory by Insulin and Glucose: Neuropsychological Observations in Alzheimer's Disease," *European Journal of Pharmacology* 490, no. 1–3 (2004): 97–113, doi:10.1016/j.ejphar.2004.02.048.

18. Watson and Craft, "Modulation of Memory."
19. Lisa Mosconi, Susan De Santi, Juan Li, Wai Hon Tsui, Yi Li, Madhu Boppana, Eugene Laska, et al., "Hippocampal Hypometabolism Predicts Cognitive Decline from Normal Aging," *Neurobiology of Aging* 29, no. 5 (2008): 676–92.
20. Ibid.
21. Ibid.
22. Hidenao Fukuyama, Masafumi Ogawa, Hiroshi Yamauchi, Shinya Yamaguchi, Jun Kimura, Yoshiaru Yonekura, and Junji Konishi, "Altered Cerebral Energy Metabolism in Alzheimer's Disease: A PET Study," *Journal of Nuclear Medicine* 35, no. 1 (1994): 1–6.
23. Samuel T. Henderson, "Ketone Bodies as a Therapeutic for Alzheimer's Disease," *Neurotherapeutics* 5, no. 3 (2008): 470–80.
24. Ibid.; Richard L. Veech, "The Therapeutic Implications of Ketone Bodies: The Effects of Ketone Bodies in Pathological Conditions: Ketosis, Ketogenic Diet, Redox States, Insulin Resistance, and Mitochondrial Metabolism," *Prostaglandins, Leukotrienes, and Essential Fatty Acids* 70 no. 3 (2004): 309–19, doi:10.1016/j.plefa.2003.09.007; and Sami A. Hashim and Theodore B. VanItallie, "Ketone Body Therapy: From the Ketogenic Diet to the Oral Administration of Ketone Ester," *Journal of Lipid Research* 55, no. 9 (2014): 1818–26, doi:10.1194/jlr.R046599.
25. Veech, "The Therapeutic Implications."
26. Stephen C. Cunnane, Alexandre Courchesne-Loyer, Camille Vandenberghe, Valérie St-Pierre, Mélanie Fortier, Marie Hennebelle, Etienne Croteau, et al., "Can Ketones Help Rescue Brain Fuel Supply in Later Life? Implications for Cognitive Health during Aging and the Treatment of Alzheimer's Disease," *Frontiers in Molecular Neuroscience* 9 (2016): 53, doi:10.3389/fnmol.2016.00053.
27. Ibid.
28. Henderson, "Ketone Bodies"; Samuel T. Henderson, Janet L. Vogel, Linda J. Barr, Fiona Garvin, Julie J. Jones, and Lauren C. Costantini, "Study of the Ketogenic Agent AC-1202 in Mild to Moderate Alzheimer's Disease: A Randomized, Double-Blind, Placebo-Controlled, Multicenter Trial," *Nutrition and Metabolism* (London) 6 (2009): 31, doi:10.1186/1743-7075-6-31; Mark A. Reger, Samuel T. Henderson, Cathy Hale, Brenna Cholerton, Laura D. Baker, G. S. Watson, Karen Hyde, et al., "Effects of Beta-hydroxybutyrate on Cognition in Memory-Impaired Adults," *Neurobiology of Aging* 25, no. 3 (2004): 311–4. doi:10.1016/S0197-4580(03)00087-3; and Mary T. Newport, Theodore B. VanItallie, Yoshihiro

Kashiwaya, Michael T. King, and Richard L. Veech, "A New Way to Produce Hyperketonemia: Use of Ketone Ester in a Case of Alzheimer's Disease," *Alzheimer's and Dementia* 11, no. 1 (2015): 99–103, doi:10.1016/j.jalz.2014.01.006.

29. Hashim and VanItallie, "Ketone Body Therapy."

30. Alexandre Courchesne-Loyer, Etienne Croteau, Christian-Alexandre Castellano, Valérie St-Pierre, Marie Hennebelle, and Stephen C. Cunnane, "Inverse Relationship Between Brain Glucose and Ketone Metabolism in Adults During Short-Term Moderate Dietary Ketosis: A Dual Tracer Quantitative PET Study," *Journal of Cerebral Blood Flow Metabolism* (September 14, 2016), doi:10.1177/0271678X16669366.

31. Cunnane et al., "Can Ketones Help Rescue."

32. Ibid.

33. Jeff Volek and Stephen Phinney, *The Art and Science of Low Carbohydrate Performance* (Lexington, KY: Beyond Obesity LLC, 2012), 35.

34. Maciej Gasior, Michael A. Rogawski, and Adam L. Hartman, "Neuroprotective and Disease-Modifying Effects of the Ketogenic Diet," *Behavioural Pharmacology* 17, no. 5-6 (2006): 431–39; and Antonio Paoli, Antonino Bianco, Ernesto Damiani, and Gerardo Bosco, "Ketogenic Diet in Neuromuscular and Neurodegenerative Diseases," *BioMed Research International* 2014 (2014): 474296, doi:10.1155/2014/474296.

35. Theodore B. VanItallie and Thomas H. Nufert, "Ketones: Metabolism's Ugly Duckling," *Nutrition Reviews* 61, no. 10 (2003): 327–41, doi:10.1301/nr.2003.oct.327-341.

36. Jeff Volek and Stephen Phinney, *Art and Science of Low Carbohydrate Living: An Expert Guide to Making the Life-Saving Benefits of Carbohydrate Restriction Susstainable and Enjoyable* (Lexington, KY: Beyond Obesity, 2011), 164.

37. VanItallie and Nufert, "Ketones: Metabolism's Ugly Duckling."

38. George F. Cahill and Richard L. Veech, "Ketoacids? Good Medicine?" *Transactions of the American Clinical and Climatological Association* 114 (2003): 149–63.

39. Volek and Phinney, *Art and Science of Low Carbohydrate Living*, 5.

40. Csaba Tóth and Zsófia Clemens, "Type 1 Diabetes Mellitus Successfully Managed with the Paleolithic Ketogenic Diet," *International Journal of Case Reports and Images* 5, no. 10 (2014): 699–703, doi:10.5348/ijcri-2014124-CR-10435.

41. Keith Runyan, "Ketogenic Diabetic Athlete," *Ketogenic Diabetic Athlete*, last modified September 12, 2016, https://ketogenicdiabeticathlete.wordpress.com/about; and Ellen Davis and Keith Runyan, *The Ketogenic Diet for Type 1 Diabetes* (Ellen Davis, MS, and Keith Runyan, MD, 2015), http://www.ketogenic-diet-resource.com/treatment-for-diabetes.html.

42. Volek and Phinney, *Art and Science of Low Carbohydrate Living*, 196.

43. Thomas M. Devlin, ed., *Textbook of Biochemistry with Clinical Correlations* (Hoboken, NJ: John Wiley & Sons, 2011), 612.

44. Ibid., 699.

45. Jimmy Moore and Eric Westman, *Keto Clarity* (Las Vegas, NV: Victory Belt, 2014), 171.

46. Henderson, "Ketone Bodies."

47. Volek and Phinney, *Art and Science of Low Carbohydrate Performance*, 53.

48. Food and Nutrition Board, Institute of Medicine, and National Academies of Sciences, *Dietary Reference Intakes for Energy, Carbohydrate, Fiber, Fat, Fatty Acids, Cholesterol, Protein, and Amino Acids* (Washington, DC: National Academies Press, 2005), 275, http://www.nap.edu/read/10490/chapter/8#275.

49. Mary Newport, *The Coconut Oil and Low-Carb Solution for Alzheimer's, Parkinson's, and Other Diseases* (Basic Health Publications, 2015).

50. Cunnane et al., "Can Ketones Help Rescue."

51. Henderson, "Ketone Bodies"; Henderson et al., "Study of the Ketogenic Agent"; Reger et al., "Effects of Beta-hydroxybutyrate on Cognition"; and Newport et al., "A New Way to Produce Hyperketonemia."

52. Mark A. Reger, G. Stennis Watson, Pattie S. Green, Laura D. Baker, Brenna Cholerton, Mark A. Fishel, Stephen R. Plymate, et al., "Intranasal Insulin Administration Dose-Dependently Modulates Verbal Memory and Plasma β-Amyloid in Memory-Impaired Older Adults," *Journal of Alzheimer's Disease* 13, no. 3 (2008): 323–31, https://www.ncbi.nlm.nih.gov/pubmed/18430999; Amy Claxton, Laura D. Baker, Angela Hanson, Emily H. Trittschuh, Brenna Cholerton, Amy Morgan, Maureen Callaghan, et al., "Long-Acting Intranasal Insulin Detemir Improves Cognition for Adults with Mild Cognitive Impairment or Early-Stage Alzheimer's Disease Dementia," *Journal of Alzheimer's Disease* 44, no. 3 (2015): 897–906, doi:10.3233/JAD-141791; and Jessica Freiherr, Manfred Hallschmid, William H. Frey, Yvonne F. Brünner, Colin D. Chapman, Christian Hölscher, Suzanne Craft, et al., "Intranasal Insulin as a Treatment for Alzheimer's Disease: A Review of Basic Research and Clinical Evidence," *CNS Drugs* 27, no. 7 (2013): 505–14, doi:10.1007/s40263-013-0076-8.

53. Leif Hertz, Ye Chen, and Helle S. Waagepetersen, "Effects of Ketone Bodies in Alzheimer's Disease in Relation to Neural Hypometabolism, β-Amyloid Toxicity, and Astrocyte Function," *Journal of Neurochemistry* 134, no. 1 (2015): 7–20, doi:10.1111/jnc.13107.

54. Yudai Nonaka, Tetsuo Takagi, Makoto Inai, Shuhei Nishimura, Shogo Urashima, Kazumitsu Honda, Toshiaki Aoyama, et al., "Lauric Acid Stimulates Ketone Body Production in the KT-5 Astrocyte Cell Line," *Journal of Oleo Science* 65, no. 8 (2016): 693–9, doi:10.5650/jos.ess16069.

55. Manuel Guzmán and Cristina Blázquez, "Is There an Astrocyte-Neuron Ketone Body Shuttle?" *Trends in Endocrinology & Metabolism* 12, no. 4 (2001): 169–73, doi:10.1016/S1043-2760(00)00370-2.

Chapter 3: The Shape and Structure of Neurons and Their Role in Alzheimer's Disease

1. Zhiyou Cai, Yu Zhao, and Bin Zhao, "Roles of Glycogen Synthase Kinase 3 in Alzheimer's Disease," *Current Alzheimer Research* 9, no 7 (2012): 864–79.

2. Jesús Avila, Francisco Wandosell, and Félix Hernández, "Role of Glycogen Synthase Kinase-3 in Alzheimer's Disease Pathogenesis and Glycogen Synthase Kinase-3 Inhibitors," *Expert Review of Neurotherapeutics* 10, no. 5 (2010): 703–10, doi:10.1586/ern.10.40; and Ana Martinez and Daniel I. Perez, "GSK-3 Inhibitors:

A Ray of Hope for the Treatment of Alzheimer's Disease?" *Journal of Alzheimer's Disease* 15, no. 2 (2008): 181–91.

3. Eduardo E. Benarroch, "Brain Cholesterol Metabolism and Neurologic Disease," *Neurology* 71, no. 17 (2008): 1368–73, doi:10.1212/01.wnl.0000333215.93440.36.

4. Roger M. Lane and Martin R. Farlow, "Lipid Homeostasis and Apolipoprotein E in the Development and Progression of Alzheimer's Disease," *Journal of Lipid Research* 46, no. 5 (2005): 949–68, doi:10.1194/jlr.M400486-JLR200.

5. Geraldine J. Cuskelly, Kathleen M. Moone, and Ian S. Young, "Folate and Vitamin B_{12}: Friendly or Enemy Nutrients for the Elderly," *Proceedings of the Nutrition Society* 66, no. 4 (2007): 548–58, doi:10.1017/S0029665107005873; and Ellen M. Whyte, Benoit H. Mulsant, Meryl A. Butters, Moshin Qayyum, Adele Towers, Robert A. Sweet, William Klunk et al., "Cognitive and Behavioral Correlates of Low Vitamin B_{12} Levels in Elderly Patients with Progressive Dementia," *American Journal of Geriatric Psychiatry* 10, no 3 (2002): 321–7.

6. A. Vogiatzoglou, H. Refsum, C. Johnston, S. M. Smith, K. M. Bradley, C. de Jager, M. M. Budge, et al., "Vitamin B_{12} Status and Rate of Brain Volume Loss in Community-Dwelling Elderly," *Neurology* 71, no. 11 (2008): 826–32, doi:10.1212/01.wnl.0000325581.26991.f2.

7. Ibid.

8. David Brownstein, *Vitamin B-12 for Health* (West Bloomfield, MI: Medical Alternatives Press, 2012).

Chapter 5: Mitochondrial Function and Dysfunction

1. Paula I. Moreira, Maria S. Santos, Raquel Seiça, and Catarina R. Oliveira, "Brain Mitochondrial Dysfunction as a Link Between Alzheimer's Disease and Diabetes," *Journal of the Neurological Sciences* 257, no, 1-2 (2007): 206–14, doi:10.1016/j.jns.2007.01.017.

2. Moreira et al., "Brain Mitochondrial Dysfunction"; Rita Perfeito, Teresa Cunha-Oliveira, and Ana Cristina Carvalho Rego, "Revisiting Oxidative Stress and Mitochondrial Dysfunction in the Pathogenesis of Parkinson Disease—Resemblance to the Effect of Amphetamine Drugs of Abuse," *Free Radical Biology and Medicine* 62 (2013): 186–201, doi:10.1016/j.freeradbiomed.2013.05.042; Giovanni Manfredi and Zuoshang Xu, "Mitochondrial Dysfunction and Its Role in Motor Neuron Degeneration in ALS," *Mitochondrion* 5, no 2 (2005): 77–87, doi:10.1016/j.mito.2005.01.002; Peizhong Maoa and P. Hemachandra Reddy, "Is Multiple Sclerosis a Mitochondrial Disease?" *Biochimica et Biophysica Acta* 1802, no. 1 (2010): 66–79, doi:10.1016/j.bbadis.2009.07.002; and Pradip K. Kamat, Anuradha Kalani, Philip Kyles, Suresh C. Tyagi, and Neetu Tyagi, "Autophagy of Mitochondria: A Promising Therapeutic Target for Neurodegenerative Disease," *Cell Biochemistry and Biophysics* 70, no. 2 (2014): 707–19, doi:10.1007/s12013-014-0006-5.

3. National Heart, Lung, and Blood Institute, "What Is Metabolic Syndrome?," *National Heart, Lung, and Blood Institute*, last modified June 22, 2016, http://www.nhlbi.nih.gov/health/health-topics/topics/ms/; Se Eun Park, Eun-Jung Rhee, Cheol-Young Park, Ki Won Oh, Sung-Woo Park, Sun-Woo Kim, and Won-Young

Lee, "Impact of Hyperinsulinemia on the Development of Hypertension in Normotensive, Nondiabetic Adults: A 4-Year Follow-Up Study," *Metabolism* 62, no. 4 (2013): 532–8, doi:10.1016/j.metabol.2012.09.013; and James R. Sowers, P. R. Standley, J. L. Ram, S. Jacober, L. Simpson, and K. Rose, "Hyperinsulinemia, Insulin Resistance, and Hyperglycemia: Contributing Factors in the Pathogenesis of Hypertension and Atherosclerosis," *American Journal of Hypertension* 6, no. 7, Pt 2 (1993): 260S–270S, doi:10.1093/ajh/6.7.260S.

4. Xukai Wang, Changqing Yu, Bo Zhand, and Yan Wang, "The Injurious Effects of Hyperinsulinism on Blood Vessels," *Cell Biochemistry and Biophysics* 69, no. 2 (2014): 213–8, doi:10.1007/s12013-013-9810-6; Enzo Bonora, Stefan Kiechl, Johann Willeit, Friedrich Oberhollenzer, Georg Egger, James B. Meigs, Riccardo C. Bonadonna, et al., "Insulin Resistance as Estimated by Homeostasis Model Assessment Predicts Incident Symptomatic Cardiovascular Disease in Caucasian Subjects from the General Population: The Bruneck Study," *Diabetes Care* 30, no. 2 (2007): 318–24, doi:10.2337/dc06-0919; and Motonobu Nakamura, Nobuhiko Satoh, Masashi Suzuki, Haruki Kume, Yukio Homma, George Seki, and Shoko Horita, "Stimulatory Effect of Insulin on Renal Proximal Tubule Sodium Transport Is Preserved in Type 2 Diabetes with Nephropathy," *Biochemical and Biophysical Research Communications* 461, no. 1 (2015): 154–8, doi:10.1016/j.bbrc.2015.04.005.

5. Stephanie Seneff, Glyn Wainwright, and Luca Mascitelli, "Nutrition and Alzheimer's Disease: The Detrimental Role of a High Carbohydrate Diet," *European Journal of Internal Medicine* 22, no. 2 (2011): 134–40, doi:10.1016/j.ejim.2010.12.017.

6. Moreira et al., "Brain Mitochondrial Dysfunction."

7. Mortimer Mamelak, "Alzheimer's Disease, Oxidative Stress and Gammahydroxybutyrate," *Neurobiology of Aging* 28, no. 9 (2007): 1340–60, doi:10.1016/j.neurobiolaging.2006.06.008.

Chapter 6: Beta-Amyloid as a Cause of Alzheimer's: Guilty Party or Wrongly Accused?

1. Dale E. Bredesen, *Cognitive Health: Dawn of the Era of Treatable Alzheimer's Disease*, film, 56:21, August 4, 2016, https://vimeo.com/173061978.

2. Samuel T. Henderson, "Ketone Bodies as a Therapeutic for Alzheimer's Disease," *Neurotherapeutics* 5, no. 3 (2008): 470–80.

3. Sónia C. Correia, Renato X. Santos, Cristina Carvalho, Susana Cardoso, Emanuel Candeias, Maria S. Santos, Catarina R. Oliveira, et al., "Insulin Signaling, Glucose Metabolism and Mitochondria: Major Players in Alzheimer's Disease and Diabetes Interrelation," *Brain Research* 1441 (2012): 64–78, doi:10.1016/j.brainres.2011.12.063.

4. Ibid.

5. Mortimer Mamelak, "Alzheimer's Disease, Oxidative Stress and Gammahydroxybutyrate," *Neurobiology of Aging* 28, no. 9 (2007): 1340–60, doi:10.1016/j.neurobiolaging.2006.06.008.

6. Uday Saxena, "Alzheimer's Disease Amyloid Hypothesis at Crossroads: Where Do We Go from Here?" *Expert Opinion on Therapeutic Targets* 14, no. 12 (2010): 1273–7, doi:10.1517/14728222.2010.528285.

7. Michael A. Castello and Salvador Soriano, "On the Origin of Alzheimer's Disease. Trials and Tribulations of the Amyloid Hypothesis," *Ageing Research Reviews* 13 (2014): 10–12, doi:10.1016/j.arr.2013.10.001; and Michael A. Castello, John D. Jeppson, and Salvador Soriano, "Moving Beyond Anti-Amyloid Therapy for the Prevention and Treatment of Alzheimer's Disease," *BMC Neurology* 14 (2014): 169, doi:10.1186/s12883-014-0169-0.
8. Theodore B. VanItallie, "Biomarkers, Ketone Bodies, and the Prevention of Alzheimer's Disease," *Metabolism* 64, no. 3 (Suppl 1) (2015): S51–S57, doi:10.1016/j.metabol.2014.10.033.

Chapter 7: ApoE4: Is There an Alzheimer's Gene?

1. Veena Theendakara, Claire A. Peters-Libeu, Patricia Spilman, Karen S. Poksay, Dale E. Bredesen, and Rammohan V. Rao, "Direct Transcriptional Effects of Apolipoprotein E," *The Journal of Neuroscience*. 36, no. 3 (2016): 685–700, doi:10.1523/JNEUROSCI.3562-15.2016.
2. Stephanie Seneff, Glyn Wainwright, and Luca Mascitelli, "Nutrition and Alzheimer's Disease: The Detrimental Role of a High Carbohydrate Diet," *European Journal of Internal Medicine* 22, no. 2 (2011): 134–40, doi:10.1016/j.ejim.2010.12.017.
3. Eric M. Reiman, Kewel Chen, Gene Alexander, Richard J. Caselli, Daniel Bandy, David Osborne, Ann M. Saunders, et al., "Functional Brain Abnormalities in Young Adults at Genetic Risk for Late-Onset Alzheimer's Dementia," *Proceedings of the National Academy of Sciences of the United States of America* 101, no. 1 (2004): 284–89, doi:10.1073/pnas.2635903100; and M. I. Kamboh, "Apolipoprotein E Polymorphism and Susceptibility to Alzheimer's Disease," *Human Biology* 67, no. 2 (1995): 195–215.
4. Reiman et al., "Functional Brain Abnormalities."
5. Ibid.
6. W. Q. Qiu and M. F. Folstein, "Insulin, Insulin-Degrading Enzyme and Amyloid-β Peptide in Alzheimer's Disease: Review and Hypothesis," *Neurobiology of Aging* 27, no. 2 (2006): 190–98, doi:10.1016/j.neurobiolaging.2005.01.004.
7. Robert Krikorian, Marcelle D. Shidler, Krista Dangelo, Sarah C. Couch, Stephen C. Benoit, and Deborah J. Clegg, "Dietary Ketosis Enhances Memory in Mild Cognitive Impairment," *Neurobiology of Aging* 33, no. 425 (2012): 425e19-425e27.
8. Jose A. Luchsinger, Ming-Xin Tang, Steven Shea, and Richard Mayeux, "Hyper-insulinemia and Risk of Alzheimer Disease," *Neurology* 63, no. 7 (2004): 1187–92.
9. Alzheimer's Association, "The Search for Alzheimer's Causes and Risk Factors," *Alzheimer's Association*, http://www.alz.org/research/science/alzheimers_disease_causes.asp#genetics.
10. Roger M. Lane and Martin R. Farlow, "Lipid Homeostasis and Apolipoprotein E in the Development and Progression of Alzheimer's Disease," *Journal of Lipid Research* 46, no. 5 (2005): 949–68, doi:10.1194/jlr.M400486-JLR200.
11. Samuel T. Henderson, "High Carbohydrate Diets and Alzheimer's Disease," *Medical Hypotheses* 62 (2004): 689–700, doi:10.1016/j.mehy.2003.11.028.

12. Lane and Farlow, "Lipid Homeostasis and Apolipoprotein E."
13. R. M. Corbo and R. Scacchi, "Apolipoprotein E (APOE) Allele Distribution in the World. Is APOE*4 a 'Thrifty' Allele?" *Annals of Human Genetics* 63, no. 4 (1999): 301–10.
14. Henderson, "High Carbohydrate Diets."
15. Ibid.
16. Ibid.
17. US National Library of Medicine Genetics Home Reference, "APOE," US National Institutes of Health, https://ghr.nlm.nih.gov/gene/APOE#conditions (July 20, 2016).
18. A. S. Henderson, S. Easteal, A. F. Jorm, A. J. Mackinnon, A. E. Korten, H. Christensen, L. Croft, et al., "Apolipoprotein E Allele Epsilon 4, Dementia, and Cognitive Decline in a Population Sample," *Lancet* 346, no. 8987 (1995): 1387–90, http://www.ncbi.nlm.nih.gov/pubmed/7475820.
19. Richard L. Veech, "The Therapeutic Implications of Ketone Bodies: The Effects of Ketone Bodies in Pathological Conditions: Ketosis, Ketogenic Diet, Redox States, Insulin Resistance, and Mitochondrial Metabolism," *Prostaglandins, Leukotrienes, and Essential Fatty Acids* 70, no. 3 (2004): 309–19, doi:10.1016/j.plefa.2003.09.007.
20. Alex Ward, Sheila Crean, Catherine J. Mercaldi, Jenna M. Collins, Dylan Boyd, Michael N. Cook, and H. Michael Arrighi, "Prevalence of Apolipoprotein E4 Genotype and Homozygotes (APOE e4/4) Among Patients Diagnosed with Alzheimer's Disease: A Systematic Review and Meta-Analysis," *Neuroepidemiology* 38, no. 1 (2012): 1–17, doi:10.1159/000334607; and Sheila Crean, Alex Ward, Catherine J. Mercaldi, Jenna M. Collins, Michael N. Cook, Nicole L. Baker, and H. Michael Arrighi, "Apolipoprotein E ε4 Prevalence in Alzheimer's Disease Patients Varies Across Global Populations: A Systematic Literature Review and Meta-Analysis," *Dementia and Geriatric Cognitive Disorders* 31, no. 1 (2011): 20–30, doi:10.1159/000321984.
21. Uffe Ravnskov, David M. Diamond, Rokura Hama, Tomohito Hamazaki, Björn Hammarskjöld, Niamh Hynes, Malcolm Kendrick et al., "Lack of an Association or an Inverse Association Between Low-Density-Lipoprotein Cholesterol and Mortality in the Elderly: A Systematic Review," *BMJ Open* 6, no. 6 (2016): e010401, doi:10.1136/bmjopen-2015-010401.
22. Ravnskov et al., "Lack of an Association"; and Nicole Schupf, Rosann Costa, Jose Luchsinger, Ming-Xin Tang, Joseph H. Lee, and Richard Mayeux, "Relationship Between Plasma Lipids and All-Cause Mortality in Nondemented Elderly," *Journal of the American Geriatrics Society* 53, no. 2 (2005): 219–26, doi:10.1111/j.1532-5415.2005.53106.x.
23. Ancestry Foundation, "AHS16—Steven Gundry—Dietary Management of the Apo E 4," YouTube video, 38:46, posted August 17, 2016, https://www.youtube.com/watch?v=Bfr9RPq0HFg.
24. Dale E. Bredesen, "Ancestral Health Symposium," presentation, Ancestral Health Symposium, Boulder, Colorado, August 11, 2016.
25. Ancestry Foundation, "AHS16—Steven Gundry."

Chapter 8: Low-Carbohydrate Diet Basics

1. Samuel T. Henderson, "High Carbohydrate Diets and Alzheimer's Disease," *Medical Hypotheses* 62 (2004): 689–700, doi:10.1016/j.mehy.2003.11.028.

Chapter 9: Cholesterol: The Brain's Best Friend

1. Roger M. Lane and Martin R. Farlow, "Lipid Homeostasis and Apolipoprotein E in the Development and Progression of Alzheimer's Disease," *Journal of Lipid Research* 46, no. 5 (2005): 949–68, doi:10.1194/jlr.M400486-JLR200.
2. Joseph Kraft, *Diabetes Epidemic & You* (Bloomington, IN: Trafford Publishing, 2011), 69.
3. Jimmy Moore and Eric Westman, *Cholesterol Clarity* (Las Vegas: Victory Belt, 2013), 158.
4. Natasha Campbell-McBride, *Put Your Heart in Your Mouth* (Cambridge: Medinform Publishing, 2007), 38.
5. Moore and Westman, *Cholesterol Clarity*, 134.
6. Campbell-McBride, *Put Your Heart in Your Mouth*, 38.
7. Moore and Westman, *Cholesterol Clarity*, 34.
8. M. M. Mielke, P. P. Zandi, M. Sjogren, D. Gustafson, S. Ostling, B. Steen, and I. Skoog, "High Total Cholesterol Levels in Late Life Associated with a Reduced Risk of Dementia," *Neurology* 64, no. 10 (2005): 1689–95. doi:10.1212/01.WNL .0000161870.78572.A5.
9. M. Mulder, R. Ravid, D. F. Swaab, E. R. de Kloet, E. D. Haasdijk, J. Julk, J. van der Boom et al., "Reduced Levels of Cholesterol, Phospholipids, and Fatty Acids in Cerebrospinal Fluid of Alzheimer Disease Patients Are Not Related to Apolipoprotein E4," *Alzheimer Disease and Associated Disorders* 12, no. 3 (1998): 198–203, http://www.ncbi.nlm.nih.gov/pubmed/9772023.
10. Y.-B. Lv, Z.-X. Yin, C.-L. Chei, M. S. Brasher, J. Zhang, V. B. Kraus, F. Qian, et al., "Serum Cholesterol Levels within the High Normal Range Are Associated with Better Cognitive Performance Among Chinese Elderly," *The Journal of Nutrition, Health & Aging* 20, no. 3 (2016): 280–7, doi:10.1007/s12603-016-0701-6.
11. Sonia Brescianini, Stefania Maggi, Gino Farchi, Sergio Mariotti, Antonio Di Carlo, Marzia Baldereschi, and Domenico Inzitari, "Low Total Cholesterol and Increased Risk of Dying: Are Low Levels Clinical Warning Signs in the Elderly? Results from the Italian Longitudinal Study on Aging," *Journal of the American Geriatrics Society* 51, no. 7 (2003): 991–6; and Nicole Schupf, Rosann Costa, Jose Luchsinger, Ming-Xin Tang, Joseph H. Lee, and Richard Mayeux, "Relationship Between Plasma Lipids and All-Cause Mortality in Nondemented Elderly," *Journal of the American Geriatrics Society* 53, no. 2 (2005): 219–26, doi:10.1111/j.1532-5415.2005.53106.x.
12. Yue-Bin Lv, Zhao-Xue Yin, Choy-Lye Chei, Han-Zhu Qian, Virgina Byers Kraus, Juan Zhang, Melanie Sereny Brasher, et al., "Low-Density Lipoprotein Cholesterol was Inversely Associated with 3-Year All-Cause Mortality Among Chinese Oldest Old: Data from the Chinese Longitudinal Healthy Longevity Survey," *Atherosclerosis* 239, no. 1 (2015): 137–42, doi:10.1016/j.atherosclerosis.2015.01.002.

13. Uffe Ravnskov, David M. Diamond, Rokura Hama, Tomohito Hamazaki, Björn Hammarskjöld, Niamh Hynes, Malcolm Kendrick, et al., "Lack of an Association or an Inverse Association between Low-Density-Lipoprotein Cholesterol and Mortality in the Elderly: A Systematic Review," *BMJ Open* 6, no. 6 (2016): e010401, doi:10.1136/bmjopen-2015-010401.

14. Seyed-Foad Ahmadi, Elani Streja, Golara Zahmatkesh, Dan Streja, Moti Kashyap, Hamid Moradi, Miklos Z. Molnar, et al., "Reverse Epidemiology of Traditional Cardiovascular Risk Factors in the Geriatric Population," *Journal of the American Medical Directors Association* 16, no. 11 (2015): 933–9, doi:10.1016/j.jamda .2015.07.014.

15. Mary Enig, *Know Your Fats* (Silver Spring, MD: Bethesda Press, 2000), 56–57.

16. Moore and Westman, *Cholesterol Clarity*, 153.

17. Enig, *Know Your Fats*, 64.

18. Barry Groves, *Trick and Treat* (London: Hammersmith Press Ltd., 2008), 89.

19. Paula I. Moreira, Maria S. Santos, Raquel Seiça, and Catarina R. Oliveira, "Brain Mitochondrial Dysfunction as a Link Between Alzheimer's Disease and Diabetes," *Journal of the Neurological Sciences* 257, no. 1–2 (2007): 206–14, doi:10.1016/j.jns .2007.01.017.

20. Anjaneyulu Kowluru, "Protein Prenylation in Glucose-Induced Insulin Secretion from the Pancreatic Islet β Cell: A Perspective," *Journal of Cellular and Molecular Medicine* 12, no. 1 (2008): 164–73, doi:10.1111/j.1582-4934.2007.00168.x; Anjaneyulu Kowluru, "Regulatory Roles for Small G Proteins in the Pancreatic β-Cell: Lessons from Models of Impaired Insulin Secretion," *American Journal of Physiology Endocrinology and Metabolism* 285, no. 4 (2003): E669–84; Rajesh Amin, Hai-Qing Chen, Marie Tannous, Richard Gibbs, and Anjaneyulu Kowluru, "Inhibition of Glucose- and Calcium-Induced Insulin Secretion from βTC3 Cells by Novel Inhibitors of Protein Isoprenylation," *The Journal of Pharmacology and Experimental Therapeutics* 303, no. 1 (2002): 82–8, doi:10.1124/jpet.102.036160; and Anjaneyulu Kowluru and Rajesh Amin, "Inhibitors of Post-Translational Modifications of G-Proteins as Probes to Study the Pancreatic Beta Cell Function: Potential Therapeutic Implications," *Current Drug Targets. Immune, Endocrine and Metabolic Disorders* 2, no. 2 (2002): 129–39.

21. Ravi V. Shah and Allison B. Goldfine, "Statins and Risk of New-Onset Diabetes Mellitus," *Circulation* 126, no. 18 (2012): e282-4, doi:10.1161/CIRCULATIONAHA .112.122135; and Henna Cederberg, Alena Stančáková, Nagendra Yaluri, Shalem Modi, Johanna Kuusisto, and Markku Laakso, "Increased Risk of Diabetes with Statin Treatment Is Associated with Impaired Insulin Sensitivity and Insulin Secretion: A 6 Year Follow-Up Study of the METSIM Cohort," *Diabetologia* 58, no. 5 (2015): 1109–17, doi:10.1007/s00125-015-3528-5.

22. Henna Cederberg et al., "Increased Risk of Diabetes."

23. Moore and Westman, *Cholesterol Clarity*, 118.

24. Mayo Clinic Staff, "Statin Side Effects: Weigh the Benefits and Risks," Mayo Clinic, http://www.mayoclinic.org/diseases-conditions/high-blood-cholesterol /in-depth/statin-side-effects/art-20046013 (August 3, 2016).

25. US Food & Drug Administration, "FDA Expands Advice on Statin Risks," US Food & Drug Administration, http://www.fda.gov/ForConsumers/Consumer Updates/ucm293330.htm (September 5, 2016).

26. US Food & Drug Administration, "FDA Drug Safety Communication: Important safety label changes to cholesterol-lowering statin drugs," US Food & Drug Administration, http://www.fda.gov/Drugs/DrugSafety/ucm293101.htm (September 5, 2016).

27. Chris Kresser, "RHR: Prevention and Treatment of Alzheimer's from a Functional Perspective—with Dr. Dale Bredesen," *Chris Kresser*, posted July 14, 2016, http://chriskresser.com/prevention-and-treatment-of-alzheimers-from-a-functional-perspective-with-dr-dale-bredesen.

28. Moore and Westman, *Cholesterol Clarity*, 117.

29. Ibid., 97.

30. Ash Simmonds, *Principia Ketogenica: Compendium of Science Literature on the Benefits of Low Carbohydrate and Ketogenic Diets* (CreateSpace, 2014).

31. Nicole Schupf et al., "Relationship Between Plasma Lipids"; Lv et al., "Low-Density Lipoprotein Cholesterol was Inversely Associated with 3-Year All-Cause Mortality Among Chinese Oldest Old"; Ravnskov et al., "Lack of an Association or an Inverse Association between Low-Density-Lipoprotein Cholesterol and Mortality in the Elderly"; Ahmadi et al., "Reverse Epidemiology of Traditional Cardiovascular Risk Factors in the Geriatric Population"; Tore Scherstén, Paul John Rosch, Karl E. Arfors, and Ralf Sundberg, "The Cholesterol Hypothesis: Time for the Obituary?" *Scandinavian Cardiovascular Journal* 45, no. 6 (2011): 322–3, doi:10.3109/14017431.2011.613203; and Christopher E. Ramsden, Daisy Zamora, Sharon Majchrzak-Hong, Keturah R. Faurot, Steven K. Broste, Robert P. Frantz, John M. Davis et al., "Re-Evaluation of the Traditional Diet-Heart Hypothesis: Analysis of Recovered Data from Minnesota Coronary Experiment (1968–73)," *BMJ* 353 (2016): i1246, doi:10.1136/bmj.i1246.

32. Thomas Dayspring, Twitter post, November 10, 2014, 8:02 p.m., https://twitter.com/Drlipid/status/531975228109627392.

33. Moore and Westman, *Cholesterol Clarity*, 34.

34. Ibid., 136.

35. Jeff Volek and Stephen Phinney, *The Art and Science of Low Carbohydrate Living* (Lexington, KY: Beyond Obesity LLC, 2011), 102.

Chapter 10: Carbohydrates: Starchy, Nonstarchy, and Not as "Complex" as You Think

1. Jimmy Moore and Eric Westman, *Keto Clarity* (Las Vegas: Victory Belt, 2014), 72.

Chapter 11: Protien: Primary Player in Our Bodies and on Our Plates

1. William F. Martin, Lawrence E. Armstrong, and Nancy Rodriguez, "Dietary Protein Intake and Renal Function," *Nutrition & Metabolism* 2 (2005): 25, doi:10.1186/1743-7075-2-25; and Claire E. Berryman, Sanjiv Agarwal, Harris R. Lieberman, Victor L. Fulgoni III, and Stefan M. Pasiakos, "Diets Higher in

Animal and Plant Protein Are Associated with Lower Adiposity and Do Not
Impair Kidney Function in US Adults," *American Journal of Clinical Nutrition*
104, no. 3 (2016): 743–9, doi:10.3945/ajcn.116.133819.

2. Wayne W. Campbell, Rodd A. Trappe, Robert R. Wolfe, and William J. Evans,
"The Recommended Dietary Allowance for Protein May Not Be Adequate for
Older People to Maintain Skeletal Muscle," *The Journals of Gerontology. Series
A, Biological Sciences and Medical Sciences* 56, no. 6 (2001): M373–M380,
doi:10.1093/gerona/56.6.M373; Wayne W. Campbell, Marilyn C. Crim, Gerard E.
Dallal, Vernon R. Young, and William J. Evans, "Increased Protein Requirements
in Elderly People: New Data and Retrospective Reassessments," *American Journal
of Clinical Nutrition* 60, no. 4 (1994): 501–9; and José A. Morais, Stéphanie
Chevalier, and Rejeanne Gougeon, "Protein Turnover and Requirements in the
Healthy and Frail Elderly," *The Journal of Nutrition, Health & Aging* 10, no. 4
(2006): 272–83.

3. Thomas Remer and Friedrich Manz, "Potential Renal Acid Load of Foods and Its
Influence on Urine pH," *Journal of the Academy of Nutrition and Dietetics* 95, no.
7 (1995): 791–7, doi:10.1016/S0002-8223(95)00219-7.

4. Jay J. Cao, LuAnn K. Johnson, and Janet R. Hunt, "A Diet High in Meat Protein
and Potential Renal Acid Load Increases Fractional Calcium Absorption and
Urinary Calcium Excretion Without Affecting Markers of Bone Resorption
or Formation in Postmenopausal Women," *The Journal of Nutrition* 141, no. 3
(2011): 391–7, doi:10.3945/jn.110.129361; and Jay J. Cao and Forrest H. Nielsen,
"Acid Diet (High-Meat Protein) Effects on Calcium Metabolism and Bone
Health," *Current Opinion in Clinical Nutrition and Metabolic Care* 13, no. 6 (2010):
698–702, doi:10.1097/MCO.0b013e32833df691.

5. Jane E. Kerstetter, Kimberly O. O'Brien, and Karl L. Insogna, "Low Protein
Intake: The Impact on Calcium and Bone Homeostasis in Humans," *The Journal
of Nutrition* 133, no. 3 (2003): 855S–861S; and Jane E. Kerstetter, Kimberly O.
O'Brien, and Karl L. Insogna, "Dietary Protein, Calcium Metabolism, and Skeletal
Homeostasis Revisited," *American Journal of Clinical Nutrition* 78, 3 Suppl (2003):
584S–592S.

6. Food and Nutrition Board, Institute of Medicine, and National Academies,
"Dietary Reference Intakes (DRIs): Recommended Dietary Allowances and
Adequate Intakes, Total Water and Macronutrients," accessed September 9, 2016,
http://fnic.nal.usda.gov/sites/fnic.nal.usda.gov/files/uploads/recommended
_intakes_individuals.pdf.

7. Berna Rahi, Zoé Colombet, Magali Gonzalez-Colaço Harmand, Jean-François
Dartigues, Yves Boirie, Luc Letenneur, and Catherine Feart, "Higher Protein
but Not Energy Intake Is Associated with a Lower Prevalence of Frailty Among
Community-Dwelling Older Adults in the French Three-City Cohort," *Journal
of the American Medical Directors Association* 17, no. 7 (2016): 672.e7–672.e11,
doi:10.1016/j.jamda.2016.05.005; and Helena Sandoval-Insausti, Raúl F. Pérez-
Tasigchana, Esther López-García, Esther García-Esquinas, Fernando Rodríguez-
Artalejo, and Pilar Guallar-Castillón, "Macronutrients Intake and Incident Frailty

in Older Adults: A Prospective Cohort Study," *The Journals of Gerontology. Series A, Biological Sciences and Medical Sciences* 71, no. 10 (October 2016): 1329–1334, http://www.ncbi.nlm.nih.gov/pubmed/26946103.

8. Mary Ann Binnie, Karine Barlow, Valerie Johnson, and Carol Harrison, "Red Meats: Time for a Paradigm Shift in Dietary Advice," *Meat Science* 98, no. 3 (2014): 445–51, doi:10.1016/j.meatsci.2014.06.024; and Neil Mann, "Dietary Lean Red Meat and Human Evolution: *European Journal of Nutrition* 39, no. 2 (2000): 71–9.

9. Loren Cordain, S. B. Eaton, J. C. Brand-Miller, N. Mann, and K. Hill, "The Paradoxical Nature of Hunter-Gatherer Diets: Meat-Based, Yet Non-Atherogenic," *European Journal of Clinical Nutrition* 56, Suppl 1 (2002): S42–S52, doi:10.1038 /sj.ejcn.1601353.

10. Loren Cordain, B. A. Watkins, G. L. Florant, M. Kelher, L. Robers, and Y. Li, "Fatty Acid Analysis of Wild Ruminant Tissues: Evolutionary Implications for Reducing Diet-Related Chronic Disease," *European Journal of Clinical Nutrition* 56, no. 3 (2002): 181–91, doi:10.1038/sj.ejcn.1601307; and Cynthia A. Daley, Amber Abbott, Patrick S. Doyle, Glenn A. Nader, and Stephanie Larson, "A Review of Fatty Acid Profiles and Antioxidant Content in Grass-Fed and Grain-Fed Beef," *Nutrition Journal* 9 (2010): 10, doi:10.1186/1475-2891-9-10.

11. Duo Li, Sirithon Siriamornpun, Mark L. Wahlqvist, Neil J. Mann, and Andrew J. Sinclair, "Lean Meat and Heart Health," *Asia Pacific Journal of Clinical Nutrition* 14, no. 2 (2005): 113–9; Alison J. McAfee, Emeir M. McSorely, Geraldine J. Cuskelly, Bruce W. Moss, Julie M. W. Wallace, Maxine P. Bonham, and Anna M. Fearon, "Red Meat Consumption: An Overview of the Risks and Benefits," *Meat Science* 84, no. 1 (2010): 1–13, doi:10.1016/j.meatsci.2009.08.029; and Shalene H. McNeill, "Inclusion of Red Meat in Healthful Dietary Patterns," *Meat Science* 98, no. 3 (2014): 452–60, doi:10.1016/j.meatsci.2014.06.028.

12. Richard D. Feinman, *The World Turned Upside Down* (Brooklyn, NY: NMS Press, 2014), 287, 296.

Chapter 12: Fat Is Not a Four Letter Word! The Critical Importance of Fat in the Body

1. Robb Wolf, *The Paleo Solution* (Las Vegas: Victory Belt, 2010), 105.

2. Jimmy Moore and Eric Westman, *Cholesterol Clarity* (Las Vegas: Victory Belt, 2013), 97.

3. Glen D. Lawrence, "Dietary Fats and Health: Dietary Recommendations in the Context of Scientific Evidence," *Advances in Nutrition* 4, no. 3 (2013): 294–302.

4. Moore and Westman, *Cholesterol Clarity*, 163.

5. Jimmy Moore and Eric Westman, *Keto Clarity* (Las Vegas: Victory Belt, 2014): 88, 114.

6. Riya Ganguly and Grant N. Pierce, "The Toxicity of Dietary Trans Fats," *Food and Chemical Toxicology* 78 (2015): 170–6, doi:10.1016/j.fct.2015.02.004; Dariush Mozaffarian, A. Aro , and Walter C. Willett, "Health Effects of Trans-Fatty Acids: Experimental and Observational Evidence," *European Journal of Clinical Nutrition* 63, Suppl 2 (2009): S5–S21, doi:10.1038/sj.ejcn.1602973; Paul Nestel, "Trans Fatty Acids: Are Its Cardiovascular Risks Fully Appreciated?" *Clinical*

Therapeutics 36, no. 3 (2014): 315–21, doi:10.1016/j.clinthera.2014.01.020; and Dariush Mozaffarian, "Trans Fatty Acids—Effects on Systemic Inflammation and Endothelial Function," *Atherosclerosis Supplements* 7, no. 2 (2006): 29–32, doi:10.1016/j.atherosclerosissup.2006.04.007.

7. Nestel, "Trans Fatty Acids."
8. A. Phivilay, C. Julien, C. Tremblay, L. Berthiaume, P. Julien, Y. Giguère, and F. Calon, "High Dietary Consumption of Trans Fatty Acids Decreases Brain Docosahexaenoic Acid But Does Not Alter Amyloid-β and Tau Pathologies in the 3xTg-AD Model of Alzheimer's Disease," *Neuroscience* 159, no. 1 (2009): 296–307, doi:10.1016/j.neuroscience.2008.12.006.
9. Ganguly and Pierce, "The Toxicity of Dietary Trans Fats"; Jean-Charles Martin and Karine Valeille, "Conjugated Linoleic Acids: All the Same or to Everyone Its Own Function?" *Reproduction, Nutrition, Development* 42, no. 6 (2002): 525–36; and Klaus W. J. Wahle, Steven D. Heys, and Dino Rotondo, "Conjugated Linoleic Acids: Are They Beneficial or Detrimental to Health?" *Progress in Lipid Research* 43, no. 6 (2004): 553–87, doi:10.1016/j.plipres.2004.08.002.
10. Wahle et al., "Conjugated Linoleic Acids"; and Arunabh Bhattacharya, Jameela Banu, Mizanur Rahman, Jennifer Causey, and Gabriet Fernandes, "Biological Effects of Conjugated Linoleic Acids in Health and Disease," *The Journal of Nutritional Biochemistry* 17, no. 12 (2006): 789–810, doi:10.1016/j.jnutbio.2006.02.009.
11. T. R. Dhiman, G. R. Anand, L. D. Satter, and M. W. Pariza, "Conjugated Linoleic Acid Content of Milk from Cows Fed Different Diets," *Journal of Dairy Science* 82, no. 10 (1999): 2146–56, doi:10.3168/jds.S0022-0302(99)75458-5.
12. Patty W. Siri-Tarino, Qi Sun, Frank B. Hu, and Ronald M. Krauss, "Meta-Analysis of Prospective Cohort Studies Evaluating the Association of Saturated Fat with Cardiovascular Disease," *American Journal of Clinical Nutrition* 91, no. 3 (2010): 535–46, doi:10.3945/ajcn.2009.27725.
13. Ibid.
14. Ibid.
15. Ibid.
16. James D. DiNicolantonio, Sean Lucan, and James H. O'Keefe, "The Evidence for Saturated Fat and for Sugar Related to Coronary Heart Disease," *Progress in Cardiovascular Diseases* 58, no. 5 (2016): 464–72, doi:10.1016/j.pcad.2015.11.006.
17. Tanja K. Thorning, Farinaz Raziani, Nathalie T. Bendsen, Arne Astrup, Tine Tholstrup, and Anne Raben, "Diets with High-Fat Cheese, High-Fat Meat, or Carbohydrate on Cardiovascular Risk Markers in Overweight Postmenopausal Women: A Randomized Crossover Trial," *The American Journal of Clinical Nutrition* 102, no. 3 (2015): 573–81, doi:10.3945/ajcn.115.109116.
18. Patty W. Siri-Tarino, Qi Sun, Frank B. Hu, and Ronald M. Krauss, "Saturated Fat, Carbohydrate, and Cardiovascular Disease," *The American Journal of Clinical Nutrition* 91, no. 3 (2010): 502–9, doi:10.3945/ajcn.2008.26285.
19. Lawrence, "Dietary Fats and Health."
20. Ibid.
21. Moore and Westman, *Cholesterol Clarity*, 141.

22. Christopher E. Ramsden, Daisy Zamora, Sharon Majchrzak-Hong, Keturah R. Faurot, Steven K. Broste, Robert P. Frantz, John M. Davis, et al., "Re-Evaluation of the Traditional Diet-Heart Hypothesis: Analysis of Recovered Data from Minnesota Coronary Experiment (1968–73)," *BMJ* 353 (2016): i1246, doi:10.1136/bmj.i1246.

Chapter 13: Special Fats for the Brain

1. Jeff Volek and Stephen Phinney, *The Art and Science of Low Carbohydrate Performance* (Lexington, KY: Beyond Obesity, 2012): 95.
2. Artemis P. Simopoulos, "Evolutionary Aspects of Diet: The Omega-6/Omega-3 Ratio and the Brain," *Molecular Neurobiology* 44, no. 2 (2011): 203–15, doi:10.1007/s12035-010-8162-0.
3. Samuel T. Henderson, "High Carbohydrate Diets and Alzheimer's Disease," *Medical Hypotheses* 62 (2004): 689–700: doi: 10.1016/j.mehy.2003.11.028.
4. Roger M. Lane and Martin R. Farlow, "Lipid Homeostasis and Apolipoprotein E in the Development and Progression of Alzheimer's Disease," *Journal of Lipid Research*, 46, no. 5 (2005): 949–68, doi:10.1194/jlr.M400486-JLR200.
5. Stephen C. Cunnane, Scott Nugent, Maggie Roy, Alexandre Courchesne-Loyer, Etienne Croteau, Sébastien Tremblay, Alex Castellano, et al., "Brain Fuel Metabolism, Aging and Alzheimer's Disease," *Nutrition* 27, no. 1 (2011): 3–20, doi:10.1016/j.nut.2010.07.021.
6. Lane and Farlow, "Lipid Homeostasis and Apolipoprotein E."
7. Z. S. Tan, W. S. Harris, A. S. Beiser, R. Au, J. J. Himali, S. Debette, A. Pikula, et al., "Red Blood Cell Omega-3 Fatty Acid Levels and Markers of Accelerated Brain Aging," *Neurology* 78, no. 9 (2012): 658–64, doi:10.1212/WNL.0b013e318249f6a9.
8. James V. Pottala, Kristine Yaffe, Jennifer G. Robinson, Mark A. Espeland, Robert Wallace, and William S. Harris, "Higher RBC EPA + DHA Corresponds with Larger Total Brain and Hippocampal Volumes: WHIMS-MRI Study," *Neurology* 82, no. 5 (2014): 435–42, doi10.1212/WNL.0000000000000080.
9. University of Maryland Medical Center, Complementary and Alternative Medicine Guide, "Omega-6 Fatty Acids," last reviewed on August 5, 2015, http://umm.edu/health/medical/altmed/supplement/omega6-fatty-acids.
10. Dwight Lundell, "World Renowned Heart Surgeon Speaks Out on What Really Causes Heart Disease," *My Science Academy*, posted August 19, 2012, http://myscienceacademy.org/2012/08/19/world-renown-heart-surgeon-speaks-out-on-what-really-causes-heart-disease.
11. Loren Cordain, S. Boyd Eaton, Anthony Sebastian, Neil Mann, Staffan Lindeberg, Bruce A. Watkins, James H. O'Keefe, et al., "Origins and Evolution of the Western Diet: Health Implications for the 21st Century," *American Journal of Clinical Nutrition* 81 (2005): 341–54.
12. Katherine Denniston, Joseph Topping, and Robert Caret, *General, Organic, and Biochemistry*, 7th Edition (New York: McGraw-Hill, 2011): 574, 772–73.
13. Food and Nutrition Board, Institute of Medicine, and National Academies, "Dietary Reference Intakes (DRIs): Recommended Dietary Allowances and Adequate Intakes, Total Water and Macronutrients," accessed September 9, 2016,

http://fnic.nal.usda.gov/sites/fnic.nal.usda.gov/files/uploads/recommended
_intakes_individuals.pdf.

14. Henderson, "High Carbohydrate Diets and Alzheimer's Disease."

15. Cynthia A. Daley, Amber Abbott, Patrick S. Doyle, Glenn A. Nader, and Stephanie Larson, "A Review of Fatty Acid Profiles and Antioxidant Content in Grass-Fed and Grain-Fed Beef," *Nutrition Journal* 9 (2010): 10, doi:10.1186/1475-2891-9-10; and Alison J. McAfee, E. M. Mcsorley, G. J. Cuskelly, A. M. Fearon, B. W. Moss, J. A. M. Beattie, J. M. W. Wallace, et al., "Red Meat from Animals Offered a Grass Diet Increases Plasma and Platelet *n*-3 PUFA in Healthy Consumers," *British Journal of Nutrition* 105 no. 1 (2011): 80–9, doi:10.1017/S0007114510003090.

16. Muhammad Imran, Faqir Muhammad Anjum, Muhammad Nadeem, Nazir Ahmad, Muhammad Kamran Khan, Zarina Mushtaq, and Shahzad Hussain, "Production of Bio-Omega-3 Eggs Through the Supplementation of Extruded Flaxseed Meal in Hen Diet," *Lipids in Health and Disease* 14 (2015): 126, doi:10.1186/s12944-015-0127-x; Ranil Coorey, Agnes Novinda, Hannah Williams, and Vijay Jayasena, "Omega-3 Fatty Acid Profile of Eggs from Laying Hens Fed Diets Supplemented with Chia, Fish Oil, and Flaxseed," *Journal of Food Science* 80, no. 1 (2015): S180–S187, doi:10.1111/1750-3841.12735; A. Antruejo, J. O. Azcona, P. T. Garcia, C. Gallinger, M. Rosmini, R. Ayerza, W. Coates, et al., "Omega-3 Enriched Egg Production: The Effect of α-linolenic ω-3 Fatty Acid Sources on Laying Hen Performance and Yolk Lipid Content and Fatty Acid Composition," *British Poultry Science* 52, no. 6 (2011): 750–60, doi:10.1080/00071668.2011.638621; and N. M. Lewis, S. Seburg, and N. L. Flanagan, "Enriched Eggs as a Source of N-3 Polyunsaturated Fatty Acids for Humans," *Poultry Science* 79, no. 7 (2000): 971–4, doi:10.1093/ps/79.7.971.

Chapter 14: Additional Dietary Considerations:
Dos and Don'ts on Dairy, Gluten, Sweeteners, and Sugar Alcohols

1. Jeff Volek and Stephen Phinney, *The Art and Science of Low Carbohydrate Performance* (Lexington, KY: Beyond Obesity LLC, 2012), 57–8.

2. Jessica R. Jackson, William W. Eaton, Nicola G. Cascella, Alessio Fasano, and Deanna L. Kelly, "Neurologic and Psychiatric Manifestations of Celiac Disease and Gluten Sensitivity," *The Psychiatric Quarterly* 83, no. 1 (2012): 91–102, doi:10.1007/s11126-011-9186-y; Khalafalla O. Bushara, "Neurologic Presentation of Celiac Disease," *Gastroenterology.* 128, no. 4 Suppl 1 (2005): S92–S97; Paola Bressan and Peter Kramer, "Bread and Other Edible Agents of Mental Disease," *Frontiers in Human Neuroscience* 10 (2016): 130, doi:10.3389/fnhum.2016.00130; and Marzia Caproni, Veronica Bonciolini, Antonietta D'Errico, Emiliano Antiga, and Paolo Fabbri, "Celiac Disease and Dermatologic Manifestations: Many Skin Clue to Unfold Gluten-Sensitive Enteropathy," *Gastroenterology Research and Practice* 2012 (2012): 952753, doi:10.1155/2012/952753.

3. Amanda E. Kalaydjian, William W. Eaton, Nicola Cascella, and Alessio Fasano, "The Gluten Connection: The Association Between Schizophrenia and Celiac Disease," *Acta Psychiatrica Scandinavica* 113, no. 2 (2006): 82–90, doi:10.1111/j.1600-0447.2005.00687.x; and Elena Lionetti, Salvatore Leonardi,

Chiara Franxonello, Margherita Macardi, Martino Ruggieri, and Carlo Catassi, "Gluten Psychosis: Confirmation of a New Clinical Entity," *Nutrients* 7, no. 7 (2015): 5532–39, doi:10.3390/nu7075235.

4. Pasquale Mansueto, Aurelio Seidita, Alberto D'Alcamo, and Antonio Carroccio, "Non-Celiac Gluten Sensitivity: Literature Review," *Journal of the American College of Nutrition* 33, no. 1 (2014): 39–54, doi:10.1080/07315724.2014.869 996; Anna Sapone, Julio C. Bai, Carolina Ciacci, Jernej Dolinsek, Peter H. R. Green, Marios Hadjivassiliou, Katri Kaukinen, et al., "Spectrum of Gluten-Related Disorders: Consensus on New Nomenclature and Classification," *BMC Medicine* 10 (2012): 13, doi:10.1186/1741-7015-10-13; and Alessio Fasano, Anna Sapone, Victor R. Zevallos, and Detlef Schuppan, "Nonceliac Gluten Sensitivity," *Gastroenterology* 148, no. 6 (2015): 1195–204, doi:10.1053/j.gastro.2014.12.049.

5. Jean-Claude Henquin, "Do Pancreatic β Cells 'Taste' Nutrients to Secrete Insulin?" *Science Signaling* 2012 5, no. 239 (2012): pe36, doi:10.1126/scisignal.2003325; and Willy J. Malaisse, "Insulin Release: The Receptor Hypothesis," *Diabetologia* 57, no. 7 (2014): 1287–90, doi:10.1007/s00125-014-3221-0.

6. M. Yanina, "Metabolic Effects of Non-Nutritive Sweeteners," *Physiology & Behavior* 152, Pt B (2015): 450–5, doi:10.1016/j.physbeh.2015.06.024.

7. Andrew G. Renwick and Samuel V. Molinary, "Sweet-Taste Receptors, Low-Energy Sweeteners, Glucose Absorption and Insulin Release," *British Journal of Nutrition* 104, no. 10 (2010): 1415–20, doi:10.1017/S0007114510002540; and Yukihiro Fujita, Rhonda D. Wideman, Madeleine Speck, Ali Asadi, David S. King, Travis D. Webber, Masakazu Haneda, et al., "Incretin Release from Gut Is Acutely Enhanced by Sugar but Not by Sweeteners in Vivo," *American Journal of Physiology–Endocrinology and Metabolism* 293, no. 3 (2009): E473–E479, doi:10.1152/ajpendo.90636.2008.

Chapter 16: A Primer on Food Quality

1. Ranil Coorey, Agnes Novinda, Hannah Williams, and Vijay Jayasena, "Omega-3 Fatty Acid Profile of Eggs from Laying Hens Fed Diets Supplemented with Chia, Fish Oil, and Flaxseed," *Journal of Food Science* 80, no. 1 (2015): S180–S187, doi:10.1111/1750-3841.12735; A. Antruejo, J. O. Azcona, P. T. Garcia, C. Gallinger, M. Rosmini, R. Ayerza, W. Coates, et al., "Omega-3 Enriched Egg Production: The Effect of α-linolenic ω-3 Fatty Acid Sources on Laying Hen Performance and Yolk Lipid Content and Fatty Acid Composition," *British Poultry Science* 52, no. 6 (2011): 750–60, doi:10.1080/00071668.2011.638621; and N. M. Lewis, S. Seburg, and N. L. Flanagan, "Enriched Eggs as a Source of N-3 Polyunsaturated Fatty Acids for Humans," *Poultry Science* 79, no. 7 (2000): 971–4, doi:10.1093/ps/79.7.971.

2. Cynthia A. Daley, Amber Abbott, Patrick S. Doyle, Glenn A. Nader, and Stephanie Larson, "A Review of Fatty Acid Profiles and Antioxidant Content in Grass-Fed and Grain-Fed Beef," *Nutrition Journal* 9 (2010): 10, doi:10.1186/1475-2891-9-10.

3. Alison J. McAfee, E. M. Mcsorley, G. J. Cuskelly, A. M. Fearon, B. W. Moss, J. A. M. Beattie, J. M. W. Wallace, et al., "Red Meat from Animals Offered a Grass

Diet Increases Plasma and Platelet *n*-3 PUFA in Healthy Consumers," *British Journal of Nutrition* 105, no. 1 (2-11): 80–9, doi:10.1017/S0007114510003090; and J. M. Leheska, L. D. Thompson, J. C. Howe, E. Hentges, J. Boyce, J. C. Brooks, B. Shriver, et al., "Effects of Conventional and Grass-Feeding Systems on the Nutrient Composition of Beef," *Journal of Animal Science* 86, no. 12 (2008): 3575–85, doi:10.2527/jas.2007-0565.

4. Andrew P. Han, "Ever Wondered: Why Is Wild Salmon a Deeper Red Than Farmed Salmon?," *Science Line*, posted September 11, 2013, http://scienceline.org /2013/09/ever-wondered-why-is-wild-salmon-a-deeper-red-than-farmed-salmon.

Chapter 17: The Importance of Exercise

1. Stephen C. Cunnane, Scott Nugent, Maggie Roy, Alexandre Courchesne-Loyer, Etienne Croteau, Sébastien Tremblay, Alex Castellano, et al., "Brain Fuel Metabolism, Aging and Alzheimer's Disease," *Nutrition* 27, no. 1 (2011): 3–20, doi:10.1016/j.nut.2010.07.021.

2. Ibid.

3. David A. Hood, Giulia Uguccioni, Anna Vainshtein, and Donna D'souza, "Mechanisms of Exercise-Induced Mitochondrial Biogenesis in Skeletal Muscle: Implications for Health and Disease," *Comprehensive Physiology* 1, no. 3 (2011): 1119–34, doi:10.1002/cphy.c100074.

4. John O. Holloszy, "Regulation by Exercise of Skeletal Muscle Content of Mitochondria and GLUT4," *Journal of Physiology Pharmacology* 59, Suppl 7 (2008): 5–18; and Isabella Irrcher, Peter J. Adhihetty, Anna-Maria Joseph, Vladimir Ljubicic, and David A. Hood, "Regulation of Mitochondrial Biogenesis in Muscle by Endurance Exercise," *Sports Medicine* 33, no. 11 (2003): 783–93.

5. Li Wang, Henrik Mascher, Niklas Psilander, Eva Blomstrand, and Kent Sahlin, "Resistance Exercise Enhances the Molecular Signaling of Mitochondrial Biogenesis Induced by Endurance Exercise in Human Skeletal Muscle," *Journal of Applied Physiology (1985)* 111, no. 5 (2011): 1335–44, doi:10.1152/japplphysiol .00086.2011.

6. Bente K. Pedersen, Maria Pedersen, Karen S. Krabbe, Helle Bruunsgaard, Vance B. Matthews, and Mark A. Febbraio, "Role of Exercise-Induced Brain-Derived Neurotrophic Factor Production in the Regulation of Energy Homeostasis in Mammals," *Experimental Physiology* 94, no. 12 (2009): 1153–60, doi:10.1113 /expphysiol.2009.048561.

7. Shoshanna Vaynman, Zhe Ying, and Fernando Gomez-Pinilla, "Hippocampal BDNF Mediates the Efficacy of Exercise on Synaptic Plasticity and Cognition," *European Journal of Neuroscience* 20, no. 10 (2004): 2580–90, doi:10.1111 /j.1460-9568.2004.03720.x.

8. Shoshanna Vaynman, Z. Ying, A. Wu, and F. Gomez-Pinella, "Coupling Energy Metabolism with a Mechanism to Support Brain-Derived Neurotrophic Factor-Mediated Synaptic Plasticity," *Neuroscience* 139 no. 4 (2006): 1221–34, doi:10.1016/j.neuroscience.2006.01.062.

9. Pedersen, "Role of Exercise-Induced Brain-Derived Neurotrophic Factor Production."

10. Sama Sleiman, Jeffrey Henry, Rami Al-Haddad, et al., "Exercise Promotes the Expression of Brain Derived Neurotrophic Factor (BDNF) through the Action of the Ketone Body β-hydroxybutyrate," Joel K. Elmquist, ed., *eLife*, no. 5 (2016): e15092. doi:10.7554/eLife.15092.

11. Ibid.

12. Vaynman et al., "Coupling Energy Metabolism"; Sleiman et al., "Exercise Promotes the Expression."

13. Roig, "The Effects of Cardiovascular Exercise on Human Memory"; Eelco V. van Dongen, Ingrid H. P. Kersten, Isabella C. Wagner, Richard G. M. Morris, and Guillén Fernández, "Physical Exercise Performed Four Hours After Learning Improves Memory Retention and Increases Hippocampal Pattern Similarity During Retrieval," *Current Biology* 26, no. 13 (2016): 1722–7, doi:10.1016/j.cub .2016.04.071; Hayley Guiney and Liana Machado, "Benefits of Regular Aerobic Exercise for Executive Functioning in Healthy Populations," *Psychonomic Bulletin & Review* 20, no. 1 (2013): 73–86, doi:10.3758/s13423-012-0345-4; Chien-Ning Tseng, Bih-Shya Gau, and Meei-Fang Lou, "The Effectiveness of Exercise on Improving Cognitive Function in Older People: A Systematic Review," *The Journal of Nursing Research* 19, no. 2 (2011): 119–31, doi:10.1097/JNR .0b013e3182198837; Ashley Carvalho, Irene Maeve Rea, Tanyalak Parimon, and Barry J. Cusack, "Physical Activity and Cognitive Function in Individuals over 60 Years of Age: A Systematic Review," *Clinical Interventions in Aging* 9 (2014): 661–82, doi:10.2147/CIA.S55520; and Rui Nouchi, Yasuyuki Taki, Hikaru Taeuchi, Atsushi Sekiguchi, Hiroshi Hashizume, Takayuki Nozawa, Haruka Nouchi et al., "Four Weeks of Combination Exercise Training Improved Executive Functions, Episodic Memory, and Processing Speed in Healthy Elderly People: Evidence from a Randomized Controlled Trial," *Age* 36, no. 2 (2014): 787–99, doi:10.1007/s11357-013-9588-x; Marc Roig, Sasja Nordbrandt, Svend Sparre Geertsen, Jens and Bo Nielsen, "The Effects of Cardiovascular Exercise on Human Memory: A Review with Meta-Analysis," *Neuroscience and Biobehavioral Reviews* 37, no. 8 (2013): 1645–66, doi:10.1016/j.neubiorev.2013.06.012.

14. Fernando Gomez-Pinilla and Charles Hillman, "The Influence of Exercise on Cognitive Abilities," *Comprehensive Physiology* 3, no. 1 (2013): 403–28, doi:10.1002/cphy.c110063.

15. Thierry Paillard, "Preventive Effects of Regular Physical Exercise Against Cognitive Decline and the Risk of Dementia with Age Advancement," *Sports Medicine—Open* 1, no. 1 (2015): 20, doi:10.1186/s40798-015-0016-x.

16. Ibid.; and Kirsten Hötting and Brigitte Röder, "Beneficial Effects of Physical Exercise on Neuroplasticity and Cognition," *Neuroscience & Biobehavioral Reviews* 37, no. 9 Pt B (2013): 2243–57, doi:10.1016/j.neubiorev.2013.04.005.

17. I. Lista and G. Sorrentino, "Biological Mechanisms of Physical Activity in Preventing Cognitive Decline," *Cellular and Molecular Neurobiology* 30, no. 4 (2010): 493–503, doi:10.1007/s10571-009-9488-x; Jasmina Pluncevic Gligoroska and Sanja Manchevska, "The Effect of Physical Activity on Cognition—Physiological Mechanisms," *Materia Socio-Medica* 24, no. 3 (2012): 198–202, doi:10.5455/msm

.2012.24.198-202; and Neva J. Kirk-Sanchez and Ellen L. McGough, "Physical Exercise and Cognitive Performance in the Elderly: Current Perspectives," *Clinical Interventions in Aging* 9 (2014): 51–62, doi:10.2147/CIA.S39506.

Chapter 18: Too Much Stress and Too Little Sleep Can Break the Brain

1. Alessandro Ieraci, Alessandra Mallei, Laura Musazzi, and Maurizio Popoli, "Physical Exercise and Acute Restraint Stress Differentially Modulate Hippocampal Brain-Derived Neurotrophic Factor Transcripts and Epigenetic Mechanisms in Mice," *Hippocampus* 25, no. 11 (2015): 1380–92, doi:10.1002/hipo.22458; and M. J. Schaaf, E. R. De Kloet, and E. Vreugdenhil, "Corticosterone Effects on BDNF Expression in the Hippocampus. Implications for Memory Formation," *Stress* 3, no. 3 (2000): 201–8.

2. Rachel Leproult and Eve Van Cauter, "Role of Sleep and Sleep Loss in Hormonal Release and Metabolism. *Endocrine Development* 17 (2010): 11–21, doi:10.1159/000262524; and G. Copinschi, "Metabolic and Endocrine Effects of Sleep Deprivation," *Essential Psychopharmacology* 6, no. 6 (2005): 341–7.

3. Lisa Morselli, Rachel Leproult, Marcella Balbo, and Karine Spiegel, "Role of Sleep Duration in the Regulation of Glucose Metabolism and Appetite," *Best Practice & Research. Clinical Endocrinology & Metabolism* 24, no. 5 (2010): 687–702, doi:10.1016/j.beem.2010.07.005; Karen A. Matthews, Ronald E. Dahl, Jane F. Owens, Laisze Lee, and Martica Hall, "Sleep Duration and Insulin Resistance in Healthy Black and White Adolescents," *Sleep* 35, no. 10 (2012): 1353–58, doi:10.5665/sleep.2112; and S. Javaheri, A. Storfer-Isser, C. L. Rosen, and S. Redline, "The Association of Short and Long Sleep Durations with Insulin Sensitivity In Adolescents," *The Journal of Pediatrics* 158, no. 4 (2011): 617–23, doi:10.1016/j.jpeds.2010.09.080.

4. Kristen L. Knutson, Karine Spiegel, Plamen Penev, and Eve Van Cauter, "The Metabolic Consequences of Sleep Deprivation," *Sleep Medicine Reviews* 11, no. 3 (2007): 163–78. doi:10.1016/j.smrv.2007.01.002.

5. Arlet V. Nedeltcheva and Frank A. J. L. Scheer, "Metabolic Effects of Sleep Disruption, Links to Obesity and Diabetes," *Current Opinion in Endocrinology, Diabetes, and Obesity* 21, no. 4 (2014): 293–98, doi:10.1097/MED.0000000000000082; and Sirimon Reutrakul and Eve Van Cauter, "Interactions Between Sleep, Circadian Function, and Glucose Metabolism: Implications for Risk and Severity of Diabetes," *Annals of the New York Academy of Sciences* 1311 (2014): 151–73, doi:10.1111/nyas.12355.

6. Esra Tasali, Babak Mokhlesi, and Eve Van Cauter, "Obstructive Sleep Apnea and Type 2 Diabetes: Interacting Epidemics," *Chest* 133, no. 2 (2008): 496–506, doi:10.1378/chest.07-0828.

7. Michael Morgenstern, Janice Wang, Norman Beatty, Tom Batemarco, Anthony L. Sica, and Harly Greenberg, "Obstructive Sleep Apnea: An Unexpected Cause of Insulin Resistance and Diabetes," *Endocrinology and Metabolism Clinics in North America* 43, no. 1 (2014): 187–204, doi:10.1016/j.ecl.2013.09.002.

8. Nadia Aalling Jessen, Anne Sofie Finmann Munk, Iben Lundgaard, and Maiken Nedergaard, "The Glymphatic System: A Beginner's Guide," *Neurochemical*

Research 40, no. 12 (2015): 2583–99, doi:10.1007/s11064-015-1581-6; and Jenna M. Tarasoff-Conway, Roxana O. Carare, Ricardo S. Osorio, Lidia Glodzik, Tracy Butler, Els Fieremans, Leon Axel, et al., "Clearance Systems in the Brain— Implications for Alzheimer Disease," *Nature Reviews. Neurology* 11, no. (8) (2015): 457–70, doi:10.1038/nrneurol.2015.119.

9. Tarasoff-Conway et al., "Clearance Systems in the Brain."

10. Erik S. Musiek, David D. Xiong, and David M. Holtzman, "Sleep, Circadian Rhythms, and the Pathogenesis of Alzheimer Disease," *Experimental & Molecular Medicine* 47, no. 3 (2015): e148, doi:10.1038/emm.2014.121.

11. Miranda M. Lim, Jason R. Gerstner, and David M. Holtzman, "The Sleep–Wake Cycle and Alzheimer's Disease: What Do We Know?" *Neurodegenerative Disease Management* 4, no. 5 (2014): 351-362, doi:10.2217/nmt.14.33; and Jee Hoon Roh, Yafei Huang, Adam W. Bero, Tom Kasten, Floy R. Stewart, Fandall J. Bateman, and David M. Holtzman, "Disruption of the Sleep-Wake Cycle and Diurnal Fluctuation of Amyloid-β as Biomarkers of Brain Amyloid Pathology," *Science Translational Medicine* 4, no. 150 (2012): 150ra122, doi:10.1126/scitranslmed.3004291.

12. Roh et al, "Disruption of the Sleep-Wake Cycle."

13. Brendan P. Lucey and Randall J. Bateman, "Amyloid-β Diurnal Pattern: Possible Role of Sleep in Alzheimer's Disease Pathogenesis," *Neurobiology of Aging* 35, Suppl 2 (2014): S29–S34, doi:10.1016/j.neurobiolaging.2014.03.035.

14. Andrew R. Mendelsohn and James W. Larrick, "Sleep Facilitates Clearance of Metabolites from the Brain: Glymphatic Function in Aging and Neurodegenerative Diseases," *Rejuvenation Research* 16, no. 6 (2013): 518–23, doi:10.1089/rej.2013.1530.

15. Hedok Lee, Lulu Xie, Mei Yu, Hongyi Kang, Tian Feng, Rashid Deane, Jean Logan et al., "The Effect of Body Posture on Brain Glymphatic Transport," *Journal of Neuroscience* 35, no. 31 (2015): 11034–44, doi:10.1523/JNEUROSCI .1625-15.2015.

Chapter 19: Intermittent Fasting: Boost Ketones and Let the Brain "Clean House"

1. Mark P. Mattson and Ruiqian Wan, "Beneficial Effects of Intermittent Fasting and Caloric Restriction on the Cardiovascular and Cerebrovascular Systems," *Journal of Nutritional Biochemistry* 16, no. 3 (2005): 129–37, doi:10.1016/j.jnutbio .2004.12.007.

2. Mark P. Mattson, "Energy Intake, Meal Frequency, and Health: A Neurobiological Perspective," *Annual Review of Nutrition* 25 (2005): 237–60, doi:10.1146/annurev .nutr.25.050304.092526.

3. Mark P. Mattson, Wenxhen Duan, Jaewon, Lee, and Zhihong Guo, "Suppression of Brain Aging and Neurodegenerative Disorders by Dietary Restriction and Environmental Enrichment: Molecular Mechanisms," *Mechanisms of Ageing and Development* 122, no. 7 (2001): 757–78, doi:10.1016/S0047-6374(01)00226-3.

4. Brownwen Martin, Mark P. Mattson, and Stuart Maudsley, "Caloric Restriction and Intermittent Fasting: Two Potential Diets for Successful Brain Aging," *Ageing Research Reviews* 5, no. 3 (2006): 332–53, doi:10.1016/j.arr.2006.04.002.

5. Mark P. Mattson, "Neuroprotective Signaling and the Aging Brain: Take Away My Food and Let Me Run," *Brain Research* 886, no 1-2 (2000): 47–53, doi:10.1016 /S0006-8993(00)02790-6; and Ángela Fontán-Lozano, Guillermo López-Lluch, José María Delgado-García, Placido Navas, and Ángel Manuel Carrión, "Molecular Bases of Caloric Restriction Regulation of Neuronal Synaptic Plasticity," *Molecular Neurobiology* 38, no. 2 (2008): 167–77, doi:10.1007/s12035-008-8040-1.

6. Mark P. Mattson, Wenzhen Duan, and Zhihong Guo, "Meal Size and Frequency Affect Neuronal Plasticity and Vulnerability to Disease: Cellular and Molecular Mechanisms," *Journal of Neurochemistry* 84, no. 3 (2003): 417–31, doi:10.1046/j.1471-4159.2003.01586.x.

Chapter 20: Your Roadmap for Making the Transition

1. A. Quiñones-Galvan and E. Ferrannini, "Renal Effects of Insulin in Man," *Journal of Nephrology* 10, no. 4 (1997): 188–91; Ralph A. DeFronzo, "The Effect of Insulin on Renal Sodium Metabolism. A Review with Clinical Implications," *Diabetologia* 21, no. 3 (1981): 165–71; and María Chávez-Canales, Juan Pablo Arroyo, Benjamin Ko, Norma Vázquez, Rocio Bautista, Maria Casteñada-Bueno, Norma A. Bobadilla, et al., "Insulin Increases the Functional Activity of the Renal NaCl Cotransporter," *Journal of Hypertension* 31, no. 2 (2013): 303–11, doi:10.1097/HJH.0b013e32835bbb83.

2. James J. DiNicolantonio and Sean Lucan, "The Wrong White Crystals: Not Salt but Sugar as Aetiological in Hypertension and Cardiometabolic Disease," *Open Heart* 1, no. 1 (2014): e000167.

3. Ellen Davis, "Who Should Not Follow a Ketogenic Diet?," Ketogenic Diet Resource, http://www.ketogenic-diet-resource.com/support-files/who-should-not -follow-a-ketogenic-diet.pdf (August 4, 2016).

4. William F. Martin, Lawrence E. Armstrong, and Nancy R. Rodriguez, "Dietary Protein Intake and Renal Function," *Nutrition & Metabolism* 2 (2005): 25, doi:10.1186/1743-7075-2-25; and Helen Kollias, "Research Review: High-Protein Diets—Safe for Kidneys," *Precision Nutrition*, http://www.precisionnutrition.com /high-protein-safe-for-kidneys (July 10, 2016).

Chapter 21: Support for Healthy Digestive Function

1. Jonathan Wright and Lane Lenard, *Why Stomach Acid Is Good for You* (Lanham, MD: M. Evans & Company, 2001).

2. Carol S. Johnston, Cindy M. Kim, and Amanda J. Buller, "Vinegar Improves Insulin Sensitivity to a High-Carbohydrate Meal in Subjects with Insulin Resistance or Type 2 Diabetes," *Diabetes Care* 27, no. 1 (2004): 281–2, doi:10.2337/diacare .27.1.281; Carol S. Johnston, Iwona Steplewska, Cindy A. Long, Lafe N. Harris, and Romina H. Ryals, "Examination of the Antiglycemic Properties of Vinegar in Healthy Adults," *Annals of Nutrition and Metabolism* 56, no. 1 (2010): 74–9, doi:10.1159/000272133; S. Liatis, S. Grammatikou, K. A. Poulia, D. Perrea, K. Makrilakis, E. Kiakoumopoulou, and N. Katsilambros, "Vinegar Reduces Postprandial Hyperglycaemia in Patients with Type II Diabetes When Added to a High, but Not to a Low, Glycaemic Index Meal," *European Journal of Clinical*

Nutrition 64, no. 7 (2010): 727–32, doi:10.1038/ejcn.2010.89; Helena Liljeberg and Inger Björck, "Delayed Gastric Emptying Rate May Explain Improved Glycaemia in Healthy Subjects to a Starchy Meal with Added Vinegar," *European Journal of Clinical Nutrition* 52, no. 5 (1998): 368–71; and E. Östman, Y. Granfeldt, L. Persson, and I. Bjorck, "Vinegar Supplementation Lowers Glucose and Insulin Responses and Increases Satiety After a Bread Meal in Healthy Subjects," *European Journal of Clinical Nutrition* 59, no. 9 (2005): 983–8, doi:10.1038/sj.ejcn.1602197.

3. David C. Williams, "You've (Hopefully) Got Some Gall," Dr. David Williams, http://www.drdavidwilliams.com/importance-of-bile-acid (August 5, 2016).

Chapter 22: Not by Diet Alone: Effective Nutritional Supplements

1. Francesco Bellia, Adriana Pietropaolo, and Giuseppe Grasso, "Formation of Insulin Fragments by Insulin-Degrading Enzyme: The Role of Zinc(II) and Cystine Bridges," *Journal of Mass Spectrometry* 48, no. 2 (2013): 135–40, doi:10.1002/jms.3060.

2. Michael Zimmermann, *Burgerstein's Handbook of Nutrition* (New York: Thieme, 2001).

3. Rosebud O. Roberts, Teresa J. Christianson, Walter K. Kremers, Michelle M. Mielk, Mary M. Machulda, Maria Vassilaka, Rabe E. Alhurani et al., "Association Between Olfactory Dysfunction and Amnestic Mild Cognitive Impairment and Alzheimer Disease Dementia," *JAMA Neurology* 73, no. 1 (2016): 93–101, doi:10.1001/jamaneurol.2015.2952; W. Lojkowska, B. Sawicka, M. Gugala, H. Sienkiewicz-Jarosz, A. Bochynska, A. Scinska, A. Korkosz, et al., "Follow-Up Study of Olfactory Deficits, Cognitive Functions, and Volume Loss of Medial Temporal Lobe Structures in Patients with Mild Cognitive Impairment," *Current Alzheimer Research* 8, no. 6 (2011): 689–98, http://www.ncbi.nlm.nih.gov/pubmed/21592056; L. Velayudhan, M. Pritchard, J. F. Powell, P. Proitsi, and S. Lovestone, "Smell Identification Function as a Severity and Progression Marker in Alzheimer's Disease," *International Psychogeriatrics* 25, no. 7 (2013): 1157–66, doi:10.1017/S1041610213000446; and J. Djordjevic, M. Jones-Gotman, K. De Sousa, and H. Chertkow, "Olfaction in Patients with Mild Cognitive Impairment and Alzheimer's Disease," *Neurobiology of Aging* 29, no. 5 (2008): 693–706, doi:10.1016/j.neurobiolaging.2006.11.014.

4. Davis W. and Steven M. Plaza, "The Safety and Efficacy of High-Dose Chromium," *Alternative Medicine Review* 7, no. 3 (2002): 218–35.

5. Kate Petersen Shay, Régis F. Moreau, Eric J. Smith, Anthony R. Smith, and Tory M. Hagen, "Alpha-Lipoic Acid as a Dietary Supplement: Molecular Mechanisms and Therapeutic Potential," *Biochimica et Biophysica Acta* 1790, no. 10 (2009): 1149–60, doi:10.1016/j.bbagen.2009.07.026; and Luc Rochette, Stéliana Ghibu, Carole Richard, Marianne Zeller, Yves Cottin, and Catherine Vergely, "Direct and Indirect Antioxidant Properties of α-Lipoic Acid and Therapeutic Potential," *Molecular Nutrition & Food Research* 57, no. 1 (2013): 114–25, doi:10.1002/mnfr.201200608.

6. Anna Gorąca, Halina Huk-Kolega, Aleksandra Piechota, Paulina Kleniewska, Elżbieta Ciejka, and Beata Skibska, "Lipoic Acid–Biological Activity and Therapeutic Potential," *Pharmacological Reports* 63, no. 4 (2011): 849–58.

7. Petya Kamenova, "Improvement of Insulin Sensitivity in Patients with Type 2 Diabetes Mellitus After Oral Administration of Alpha-Lipoic Acid," *Hormones (Athens)* 5, no. 4 (2006): 251–8; and Hadi Moini, Oren Tirosh, Young Chul Park, Kyung-Joo Cho, and Lester Packer, "R-Alpha-Lipoic Acid Action on Cell Redox Status, the Insulin Receptor, and Glucose Uptake in 3T3-L1 Adipocytes," *Archives of Biochemistry and Biophysics* 397, no. 2 (2002): 384–91, doi:10.1006/abbi.2001.2680.

8. Annette Maczurek, Lezanne Ooi, Mili Patel, and Gerald Münch, "Lipoic Acid as an Anti-inflammatory and Neuroprotective Treatment for Alzheimer's Disease," *Advanced Drug Delivery Reviews* 60, no. 13-14 (2008): 1463–70, doi:10.1016/j.addr.2008.04.015; and L. Holmquist, G. Stuchbury, K. Berbaum, S. Muscat, S. Young, K. Hager, J. Engel et al., "Lipoic Acid as a Novel Treatment for Alzheimer's Disease and Related Dementias," *Pharmacology & Therapeutics* 113, no. 1 (2007): 154–64, doi:10.1016/j.pharmthera.2006.07.001.

9. Janos Zempleni, Timothy A. Trusty, and Donald M. Mock, "Lipoic Acid Reduces the Activities of Biotin-Dependent Carboxylases in Rat Liver," *The Journal of Nutrition* 127, no. 9 (1997): 1776–81.

10. Artemis P. Simopoulos, "Evolutionary Aspects of Diet: The Omega-6/Omega-3 Ratio and the Brain," *Molecular Neurobiology* 44, no. 2 (2011): 203–15, doi:10.1007/s12035-010-8162-0.

11. Russell T. Matthews, Lichuan Yang, Susan Browne, Myong Baik, and M. Flint Beal, "Coenzyme Q10 Administration Increases Brain Mitochondrial Concentrations and Exerts Neuroprotective Effects," *Proceedings of the National Academy of Sciences of the United States of America* 95, no. 15 (1998): 8892–97; M. Flint Beal, "Mitochondrial Dysfunction and Oxidative Damage in Alzheimer's and Parkinson's Diseases and Coenzyme Q10 as a Potential Treatment," *Journal of Bioenergetics and Biomembranes* 36, no. 4 (2004): 381–6, doi:10.1023/B:JOBB.0000041772.74810.92; A. Joyce Young, Stephanie Johnson, David C. Steffens, and P. Murali Doraiswamy, "Coenzyme Q10: A Review of Its Promise as a Neuroprotectant," *CNS Spectrums* 12, no. 1 (2007): 62–8, http://www.ncbi.nlm.nih.gov/pubmed/17192765; Wendy R. Galpern and Merit E. Cudkowicz, "Coenzyme Q Treatment of Neurodegenerative Diseases of Aging," *Mitochondrion* 7, Suppl (2007): S146–S153, doi:10.1016/j.mito.2007.01.004; M. Mancuso, D. Orsucci, L. Volpi, V. Calsolaro, and G. Siciliano, "Coenzyme Q10 in Neuromuscular and Neurodegenerative Disorders," *Current Drug Targets* 11, no. 1 (2010): 111–21, http://www.ncbi.nlm.nih.gov/pubmed/20017723; and D. Orsucci, M. Mancuso, E. C. Ienco, A. Logerfo, and G. Ciciliano, "Targeting Mitochondrial Dysfunction and Neurodegeneration by Means of Coenzyme Q10 and Its Analogues," *Current Medicinal Chemistry* 18, no. 26 (2011): 4053–64, doi:10.2174/092986711796957257.

12. Xifei Yang, George Dai, Geng Li, and Edward S. Yang, "Coenzyme Q10 Reduces Beta-Amyloid Plaque in an APP/PS1 Transgenic Mouse Model of Alzheimer's Disease," *Journal of Molecular Neuroscience* 41, no. 1 (2010): 110–3, doi:10.1007/s12031-009-9297-1; Xifei Yang, Ying Yang, Geng Li, Jianzhi Wang, and Edward S.

Yang, "Coenzyme Q10 Attenuates β-Amyloid Pathology in the Aged Transgenic Mice with Alzheimer Presenilin 1 Mutation," *Journal of Molecular Neuroscience* 34, no. 2 (2008): 165–71, doi:10.1007/s12031-007-9033-7; and Magali Dumont, Khatuna Kipiani, Fangmin Yu, Elizabeth Wille, Maya Katz, Noel Y. Calingasan, and Gunnar K. Gouras, "Coenzyme Q10 Decreases Amyloid Pathology and Improves Behavior in a Transgenic Mouse Model of Alzheimer's Disease," *Journal of Alzheimer's Disease* 27, no. 1(2011): 211–23, doi:10.3233/JAD-2011-110209.

13. Igor Pravst, Katja Zmitek, and Janko Zmitek, "Coenzyme Q10 Contents in Foods and Fortification Strategies," *Critical Reviews in Food Science and Nutrition* 50, no. 4 (2010): 269–80, doi:10.1080/10408390902773037.

14. Kei Mizuno, Masaaki Tanaka, Staoshi Nozaki, Hiroshi Mizuma, Suzuka Ataka, Tsuyoshi Tahara, Tomohiro Sugino, et al., "Antifatigue Effects of Coenzyme Q10 During Physical Fatigue," *Nutrition* 24, no. 4 (2008): 293–99, doi:10.1016/j.nut .2007.12.007.

15. A. Carta, M Calvani, D. Bravi, and S. N. Bhuachalla, "Acetyl-L-Carnitine and Alzheimer's Disease: Pharmacological Considerations Beyond the Cholinergic Sphère," *Annals of the New York Academy of Sciences* 695 (1993): 324–26, doi:10.1111/j.1749-6632.1993.tb23077.x.

16. Linus Pauling Institute Micronutrient Information Center, "L-Carnitine," *Oregon State University*, accessed August 14, 2016, http://lpi.oregonstate.edu/mic/dietary -factors/L-carnitine#biosynthesis-sources.

17. A. Spagnoli, U. Lucca, G. Manasce, L. Bandera, G. Cizza, G. Forloni, M. Tettamanti, et al., "Long-Term Acetyl-L-Carnitine Treatment in Alzheimer's Disease," *Neurology* 41, no. 11 (1991): 1726–32, http://www.ncbi.nlm.nih.gov /pubmed/1944900; and Sheila A. Hudson and Naji Tabet, "Acetyl-L-Carnitine for Dementia," *Cochrane Database of Systematic Reviews* 2 (2003): CD003158, doi:10.1002/14651858.CD003158.

18. Jun Yin, Huli Xing, and Jianping Ye, "Efficacy of Berberine in Patients with Type 2 Diabetes," *Metabolism: Clinical and Experimental* 57, no. 5 (2008): 712–17, doi:10.1016/j.metabol.2008.01.013.

19. Hao Zhang, Jing Wei, Rong Xue, Jin-Dan Wu, Wei Zhao, Zi-Zheng Wang, Shu-Kui Wang, et al., "Berberine Lowers Blood Glucose in Type 2 Diabetes Mellitus Patients Through Increasing Insulin Receptor Expression," *Metabolism* 59, no. 2 (2010): 285–92, doi:10.1016/j.metabol.2009.07.029.

20. Li Liu, Yun-Li Yu, Jian-Song Yang, Yang Li, Yao-Wu Liu, Yan Liang, Xiao-Dong Liu, et al, "Berberine Suppresses Intestinal Disaccharidases with Beneficial Metabolic Effects in Diabetic States, Evidences from in Vivo and in Vitro Study," *Naunyn Schmiedeberg's Archives of Pharmacology* 381, no. 4 (2010): 371–81, doi:10.1007/s00210-010-0502-0.

21. Hyun Ah Jung, Byung-Sun Min, Takako Yokozawa, Je-Hyun Lee, Yeong Shik Kim, and Jae Sue Choi. "Anti-Alzheimer and Antioxidant Activities of Coptidis Rhizoma Alkaloids," *Biological and Pharmaceutical Bulletin* 32, no. 8 (2009): 1433–38, doi:10.1248/bpb.32.1433.

22. Ibid.

23. Hong-Fang Ji and Liang Shen, "Molecular Basis of Inhibitory Activities of Berberine against Pathogenic Enzymes in Alzheimer's Disease," *The Scientific World Journal* 2012 (2012): 823201, doi:10.1100/2012/823201.

24. Siva Sundara Kumar Durairajan, Liang-Feng Liu, Jai-Hong Lu, Lei-Lei Chen, Qiuju Yuan, Sookja K. Chung, Ling Huang, et al., "Berberine Ameliorates β-Amyloid Pathology, Gliosis, and Cognitive Impairment in an Alzheimer's Disease Transgenic Mouse Model," *Neurobiology of Aging* 33, no. 12 (2012): 2903–19, doi:10.1016/j.neurobiolaging.2012.02.016.

25. Rui Wang, Han Yan, and Zi-can Tang, "Progress in Studies of Huperzine A, a Natural Cholinesterase Inhibitor from Chinese Herbal Medicine," *Acta Pharmacologica Sinica* 27, no. 1 (2006): 1–26, doi:10.1111/j.1745-7254.2006.00255.x.

26. Ibid.; and Hai Yan Zhang, Chun Yan Zheng, Han Yan, Zhi Fei Wang, Li Li Tang, Xin Gao, and Xi Can Tang, "Potential Therapeutic Targets of Huperzine A for Alzheimer's Disease and Vascular Dementia," *Chemico-Biological Interactions* 175, no. 1–3 (2008): 396–402, doi:10.1016/j.cbi.2008.04.049.

27. Alicia R. Desilets, Jennifer J. Gickas, and Kaelen C. Dunican, "Role of Huperzine A in the Treatment of Alzheimer's Disease," *Annals of Pharmacotherapy* 43, no. 3 (2009): 514–18, doi:10.1345/aph.1L402.

28. J. Li, H. M. Wu, R. L. Zhou, G. J. Liu, and B. R. Dong, "Huperzine A for Alzheimer's Disease," *Cochrane Database of Systematic Reviews* 2 (2008): CD005592, doi:10.1002/14651858.CD005592.pub2.

29. Guoyan Yang, Yuyi Wang, Jinzhou Tian, and Hian-Ping Liu, "Huperzine A for Alzheimer's Disease: A Systematic Review and Meta-Analysis of Randomized Clinical Trials," Roberta W. Scherer, ed., *PLoS ONE* 8, no. 9 (2013): e74916, doi:10.1371/journal.pone.0074916.

30. M. S. Rafii, S. Walsh, J. T. Little, K. Behan, B. Reynolds, C. Ward, S. Jin, et al., "A Phase II Trial of Huperzine A in Mild to Moderate Alzheimer Disease," *Neurology* 76, no. 16 (2011): 1389–94, doi:10.1212/WNL.0b013e318216eb7b.

31. Winyoo Chowanadisai, Kathryn A. Bauerly, Eskouhie Tchaparian, Alice Wong, Gino A. Cortopassi, and Robert B. Rucker, "Pyrroloquinoline Quinone Stimulates Mitochondrial Biogenesis Through cAMP Response Element-binding Protein Phosphorylation and Increased PGC-1α Expression," *The Journal of Biological Chemistry* 285, no. 1 (2010): 142–52, doi:10.1074/jbc.M109.030130; Calliandra B. Harris, Winyoo Chowanadisai, Darya O. Mishchuk, Mike A. Satre, Carolyn M. Slupsky, and Robert B. Rucker, "Dietary Pyrroloquinoline Quinone (PQQ) Alters Indicators of Inflammation and Mitochondrial-Related Metabolism in Human Subjects," *The Journal of Nutritional Biochemistry* 24, no. 12 (2013): 2076–84, doi:10.1016/j.jnutbio.2013.07.008; and Kathryn Bauerly, Calliandra Harris, Winyoo Chowanadisai, James Graham, Peter J. Havel, Eskouhie Tchaparian, Mike Satre, et al., "Altering Pyrroloquinoline Quinone Nutritional Status Modulates Mitochondrial, Lipid, and Energy Metabolism in Rats," Immo A. Hansen, ed., *PLoS ONE* 6, no. 7 (2011): e21779, doi:10.1371/journal.pone.0021779.

32. Robert Rucker, Winyoo Chowanadisai, and Masahiko Nakano, "Potential Physiological Importance of Pyrroloquinoline Quinone," *Alternative Medicine*

Review 14, no. 3 (2009): 268–77; H. S. Misra, Y. S. Raipurohit, and N. P. Kharnar, "Pyrroloquinoline-Quinone and Its Versatile Roles in Biological Processes," *Journal of Biosciences* 37, no. 2 (2012): 313–25; Qi Zhang, Mi Shen, Mei Ding, Dingding Shen, and Fei Ding, "The Neuroprotective Action of Pyrroloquinoline Quinone Against Glutamate-Induced Apoptosis in Hippocampal Neurons Is Mediated Through the Activation of PI3K/Akt Pathway," *Toxicology and Applied Pharmacology* 252, no. 1 (2011): 62–72, doi:10.1016/j.taap.2011.02.006; and Jiaojiao Qin, Meilong Wu, Shu Yu, Xiaorong Gao, Jingjing Zhang, Xingyue Dong, Jinyan Ji, et al., "Pyrroloquinoline Quinone-Conferred Neuroprotection in Rotenone Models of Parkinson's Disease," *Toxicology Letters* 238, no. 3 (2015): 70–82, doi:10.1016/j.toxlet.2015.08.011.

33. Warnakulasuriya Mary Ann Dipika Binosha Fernando, Ian J. Martins, K. G. Goozee, Charles S. Brennan, V. Jayasena, and R. N. Martins, "The Role of Dietary Coconut for the Prevention and Treatment of Alzheimer's Disease: Potential Mechanisms of Action," *The British Journal of Nutrition* 114, no. 1 (2015): 1–14, doi:10.1017/S0007114515001452.

Chapter 23: Don't Go It Alone: Moral Support and Other Support Strategies for a Low-Carb Diet

1. Richard D. Feinman and Jeff Volek, "Carbohydrate Restriction as the Default Treatment for Type 2 Diabetes and Metabolic Syndrome," *Scandinavian Cardiovascular Journal* 42, no. 4 (2008): 256–63, doi:10.1080/14017430802014838; Jeff S. Volek, Stephen D. Phinney, Cassandra E. Forsythe, Erin E. Quann, Richard J. Wood, Michael J. Puglisi, William J. Kraemer, et al., "Carbohydrate Restriction Has a More Favorable Impact on the Metabolic Syndrome Than a Low Fat Diet," *Lipids* 44, no. 4 (2009): 297–309, doi:10.1007/s11745-008-3274-2; and Richard D. Feinman, Wendy K. Pogozelski, Arne Astrup, Richard K. Bernstein, Eugene J. Fine, Eric C. Westman, Anthony Accurso, et al., "Dietary Carbohydrate Restriction as the First Approach in Diabetes Management: Critical Review and Evidence Base," *Nutrition* 31, no. 1 (2015): 1–13, doi:10.1016/j.nut.2014.06.011.

2. Csaba Tóth and Zsófia Clemens, "Type 1 Diabetes Mellitus Successfully Managed with the Paleolithic Ketogenic Diet," *International Journal of Case Reports and Images* 5, no. 10 (2014): 699–703, doi:10.5348/ijcri-2014124-CR-10435.

3. Jeff Volek, Maria Luz Fernandez, Richard D. Feinman, and Stephen Phinney, "Dietary Carbohydrate Restriction Induces a Unique Metabolic State Positively Affecting Atherogenic Dyslipidemia, Fatty Acid Partitioning, and Metabolic Syndrome," *Progress in Lipid Research* 47, no. 5 (2008): 307–18, doi:10.1016/j.plipres.2008.02.003; Eric Westman, Jeff S. Volek, and Richard D. Feinman, "Carbohydrate Restriction Is Effective in Improving Atherogenic Dyslipidemia Even in the Absence of Weight Loss," *American Journal of Clinical Nutrition* 84, no. 6 (2006): 1549; Jeff Volek and Matthew J. Sharman, "Cardiovascular and Hormonal Aspects of Very-Low-Carbohydrate Ketogenic Diets," *Obesity Research* 12, Suppl 2 (2004): 115S–123S, doi:10.1038/oby.2004.276; Richard J. Wood, Maria Luz Fernandez, Matthew J. Sharman, Ricardo Silvestre, Christine M. Greene, Tosca

L. Zern, Sudeep Shrestha, et al., "Effects of a Carbohydrate-Restricted Diet with and Without Supplemental Soluble Fiber on Plasma Low-Density Lipoprotein Cholesterol and Other Clinical Markers of Cardiovascular Risk," *Metabolism* 56, no. 1 (2007): 58–67, doi:10.1016/j.metabol.2006.08.021; Matthew J. Sharman, William J. Kraemer, Dawn M. Love, Neva G. Avery, Ana L. Gómez, Timothy P. Scheett, and Jeff S. Volek, "A Ketogenic Diet Favorably Affects Serum Biomarkers for Cardiovascular Disease in Normal-Weight Men," *The Journal of Nutrition* 132, no. 7 (2002): 1879–85; and Jeff S. Volek, Matthew J. Sharman, Ana Lourdes Gomez, Timothy P. Scheett, and William J. Kraemer, "An Isoenergetic Very Low Carbohydrate Diet Improves Serum HDL Cholesterol and Triacylglycerol Concentrations, the Total Cholesterol to HDL Cholesterol Ratio and Postprandial Lipemic Responses Compared with a Low Fat Diet in Normal Weight, Normolipidemic Women," *The Journal of Nutrition* 133, no. 9 (2003): 2756–61.

4. Eric C. Westman. Richard D. Feinman, John D. Mavropoulos, Mary C. Vernon, Jeff S. Volek, James A. Wortman, William S. Yancy, et al., "Low-Carbohydrate Nutrition and Metabolism," *American Journal of Clinical Nutrition* 86, no. 2 (2007): 276–84.

5. Cassandra Forsythe, Stephen D. Phinney, Maria Luz Fernandez, Erin E. Quann, Richard J. Wood, Doug M. Bibus, William J. Kraemer, et al., "Comparison of Low Fat and Low Carbohydrate Diets on Circulating Fatty Acid Composition and Markers of inflammation," *Lipids* 43, no. 1 (2008): 65–77, doi:10.1007/s11745 -007-3132-7.

6. Jeff S. Volek, Kevin D. Ballard, Ricardo Silvestre, Daniel A. Judelson, Erin E. Quann, Cassandra E. Forsythe, Maria Luz Fernandez, et al., "Effects of Dietary Carbohydrate Restriction Versus Low-Fat Diet on Flow-Mediated Dilation," *Metabolism* 58, no. 12 (2009): 1769–77, doi:10.1016/j.metabol.2009.06.005.

7. Gregory L. Austin, Michelle T. Thiny, Eric C. Westman, William S. Yancy Jr., and Nicholas J. Shaheen, "A Very Low-Carbohydrate Diet Improves Gastroesophageal Reflux and Its Symptoms," *Digestive Diseases and Sciences* 51, no. 8 (2006): 1307–12, doi:10.1007/s10620-005-9027-7; William S. Yancy Jr., Dawn Provenzale, and Eric C. Westman, "Improvement of Gastroesophageal Reflux Disease After Initiation of a Low-Carbohydrate Diet: Five Brief Case Reports," *Alternative Therapies in Health and Medicine* 7, no. 6 (2001): 120, 116–9; and S. D. Pointer, J. Rickstrew, J. C. Slaughter, M. F. Vaezi, and H. J. Silver, "Dietary Carbohydrate Intake, Insulin Resistance and Gastro-Oesophageal Reflux Disease: A Pilot Study in European- and African-American Obese Women," *Alimentary Pharmacology & Therapeutics* (September 1, 2016), http://www.ncbi.nlm.nih.gov/pubmed/27582035.

8. John C. Mavropoulos, William S. Yancy, Juanita Hepburn, and Eric C. Westman, "The Effects of a Low-Carbohydrate, Ketogenic Diet on the Polycystic Ovary Syndrome: A Pilot Study," *Nutrition & Metabolism* 2 (2005): 35, doi:10.1186/1743 -7075-2-35; and Antonio Paoli, Alessandro Rubini, Jeff S. Volek, and Keith A. Grimaldi, "Beyond weight loss: a review of the therapeutic uses of very-low-carbohydrate (ketogenic) diets," *European Journal of Clinical Nutrition* 67, no. 8 (2013): 789–96, doi:10.1038/ejcn.2013.116.

9. James R. Phelps, Susan V. Siemers, and Rif S. El-Mallakh, "The Ketogenic Diet for Type II Bipolar Disorder," *Neurocase* 19, no. 5 (2013): 423–6, doi:10.1080/1355479 4.2012.690421; and R. S. El-Mallakh and M. E. Paskitti, "The Ketogenic Diet May Have Mood-Stabilizing Properties," *Medical Hypotheses* 57, no. 6 (2001): 724–6, doi:10.1054/mehy.2001.1446.

10. Lindsey B. Gano, Mili Patel, and Jong M. Rho, "Ketogenic Diets, Mitochondria, and Neurological Diseases," *Journal of Lipid Research* 55, no. 11 (2014): 2211–28, doi:10.1194/jlr.R048975; Carl E. Stafstrom and Jong M. Rho, "The Ketogenic Diet as a Treatment Paradigm for Diverse Neurological Disorders," *Frontiers in Pharmacology* 3 (2012): 59, doi:10.3389/fphar.2012.00059; Maciej Gasior, Michael A. Rogawski, and Adam L. Hartman, "Neuroprotective and Disease-Modifying Effects of the Ketogenic Diet," *Behavioural Pharmacology* 17, no. 5-6 (2006): 431–39; Antonio Paoli, Antonino Bianco, Ernesto Damiani, and Gerardo Bosco, "Ketogenic Diet in Neuromuscular and Neurodegenerative Diseases," *BioMed Research International* 2014 (2014): 474296, doi:10.1155/2014/474296; Zhong Zhao, Dale J. Lange, Andre Voustianiouk, Donal MacGrogan, Lap Ho, Jason Suh, Nelson Humala, et al., "A Ketogenic Diet as a Potential Novel Therapeutic Intervention in Amyotrophic Lateral Sclerosis," *BMC Neuroscience* 7 (2006): 29, doi:10.1186/1471-2202-7-29; and Mithu Storoni and Gordon T. Plant, "The Therapeutic Potential of the Ketogenic Diet in Treating Progressive Multiple Sclerosis," *Multiple Sclerosis International* 2015 (2015): 681289, doi:10.1155/2015/681289.

11. Mayumi L. Prins, "Diet, Ketones and Neurotrauma," *Epilepsia* 49, Suppl 8 (2008): 111–13, doi:10.1111/j.1528-1167.2008.01852.x; Mayumi L. Prins and Joyce H. Matsumoto, "The Collective Therapeutic Potential of Cerebral Ketone Metabolism in Traumatic Brain Injury," *Journal of Lipid Research* 55, no. 12 (2014): 2450–57, doi:10.1194/jlr.R046706; Hayden White and Balasubramanian Venkatesh, "Clinical Review: Ketones and Brain Injury," *Critical Care* 15, no. 2 (2011): 219, doi:10.1186/cc10020; and Mayumi L. Prins, "Cerebral Metabolic Adaptation and Ketone Metabolism After Brain Injury," *Journal of Cerebral Blood Flow and Metabolism* 28, no. 1 (2008): 1–16, doi:10.1038/sj.jcbfm.9600543.

12. Bryan G. Allen, Sudershan K. Bhatia, Carryn M. Anderson, Julie M. Eichenberger-Gilmore, Zita A. Sibenaller, Kranti A. Mapuskar, et al., "Ketogenic Diets as an Adjuvant Cancer Therapy: History and Potential Mechanism," *Redox Biology* 2 (2014): 963–70, doi:10.1016/j.redox.2014.08.002; Weihua Zhou, Purna Mukherjee, Michael A. Kiebish, William T. Markis, John G. Mantis, and Thomas N. Seyfried, "The Calorically Restricted Ketogenic Diet, an Effective Alternative Therapy for Malignant Brain Cancer," *Nutrition & Metabolism* 4 (2007): 5, doi:10.1186/1743-7075-4-5; Rainer Klement and Ulrike Kämmerer, "Is There a Role for Carbohydrate Restriction in the Treatment and Prevention of Cancer?" *Nutrition & Metabolism* 8 (2011): 75, doi:10.1186/1743-7075-8-75; and Thomas N. Seyfried, Roberto E. Flores, Angela Poff, and Dominic P. D'Agostino, "Cancer as a Metabolic Disease: Implications for Novel Therapeutics," *Carcinogenesis* 35, no. 3 (2014): 515–27, doi:10.1093/carcin/bgt480.

Chapter 24: Potential Prevention Strategies

1. Catherine Crofts, Caryn Zinn, Mark Wheldon, and Grant Schofield, "Hyperinsulinemia: A Unifying Theory of Chronic Disease?" *Diabesity* 1, no. 4 (2015): 34–43, doi:10.15562/diabesity.2015.19.
2. Dale E. Bredesen, *Cognitive Health: Dawn of the Era of Treatable Alzheimer's Disease*, film, 56:21, August 4, 2016, https://vimeo.com/173061978.
3. Theodore Naiman, MD, email message to author, August 8, 2016.
4. Bredesen, *Cognitive Health*, film.
5. Ibid.
6. Theodore Naiman, MD, email message to author, August 8, 2016.
7. Ibid.
8. Mayo Clinic Staff, "HDL Cholesterol: How to Boost Your 'Good' Cholesterol," Mayo Clinic, http://www.mayoclinic.org/diseases-conditions/high-blood -cholesterol/in-depth/hdl-cholesterol/ART-20046388 (September 9, 2016).
9. Theodore Naiman, MD, email message to author, August 8, 2016.
10. Jeff Volek and Stephen Phinney, *The Art and Science of Low Carbohydrate Performance* (Lexington, KY: Beyond Obesity, 2011), 102; and Jonny Bowden and Stephen Sinatra, *The Great Cholesterol Myth* (Beverly, MA: Fair Winds Press, 2012), 44.
11. William S. Harris, "The Omega-3 Index: Clinical Utility for Therapeutic Intervention," *Current Cardiology Reports*, 12, no. 6 (2010): 503–8, doi:10.1007 /s11886-010-0141-6; and True Health Diagnostics, laboratory test report provided to author, July 2015.
12. Mayo Clinic Staff, "C-Reactive Protein Test," Mayo Clinic, http://www.mayoclinic .org/tests-procedures/c-reactive-protein/basics/results/prc-20014480 (August 16, 2016).
13. University of Rochester Medical Center Health Encyclopedia, "Homocysteine," https://www.urmc.rochester.edu/encyclopedia/content.aspx?contenttypeid=167 &contentid=homocysteine (September 9, 2016).
14. Bowden and Sinatra, *The Great Cholesterol Myth*, 174.
15. Mayo Clinic Staff, "Liver Function Tests," Mayo Clinic, http://www.mayoclinic.org /tests-procedures/liver-function-tests/basics/results/prc-20012602 (August 16, 2016).
16. Theodore Naiman, MD, email message to author, August 8, 2016.
17. Bowden and Sinatra, *The Great Cholesterol Myth*, 174.
18. Mayo Clinic Staff, "Liver Function Tests."
19. Katy Bowman, *Move Your DNA: Restore Your Health Through Natural Movement* (Sequim, WA: Propriometrics Press, 2014).
20. The Washington Post, "A Workout at Work?" https://www.washingtonpost.com /graphics/health/workout-at-work (September 9, 2016).

Conclusion: Why Alzheimer's Is on the Rise and How to Repair a Broken Brain

1. Dale E. Bredesen, *Cognitive Health: Dawn of the Era of Treatable Alzheimer's Disease*, film, 56:21, August 4, 2016, https://vimeo.com/173061978.
2. Samuel T. Henderson, "High Carbohydrate Diets and Alzheimer's Disease," *Medical Hypotheses* 62 (2004): 689–700, doi:10.1016/j.mehy.2003.11.028.

RECOMMENDED RESOURCES

Low-Carbohydrate and Ketogenic Diets

Books

The Art and Science of Low Carbohydrate Living, by Jeff Volek and Stephen Phinney. 2011. Beyond Obesity, LLC: Lexington, KY.

The Art and Science of Low Carbohydrate Performance, by Jeff Volek and Stephen Phinney. 2011. Beyond Obesity, LLC: Lexington, KY.

Keto Clarity, by Jimmy Moore and Eric Westman. 2014. Victory Belt: Las Vegas, NV.

Low Carbohydrate Living, by Jonny Bowden. 2012. Sterling: New York, NY.

The New Atkins for a New You, by Eric Westman, Stephen Phinney, and Jeff Volek. 2010. Fireside: New York, NY.

Protein Power Lifeplan, by Michael Eades and Mary Dan Eades. 2001. Grand Central: New York, NY.

The World Turned Upside Down, by Richard Feinman. 2014. NMS Press: Brooklyn, NY.

Websites

Burn Fat Not Sugar (Theodore Naiman, MD): www.burnfatnotsugar.com

"Butter Bob Briggs" (YouTube channel): www.youtube.com/channel /UCiue5Soilcbqp3XS2c1P1PA

The Charlie Foundation: www.charliefoundation.org

Diagnosis Diet (Georgia Ede, MD): www.diagnosisdiet.com

Diet Doctor (Andreas Eenfeldt, MD): www.dietdoctor.com/low-carb

KetoGains: www.ketogains.com

Ketogenic Diet Resource: www.ketogenic-diet-resource.com

Low Carb Dietitian (Franziska Spritzler, RD): www.lowcarbdietitian.com

Low Carb RN (Kelley Pounds, RN): www.lowcarbrn.wordpress.com

Podcasts (all are available on iTunes)

Keto Talk, with Jimmy and the Doc: www.ketotalk.com

Ketovangelist: www.ketovangelist.com/category/podcast

The Livin' La Vida Low Carb Show, with Jimmy Moore: www.thelivinlowcarbshow .com/shownotes

Two Keto Dudes: www.2ketodudes.com/archives.aspx

Paleolithic Diets
Books

The Paleo Answer, by Loren Cordain. 2012. Houghton Mifflin Harcourt: Orlando, FL.
The Paleo Cure, by Chris Kresser. 2014. Little, Brown and Company: Boston, MA.
The Paleo Solution, by Robb Wolf. 2010. Victory Belt: Las Vegas, NV.
Practical Paleo, by Diane Sanfilippo. 2016. Victory Belt: Las Vegas, NV.
The Primal Blueprint, by Mark Sisson. 2009. Primal Nutrition: Malibu, CA.
Primal Body, Primal Mind, by Nora Gedgaudas. 2009. Primal Body—
Primal Mind: Portland, OR.

Websites

Chris Kresser, L.Ac: www.chriskresser.com
Diane Sanfilippo: www.balancedbites.com
Mark's Daily Apple: www.marksdailyapple.com
The Paleo Diet™ (Loren Cordain, PhD): www.thepaleodiet.com
Robb Wolf: www.robbwolf.com/what-is-the-paleo-diet

Podcasts (all are available on iTunes)

Balanced Bites, with Diane Sanfilippo and Liz Wolfe:
www.balancedbites.com/podcasts
The Paleo Solution, with Robb Wolf: www.robbwolf.com/podcast
Revolution Health Radio, with Chris Kresser: www.chriskresser.com/podcasts

Insulin, Diabetes, and Fasting
Books

The Complete Guide to Fasting, by Jason Fung, MD, and Jimmy Moore. 2016. Victory Belt: Las Vegas, NV.
Conquer Type 2 Diabetes with a Ketogenic Diet (e-book), by Ellen Davis and Keith Runyan. 2015. Available at: www.ketogenic-diet-resource.com/diabetes-diet.html
Diabetes Epidemic & You, by Joseph Kraft. 2001. Trafford: Bloomington, IN.
Dr. Bernstein's Diabetes Solution. 2011. Little, Brown and Company: Boston, MA.
The Obesity Code, by Jason Fung, MD. 2016. Greystone Books: Vancouver, BC Canada.

Websites

Intensive Dietary Management (Jason Fung, MD):
www.intensivedietarymanagement.com
"It's the Insulin, Stupid," multipart blog series by Amy Berger, MS, CNS, NTP:
www.tuitnutrition.com/2015/09/its-the-insulin-1.html
Optimizing Nutrition: www.optimisingnutrition.com
Type One Grit Facebook page: www.facebook.com/Type1Grit
(for individuals using very low-carb/ketogenic diets to manage type 1 diabetes)

Cholesterol
Books

Cholesterol Clarity, by Jimmy Moore and Eric Westman. 2013. Victory Belt: Las Vegas, NV.
The Cholesterol Myths, by Uffe Ravnskov. 2000. NewTrends: Washington, DC.
The Great Cholesterol Myth, by Jonny Bowden and Stephen Sinatra. 2012. Fair Winds Press: Beverly, MA.
Put Your Heart in Your Mouth, by Natasha Campbell-McBride. 2013. Medinform: Cambridge, UK.

Websites

"Cholesterol: Friend or Foe?": www.westonaprice.org/know-your-fats/cholesterol -friend-or-foe
Cholesterol and Health (Chris Masterjohn, PhD): www.cholesterol-and-health.com
The Fat Emperor: www.thefatemperor.com (Several informational videos are available at www.thefatemperor.com/latest-material or on the author's YouTube channel at www.youtube.com/channel/UCPn4FsiQP15nudug9FDhluA.)
"The Straight Dope on Cholesterol," on Eating Academy (Peter Attia, MD): www.eatingacademy.com/nutrition/the-straight-dope-on-cholesterol-part-i (This multipart series is geared toward the especially science- and technical-minded reader.)

Dietary Fats and Nutrition Controversies
Books

The Big Fat Surprise, by Nina Teicholz. 2014. Simon & Schuster: New York, NY.
Good Calories, Bad Calories, by Gary Taubes. 2007. Alfred A. Knopf: New York, NY.
Know Your Fats, by Mary Enig. 2008. Bethesda Press: Silver Spring, MD.
Nourishing Traditions, by Sally Fallon and Mary Enig. NewTrends: Washington, DC.
The Queen of Fats, by Susan Allport. 2006. University of California Press: Berkeley, CA.
Trick and Treat, by Barry Groves. 2008. Hammersmith Press: London, UK.

Websites

The Definitive Guide to Oils, by Mark Sisson: www.marksdailyapple.com/healthy-oils
Printable guide to safe cooking fats: www.balancedbites.com/PDFs/BOOK_EXTRAS /PracticalPaleo_GuidetoCookingFats.pdf
Shaking Up the Salt Myth, by Chris Kresser, L.Ac: www.chriskresser.com /specialreports/salt
The Truth About Red Meat, by Chris Kresser, L.Ac: www.chriskresser.com/the-truth -about-red-meat

Grains
Books

Dangerous Grains, by James Braly and Ron Hoggan. 2002. Avery (Penguin Group USA): New York, NY.

Fiber Menace, by Konstantin Monastyrsky. 2008. Ageless Press: Rutherford, NJ.
Grain Brain, by David Perlmutter. 2013. Little, Brown and Company: New York, NY.
Wheat Belly Total Health, by William Davis 2014. Rodale Books: Emmaus, PA.

Digestive Function

Books

Digestive Health with Real Food, by Aglaée Jacob. 2013. Paleo Media Group.
Why Stomach Acid Is Good for You, by Jonathan Wright and Lane Lenard. 2001.
Rowman & Littlefield Publishing Group: Lanham, MD.

Cookbooks and Recipes

Note: Some of these cookbooks and websites feature "Paleo" recipes. Many of these
will be suitable for low-carbohydrate and ketogenic diets, but some will not. Use your
best judgment in looking at the ingredients in order to assess whether the recipes are
appropriate for you.

Books

Fat Bombs, by Martina Slajerova. 2016. Fair Winds Press: Beverly, MA.
The KetoDiet Cookbook, by Martina Slajerova. 2016. Fair Winds Press: Beverly, MA.
The Ketogenic Cookbook, by Jimmy Moore and Maria Emmerich. 2015. Victory Belt:
Las Vegas, NV.
The Ketogenic Kitchen, by Domini Kemp and Patricia Daly. 2016. Chelsea Green:
White River Junction, VT.
Mediterranean Paleo, by Caitlin Weeks, Nabil Boumrar, and Diane Sanfilippo.
2014. Victory Belt: Las Vegas, NV.
Phase 2 Low-Carb Recipes, by Better Homes and Gardens. 2004. Meredith
Corporation: Des Moines, IA.
The Primal Blueprint Cookbook, by Mark Sisson with Jennifer Meier. 2010. Primal
Nutrition: Malibu, CA.
Any cookbooks by Dana Carpender
Any cookbooks by George Stella

Websites

All Day I Dream About Food: www.alldayidreamaboutfood.com
Carrie Brown's Recipe Index: www.marmaladeandmileposts.com/recipe-index
Caveman Keto: www.cavemanketo.com
Ditch the Carbs: www.ditchthecarbs.com
I Breathe I'm Hungry: www.ibreatheimhungry.com
Linda Sue's Low Carb Recipes: www.genaw.com/lowcarb
Nom Nom Paleo: www.nomnompaleo.net/recipeindex
Ruled.me: www.ruled.me
Sugar Free Sheila: www.sugarfreesheila.com/low-carb-recipes
Wicked Stuffed Keto: www.wickedstuffed.com

Finding Local Farms

Your local chapter of the Weston A. Price Foundation will be able to point you toward small farms in your area raising animals on grass and pasture, and/or growing produce: www.westonaprice.org/local-chapters.

Search for farms in your area on Eat Wild: www.eatwild.com/products/index.html.

Search community websites and publications to find out about farmers' markets and farmstand stores in your area.

INDEX

Note: Page numbers in *italics* refer to photographs and figures; page numbers followed by *t* refer to tables

abdominal obesity, 4
absorption of nutrients
    antacid effects on, 230, 240
    cholesterol needed for, 107–8
    importance of fat to, 135
    vitamin B_{12}, 52, 54
acetoacetate, 33, 42, 43
acetone
    keto breath from, 41, 43, 236
    measuring at home, 41
acetylcholine, 103, 250
acetylcholinesterase, 250
acid reflux, 239–240
acid residue, from proteins, 125
AD. *See* Alzheimer's disease
adipose tissue. *See* body fat
adiposity. *See* obesity
advanced glycation end-products (AGEs), 66, 74, 220
aerobic exercise, 207, 265
Afghan cuisine, tips for dining out, 188
age
    cholesterol-cognitive function connection, 98, 99
    declining levels of stomach acid, 52
    detection of brain glucose metabolism decline, 6
    MCI and AD diagnosis at younger ages, 6–7, 40
    rate of improvement and, 270
AGEs (advanced glycation end-products), 66, 74, 220·
ALA. *See* alpha-linolenic acid
alcoholic beverages, in nutritional strategy, 174
alkaline residues, 125
alliums, 83, 117
allspice, 69
almond milk, 166, 174, 245
alpha-linolenic acid (ALA), 156, 161, 234
alpha-lipoic acid, 247–48

ALT blood tests, 261
Alzheimer, Alois, xx
Alzheimer's Association, 79
Alzheimer's disease (AD). *See also* risk factors
    for Alzheimer's disease
    glucose metabolism decline, 5–8, 21–22
    hallmarks of, 5–6, 47, 49–50, 72, 250
    identifying fundamental causes of, 1–2, 80–82, 207–8
    lack of progress in treatment, xix–xx, 50
    overlap with metabolic syndrome, 4–5, 16–17
    rise in, 267–271
    type 3 diabetes concept, 16–21
American bistro cuisine, tips for dining out, 189
American Diabetes Association, 17
amino acids
    in apoE2, E3, and E4 molecules, 78
    conversion into glucose, 9, 35
    role in health, 124, 205–6
amyloid hypothesis, xii, 74–75
amyloid plaques. *See* beta-amyloid (Aß) plaques
animal fats
    conventional recommendations against, 137, 169, 267
    fatty acid composition of, 142t
    in nutritional strategy, 128, 145, 195, 197
    traditional use of, 102
animal proteins. *See also specific types*
    ApoE4 genotype considerations, 82, 83
    benefits of, 130–33, 131t
    food quality concerns, 127, 195–200
    omega-3 and-6 fats in, 159–160
    vegetarian and vegan concerns, 233
    vitamin B_{12} in, 52
antacids
    contribution to vitamin B_{12} deficiency, 52
    effects on digestion and absorption, 240–41, 244, 268
    medication precautions, 230
antioxidants, body, 68

conjugated linoleic acid (CLA), 197
constipation, 237–38
contraindications to low-carbohydrate diet, 231–33
convenience store foods, for eating on the go, 191
conventional medicine
    changing views of fat, 82, 136, 137, 144–45
    lack of progress in AD treatment, xix–xx, 50
cookbooks, 182–83, 309
cookie sheets, 186
cooking fats and oils
    ApoE4 genotype considerations, 82
    misguided views on cholesterol, 102
    oxidation concerns, 139
    recommended types, 141–46, 142t
cooking tips, 181–84, 244–45
corn oil
    cooking cautions, 146
    manufacturing concerns, 139–141
    omega-6 fats in, 160
    in processed foods, 147
coronary artery calcium scan (CAC), 115, 116
Correia, Sónia, 72–73
corticosteroid drugs, 231
cortisol, 211–12, 214, 215, 231
cost concerns
    AD-related health care, 1
    food quality, xxii, 201–2
cottonseed oil, 140, 141, 160, 166
counting carbs, 121–23
Craft, Suzanne, 19
cramps, muscle, 236
cravings for sweets, 169, 171, 192–93
C-reactive protein (CRP), 115, 261
cruciferous vegetables
    ApoE4 genotype considerations, 83
    importance of cooking, 118
    in list of recommended carbohydrates, 117–18
cubicle calisthenics, 264
Cunnane, Stephen
    on DHA, 157
    on insulin resistance, 18
    ketones research, 25, 26, 27
    on muscle loss, 206
cyanocobalamin, 54
cytoskeletons, 49–50

D'Agostino, Dominic, 106
daily activity, need for, 263–65. See also exercise
dairy foods
    ApoE4 genotype considerations, 83
    food quality concerns, 197–98
    in nutritional strategy, 164–65
    omega-3 and-6 fats in, 159–160
    permissible, 165
    types to limit or avoid, 166, 174

dairy substitutes, 166
dark chocolate, 155, 180, 193
Davis, Ellen, 122
Davis, William, 143
Dayspring, Thomas, 110, 113
dehydration, 235–36
dendrites
    normal, 45, 46, 46
    shrinking of, 48–49
depression
    from low cholesterol, 107
    from vitamin B_{12} deficiency, 53
desserts, suggestions for, 192–93
dextrose, in artificial sweeteners, 169
DHA (docosahexaenoic acid)
    from alpha-linolenic acid, 161
    in omega-3 supplements, 248
    structural role in the brain, 147, 156–57
    vegetarian and vegan concerns, 234
diabetes
    fasting precautions, 224
    glycation effects, 65–66
    medication precautions, 229
    resources about, 307
    type 3 diabetes concept, 16–21
diabetes, type 1
    diabetic ketoacidosis concerns, 31, 32
    insulin dependence, 261
    low-carbohydrate diet benefits, 231, 256
diabetes, type 2
    administration of insulin with, 101
    association with AD, 2, 4–5, 8, 20–21
    brain-derived neurotrophic factor connection, 207–8
    diabetic ketoacidosis concerns, 31, 32
    diagnosis of, 17–19
    hyperinsulinemia with, 2–3, 20, 72, 101, 261
    hypertension with, 40
    increasing rates of, 40, 136
    low-carbohydrate diet benefits, 231, 256
    sleep debt concerns, 215
    statin drug concerns, 104, 106
diabetes in-situ, as phrase, 19
diabetes of the brain, as phrase, 16
diabetic ketoacidosis, 10, 31–34, 32t
diet. See specific types
dietary cholesterol. See also cholesterol
    conventional recommendations against, 3
    limited availability of, in conventional care facilities, xxii
    need for, 54, 100
    serum cholesterol vs., 99–102
dietary fat, 134–162. See also body fat; specific types
    in animal proteins, 127
    in beef, 196, 197

318   INDEX

ABOUT THE AUTHOR

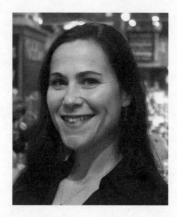

Amy Berger, MS, CNS, NTP, has a master's degree in human nutrition and is a certified nutrition specialist and nutritional therapy practitioner. She is a US Air Force veteran and spent years doing what nutrition and health experts claimed were "all the right things" to lose weight and maintain optimal health but failed to experience the expected results. Wanting to understand why the conventional advice about low-calorie, low-fat dieting and exercise did not lead to the promised outcomes, she began researching and came to learn that much of what we currently believe about "healthy diets" is misguided and, in some cases, downright incorrect. Having learned these lessons the hard way, she has dedicated her career to showing others that vibrant health does not require starvation, deprivation, or living at the gym. Men and women cannot live by lettuce alone; *real people need real food!* You can read her blog and find more of her work at www.tuitnutrition.com.